T3-BEA-559

NEW WAYS OF
MAKING BABIES

MEDICAL ETHICS SERIES

David H. Smith and Robert M. Veatch, Editors

NEW WAYS OF
MAKING BABIES

THE CASE OF
EGG DONATION

EDITED BY

Cynthia B. Cohen

COMMISSIONED BY

the National Advisory Board on Ethics in Reproduction (NABER)

INDIANA UNIVERSITY PRESS

Bloomington and Indianapolis

© 1996 by the National Advisory Board on Ethics in Reproduction (NABER)

The paper used in this publication meets the minimum requirements of American National Standard for Information Sciences—Permanence of Paper for Printed Library Materials, ANSI Z39.48-1984.

Manufactured in the United States of America

Library of Congress Cataloging-in-Publication Data

New ways of making babies : the case of egg donation / edited by
Cynthia B. Cohen ; commissioned by the National Advisory Board on
Ethics in Reproduction.
    p.   cm. — (Medical ethics series)
  Includes bibliographical references and index.
  ISBN 0-253-33058-0 (cloth : alk. paper)
  1. Human reproductive technology—Moral and ethical aspects.
  2. Ovum—Transplantation—Moral and ethical aspects.   I. Cohen,
Cynthia B.   II. National Advisory Board on Ethics in Reproduction.
III. Series.
RG133.5.N49   1996
176—dc20   95-51471

1 2 3   4   5   01   00   99   98   97   96

CONTENTS

Part B. Ethical and Policy Issues Raised by Egg Donation

SECTION IV

ACKNOWLEDGMENTS

A version of Thomas H. Murray's essay appeared in his volume, *The Worth of the Child,* published by the University of California Press in 1996.

A version of John A. Robertson's essay will appear as a contribution to *Family Building through Egg and Sperm Donation: Medical, Legal, and Ethical Issues,* ed. Machelle M. Seibel and Susan Crockin (Boston: Jones and Bartlett, 1996).

Sections II and III of Dan W. Brock's chapter draw on his paper, "Reproductive Freedom: Its Nature, Bases, and Limits," prepared for a conference on "Women, Equality, and Reproductive Technology," part of a larger project on the capabilities approach in economic development of the World Institute for Development Economics Research of the United Nations University, Helsinki, Finland. That paper is forthcoming in a collection of the conference papers to be published by Oxford University Press.

INTRODUCTION
Cynthia B. Cohen, Ph.D., J.D.

Since 1984, when the first reported oocyte or egg donation was performed in Australia, a growing number of
infertile women have brought children into the world by
this means. Today oocyte donation, in which an embryo
is created from a donated egg and sperm of the receiving
woman's partner and implanted in a woman's uterus in
hopes of achieving a pregnancy, has become an established procedure. Yet it has been a decidedly hidden procedure — until recently when headlines in newspapers
around the world proclaimed it had been used to enable
women in their 50s and early 60s, termed "granny
moms," to give birth. Soon after, the front pages declared
that investigators planned to transplant ovaries or eggs
from aborted fetuses into infertile women as a new way of
making babies. And even more recently, the media alleged
that "egg-swapping," in which donated eggs were fertilized and implanted in the wombs of other women without
the knowledge or consent of the donors, had been carried
out at one clinic in the United States.

These controversial announcements have revived concern that novel reproductive technologies are being introduced too speedily before we have had a chance to evaluate them ethically and ascertain their effects on our social
and legal fabric. We have just barely begun to consider
where the appropriate limits to the use of these techniques
lie and what values are at risk. Should these novel means
of reproduction be used eugenically, selecting donors
and recipients deliberately to produce more attractive,
brighter, or artistically gifted children? Should biological
relationships provide the key to determining the parentage of offspring born of gamete donation, or should private
contractual arrangements govern? Should children resulting from third-party donation have the right when they
reach maturity to track down their genetic parents? The
issues multiply as the technology races ahead. They com-

pound further when superimposed on recent dramatic changes in our approach to male-female relationships, family structure, and female work patterns.

As the rate at which these technological means of reproduction develop accelerates, our ability to respond to them and set ethical limits to their use seems to diminish. Today we are at a pivotal moment before positions have become so hardened that reasoned argument and thoughtful consensus in this area are impossible. This is an appropriate time in which to grapple with the fundamental ethical and policy questions raised by the new reproductive technologies.

This book addresses these questions by focusing on oocyte donation, a technique that raises many of the paradigm ethical and policy issues common to the new reproductive technologies. As a procedure in which the egg is obtained from a woman who will not bear or raise the child, fertilized *in vitro* (in a glass dish) with the sperm of a man who usually will be the rearing father, and then implanted in a woman who is expected to bear and rear the child, it also creates novel ethical issues about women, parents, and families not associated with many other forms of assisted reproduction. A focus on egg donation, therefore, allows us to be both comprehensive and particular. It enables us to draw together many of the reflections that have been generated by earlier technologies and to offer what our authors hope are useful recommendations for employing this particular procedure.

THE ROLE OF THE NATIONAL ADVISORY BOARD ON ETHICS IN REPRODUCTION (NABER)

This volume was developed by the National Advisory Board on Ethics in Reproduction (NABER), a panel in the private sector with members from the fields of ethics, theology, law, medicine, genetics, and public policy[1] established in 1991. Its basic purposes are to provide a forum for reasoned discussion of ethical and policy issues raised by the new reproductive technologies, fetal and embryo research, and fetal tissue use; and to make sound, reasoned recommendations about these issues.[2] The work of NABER is designed to assist public policymakers, physicians and nurses, and members of the public who are puzzling over the serious ethical questions raised by our growing capacity to affect the beginnings of human life.

NABER was established to step into a vacuum in American public life created by the lack of a national body to initiate and stimulate debate about ethical and policy issues arising in reproductive practice and research. The national forum that began to examine reproductive technologies was allowed to lapse early in the 1980s; efforts to develop a successor have been unsuccessful. In contrast, countries in other parts of the world, including Britain, Australia, France, and Canada have created commissions that have given considerable scrutiny to these issues and developed guidelines for their use.

Officials in this country, however, have been anxious to avoid such politically explosive subjects, and only physicians who provide these procedures have developed standards for employing them.

The American Fertility Society (AFS), now known as the American Society for Reproductive Medicine (ASRM), has been developing guidelines for the use of successively developed methods of assisted reproduction since 1986. These self-imposed professional standards have been extremely helpful to practitioners in the field of infertility. The guidelines are prefaced by overviews of ethics and the law, and provide a sense of current practice in reproductive medicine in their body. Practitioners themselves, however, realized that some guidance from an interdisciplinary group that functioned independently of physician organizations was also necessary. It was AFS and the American College of Obstetricians and Gynecologists (ACOG) that provided seed money to establish NABER as a disinterested external organization that could begin to develop comprehensive guidelines for use of methods of assisted reproduction and provide advice on research in this area. NABER is now funded by respected private foundations.[3]

The purpose of this volume is to identify and recommend ways in which to resolve some of the pressing issues created by oocyte donation and the new reproductive technologies as a whole. It provides descriptions of practices and policies at four egg donation centers, reflective papers on ethical and policy questions raised by egg donation, and a report and recommendations on the use of oocyte donation by NABER.

HOW OOCYTE DONATION IS CARRIED OUT AT FOUR CENTERS

What happens to those who, after struggling to have children coitally, learn their best hope is to seek professional help and attempt to use donated eggs? A rapidly growing number of oocyte donation centers are opening their doors to such couples. In Part A of this book, the procedures and policies at four oocyte donation centers, two of which are university affiliated nonprofit and two of which are for-profit, are presented by those who administer them. These authors describe how and why incoming couples and donors are screened and counseled and how each center has addressed some of the ethical and policy questions.

The oocyte donation program at the University of Washington described in Chapter 1 is the hub of a regional referral system in which private physicians conduct preliminary screening and testing, before sending women to the public university infertility center for a stimulation attempt. A special feature of this program is that a coordinator, who functions both as nurse-clinician and program administrator, serves to recruit and screen donors, counsel donors and recipients, and manage financial issues and outcome statistics. In Chapter 2, Barad and Cohen describe the private university-affiliated oocyte donation program at Montefiore Hospital/Albert Einstein Medical Center in the Bronx, New York, which is located in a region that attracts patients from a great variety of socioeconomic backgrounds. They discuss such matters as donor motivation and the screening of single women and reveal a remarkable flexibility and openness in their explanation of why they changed their minds about donor anonymity. Of note is the fact that this program has been continuously assisted by an ethics committee since its inception.

The egg donation programs at IVF America in Boston, Massachusetts, and the Huntington Reproductive Center in Pasadena, California, whose descriptions follow in Chapters 3 and 4, offer a sense of how programs that are arguably subject to market pressures to a greater degree than their not-for-profit counterparts address relevant ethical and policy issues. The Boston program is distinctive for at least two reasons: (1) It is one of several infertility centers run by a parent corporation, and (2) it is located in a state with some insurance coverage of IVF procedures (and therefore has access to a larger pool of women with the means to utilize egg donation than programs in states with no such coverage). Among the interesting features of this program are its policies of not accepting student donors or allowing couples to advertise for their own donors. The description of the program at the Huntington Reproductive Center in California, which is a free-standing infertility center, frankly addresses such questions as whether multiple births present an insurmountable safety problem to recipients and children and whether egg donation within the family is advisable. Serafini and his colleagues place special emphasis on questions related to quality control and outcome measurement, carefully detailing the factors that lead to variation in reports of pregnancy and delivery rates.

ETHICAL, LEGAL, AND POLICY ISSUES

Reflective articles on major ethical and policy issues that arise in the use of egg donation and the new reproductive technologies by leading scholars appear in Part B of this volume. The most fundamental ethical issue, of course, is whether methods of artificial conception—egg donation in particular—are ethically acceptable at all. Many people reject them as undermining long-held beliefs in love, marriage, the family, and lineage. Others defend them as humanitarian ways of bringing children to people desperate to have them. Our papers begin with two that raise a concern about whether the language of liberty and choice is sufficient to provide ethical grounding for the new reproductive technologies.

Thomas Murray suggests in Chapter 5 that the uneasiness we feel about some new ways of making babies indicates that we need to reframe our ethical questions in terms of the whys and wherefores of families, rather than retain the language of production, commerce, and control. The question we should ask about these novel means of reproduction, he maintains, is whether they create not just individual parent-child relationships, but the kinds of relationships that foster mutuality, loyalty, trust, and love within families. Do they help build social attitudes and institutions that support the flourishing of children and adults within families? He concludes that if practices associated with these new techniques, such as the payment of gamete donors, threaten cultural meanings and institutions, they are not ethically acceptable.

In a related vein, Lisa Cahill in Chapter 6 highlights certain areas of ethical concern that can be neglected by an emphasis on individuality, liberty, and autonomy. The modern ideal of self-creating individuality can slide into subjectivism, and finally nihilism, if these other areas are not considered. Cahill stresses the significance of biological kinship for the social meaning of parenthood. As the mother of three adopted and two biological children, she recognizes that in exceptional situations the social dimension of parenthood can outweigh the biological. She offers four criteria for when this is generally justified, and maintains that ethically these permit adoption and stepparenting, but not gamete donation. She concludes with a sympathetic examination of the radical feminist critique of a culture that presents women with images of mothering as critical to their identity, pregnancy as the culmination of their sexuality, and fertility as a sign of youthfulness and worth.

The thrust of the next four articles in Part B is toward investigation of specific ethical and policy issues related to the clinical setting, beginning with those about donors and then moving to those that arise about recipients as well.

Cynthia Cohen focuses on the role of gamete donors in Chapter 7, and asks what, if anything, do these individuals owe to their biological children? Through an exploration of arguments frequently given for and against gamete donor anonymity, she finds two fundamentally different—and conflicting—moral views of egg donation that are assumed in our society. Each of these implies different roles for gamete donors. The vision of egg donation that we want to encourage, that of a life-creating gift from one individual in response to a basic human need of another, entails certain obligations on the part of recipients and donors to each other and to the children who result. Cohen provides an ethical and policy framework to enable participants in egg donation to meet these obligations and to relate to one another after birth of the child. Among her recommendations are that donors and recipients be "matched" according to their willingness to be identified, and that either identifying or nonidentifying information about the donor be provided to recipients before conception and to the resulting children when they reach maturity.

Whether gamete donors should be paid has been a prime point of controversy. In Chapter 8, Ruth Macklin explores the arguments surrounding the practice of paying egg donors and finds payment for the donor's time, risk, and inconvenience—but not for her egg—ethically acceptable. Macklin explores the charge of exploitation of women, which she finds dubious, and goes on to consider various ethical principles that might be violated by the practice of paying egg donors. She concludes that while commodification of oocyte donation is "unsavory," this is not a category of moral disvalue strong enough to warrant its prohibition. She considers regulation of this practice a reasonable middle ground between free-market commercialization and outright prohibition of payment.

In Chapter 9, Carson Strong explores several ethical and legal issues raised by genetic testing of donors and recipients in clinical practice. Current professional guidelines for genetic screening of donors, he finds, omit important considerations, including the ethical principles upon which they are based. He offers an ethical framework for genetic screening of donors and recipients that allows use of more than minimalist standards and provides criteria for assessing when routine screening should—and should not—be employed. Strong concludes that the ethical arguments in favor of enhancing the genetic quality of offspring outweigh those against, and maintains that this should be legally permitted.

What would a feminist egg donation policy look like, taking the clinical setting into account? Rosemarie Tong in Chapter 10 can find no single feminist position on egg donation. Undaunted, she first outlines alternative feminist approaches and discusses the reasons for disagreement among these. She then sketches a policy for gamete donation and reception that incorporates the values and concerns of many different sorts of feminists. Such a policy would include paid donors and multiparented families, but would exclude certain forms of donor screening and deliberate enhancement of the characteristics of children.

The final four articles in Part B are directed more to questions of general policy than to issues that arise in the clinical setting. They consider who should be in charge of regulating oocyte donation, the current legal status of the procedure, how race, ethnicity, and socioeconomic status affect access to oocyte donation, and whether reproductive technologies such as oocyte donation should be covered in health insurance benefit packages.

Andrea Bonnicksen assesses whether some of the major ethical and policy issues raised by egg donation are best addressed by policy responses in the private or public sector in Chapter 11. The issues on which she focuses relate to the protection of donors and recipients, compensation, and the definition of parenthood. Bonnicksen highlights a policy tension that also arises in other forms of assisted reproduction: Reproduction is a private activity in which government involvement is not necessarily advisable or constitutional; yet self-monitoring in the private sector may not lead to sufficiently strict oversight to protect those who are involved in egg donation. She concludes that accelerated self-monitoring in the private sector is needed and that narrowly crafted public policies are advisable.

John Robertson, in Chapter 12, notes that except for five states, there is no legislation or court decision that directly addresses egg donation. Consequently, a myriad of legal questions about this procedure—ranging from whether the parties' intentions to exclude the donor from rearing rights in offspring will have legal effect to whether egg donation to women past the normal age of childbearing can be banned—remain unanswered. These uncertainties, however, present no insuperable barrier to performing egg donation, he indicates, and he suggests reasonable steps to take with regard to rearing rights and duties, risks to donors, payment to donors, and offspring welfare, until the law is clarified.

What impact has egg donation on poor women and members of various racial and ethnic groups, and what ethical and policy challenges does this raise? In Chapter 13, Heitman and Schlachtenhaufen first consider who counts in classification schemes for race, ethnicity, and socioeconomic status, noting certain difficulties this raises for the development of meaningful policy on egg donation. They go on to explore how differences in cultural perspectives affect the perceived meaning of infertility for members of various groupings and how these impinge on their participation in egg donation. Of special interest is their interpretation of the religious meaning of infertility for women who struggle to find meaning in this condition. They claim that poor and nonwhite women are unlikely to become the victims of commodification or exploitation from egg donation, but that—despite ethical debate about just distribution of health care resources—their exclusion from access to this technique is reinforced by current practices. Ironically, they maintain, whether this exclusion is an exclusively negative consequence is very much in question. They recommend a preventive and primary care program of education, preventive services, and treatment for sexually transmitted diseases (STDs) to empower poor and nonwhite women to safeguard their fertility and reproductive health.

Should new reproductive technologies such as oocyte donation be included in health insurance benefit packages? In Chapter 14, Dan Brock first analyzes the right to reproductive freedom to maintain that access to the new reproductive technologies is appropriately considered part of that right. He goes on to present arguments that support assigning high moral importance to these technologies in comparison with other health care services. Special features of oocyte donation and other methods of assisted reproduction that he cites do not justify excluding them from insurance coverage, he claims. He concludes that the new reproductive technologies ought, as a matter of justice, to be included within health care benefit packages that should be available to all.

REPORT AND RECOMMENDATIONS OF THE NATIONAL ADVISORY BOARD ON ETHICS IN REPRODUCTION (NABER)

Part C of this book presents the Report and Recommendations on the Use of Oocyte Donation developed by the National Advisory Board on Ethics in Reproduction (NABER). This is divided into four sections. In the first, the board looks at whether oocyte donation is ethically acceptable in principle and delineates the values that inform the report, in the second at ethical and policy considerations relevant to the recipient, in the third at ethical and policy considerations relevant to the donor, and in the last, at whether groups in the private or public sector should regulate further development and applications of oocyte donation. Among the major recommendations of this report are that

—a wider range of information should be offered to potential oocyte recipients and donors

—counseling of potential recipients and donors by trained personnel functioning independently of practitioners should be an essential element in all programs

—screening of recipients and donors should be kept distinct from counseling

—the practice of oocyte donation in women of advanced reproductive age should be pursued only with extreme caution

—single women should be granted access to this procedure with counseling about special considerations

—oocyte donation programs should offer standard measures of reimbursement

—arrangements in which poor women donate eggs to those who are well-to-do in exchange for coverage of their own IVF procedure should be discouraged

—donors should be screened for voluntariness with special review in cases of intrafamilial donation

—programs should purchase insurance to compensate donors who suffer injury or disability due to their participation

—donors and recipients should be matched on the basis of whether they want to relate as known persons or as nonidentified persons

—a broadly constituted task force should develop intercenter guidelines for many facets of oocyte donation

—a centrally coordinated network of registries should be established in this country with permanent records containing medical, genetic, and certain social information about donors in either identifiable or coded form.

FOR WHOM THIS BOOK IS WRITTEN

This book is intended for several audiences. The first is the community of practitioners in infertility and the second patients who seek their assistance in countering infertility. For these audiences, we seek to give guidance about the ways in which the ethical aspects of infertility treatment can be incorporated into patient care in the clinical setting. Thus, descriptions of the policies and procedures at several different oocyte donation programs are provided, as well as a report that addresses the policies and practices of clinics from the perspective of both practitioners and patients.

A third audience is the body of policymakers on the national and state levels who must risk addressing this politically explosive topic. For them, we offer deliberations by distinguished experts on many of the pressing policy issues and recommendations in the report that we believe represent a consensus not only among members of NABER, but in the larger society.

Yet another audience is the diverse group of laypeople and professionals interested in the ethics of reproductive technology, but not directly involved in providing or receiving these services. For this audience, we offer not only a way of becoming aware of what goes on in a variety of programs, but arguments and positions in the papers that are collected in this volume and the report with its emphasis on clinical and policy recommendations. By thus separating to a degree the practical and policy guidelines from some of the detailed philosophical considerations at their foundation, we hope to produce a clearer presentation of the issues for each audience. We also hope that each of these audiences will profit by reading all parts.

NOTES

1. Members of NABER at the time this volume was developed were Albert R. Jonsen, Ph.D., Professor and Chair, Medical History and Ethics, University of Washington, Seattle, WA, Chair; Ruth Macklin, Ph.D., Professor of Bioethics, Albert Einstein College of Medicine, Bronx, NY, Vice Chair; Ezra Davidson, Jr., M.D., Professor and Chair, Department of Obstetrics and Gynecology, King-Drew Medical Center, Los Angeles, CA, Treasurer; Lisa Sowle Cahill, Ph.D., Professor of Theology, Boston College, Boston, MA; Thomas E. Elkins, M.D., Professor and Chair, Department of Obstetrics and Gynecology, Louisiana State University, New Orleans, LA; Clifford Grobstein, Ph.D., Professor Emeritus in Science, Technology, and Public Affairs, University of California School of Medicine, San Diego, CA; John S. Hoff, J.D., Swidler and Berlin, Chartered, Washington, DC; Patricia King, J.D., Professor of Law, Georgetown Law Center, Washington, DC; Mildred T. Stahlman, M.D., Professor of Pediatrics and Pathology, Vanderbilt University School of Medicine, Nashville, TN; Moses Tendler, Ph.D., Professor of Biology, Talmudic Law, and Jewish Medical Ethics, Yeshiva University, New York, NY; and Walter J. Wadlington, LLB., Professor, University of Virginia School of Law, Charlottesville, VA; Cynthia B. Cohen, Ph.D., J.D., Executive Director.

2. See Cynthia B. Cohen and Albert R. Jonsen, "The Future of the Fetal Tissue Bank," *Science* 262 (1993): 1663–65; NABER, "Report on Human Cloning through Embryo Splitting: An Amber Light," in "Special Issue: Ethics and the Cloning of Human Embryos," ed. Cynthia B. Cohen, *Kennedy Institute of Ethics Journal* 4 (1994): 251–82.

3. The Ford Foundation, the Greenwall Foundation, the Walter and Elise Haas Fund, the Josiah Macy, Jr. Foundation, and the Rockefeller Foundation.

PART A

Procedures and Policies at
Four Oocyte Donation Centers

ONE

DONOR OOCYTE PROGRAM AT UNIVERSITY OF WASHINGTON MEDICAL CENTER

Nancy A. Klein, M.D.,
Gretchen Sewall, R.N., M.S.W., and
Michael R. Soules, M.D.

BACKGROUND

In 1988, the University of Washington Medical Center (UWMC) Donor Oocyte Program was established to provide assisted reproductive technology services to women with premature or impending ovarian failure. The initial cases involved recipient women whose oocyte donors were known to them; however, since that time we have developed an anonymous donor program for recruitment and screening of young women willing to serve as oocyte donors. Since the beginning of the program, we have performed over 200 cycles of *in vitro* fertilization (IVF) through the Donor Oocyte Program. We will outline the indications, procedures, and outcome of the program at the University of Washington.

INDICATIONS FOR DONOR OOCYTE IVF

The classic indication for donor oocyte IVF is premature ovarian failure (e.g., gonadal dysgenesis). Currently, donor oocyte IVF is also offered to women at risk for transmitting certain genetic diseases, women with poor response to ovarian hyperstimulation, and women with multiple failed attempts at the use of assisted reproductive technology. Because of the poor pregnancy rates achieved through assisted reproductive technology in women aged 40 and older (especially when they exhibit elevated baseline follicle stimulating hormone levels), these women may also be candidates for elective primary treatment with donor oocyte IVF. Through oocyte donation, women of advanced reproductive age are not only offered significantly improved cycle fecundity rates but also reduced spontaneous abortion rates compared to the respective expected rates for their age group. Even women who have experienced a natural menopause (up to age 50 years) may elect to conceive via donor oocyte IVF. Indications for the UWMC Donor Oocyte Program include the following:

1) premature ovarian failure
2) premenopausal oophorectomy (ovary removal)
3) genetic indications
4) poor response to ovarian stimulation
5) natural menopause
6) multiple failed assisted reproductive technology attempts
7) persistently abnormal oocytes obtained at IVF
8) assisted reproductive technology candidates ≥40 years old wishing to optimize their pregnancy rate and decrease their rate of spontaneous abortion and chromosome abnormalities

DONOR OOCYTE PROGRAM COORDINATOR

A special feature of the UWMC DOP is the presence of a dedicated full-time professional staff member to act as coordinator. Currently serving in this capacity is a reproductive endocrinology nurse with an advanced degree in clinical social work who functions under the direct supervision of the Assisted Reproductive Technology director and clinic manager. The coordinator functions both as a clinician and as a program administrator.

As a clinician, she provides nursing care and counseling service to donors and recipients prior to and immediately following active oocyte donation cycles. Specific clinical tasks include recruiting, screening, and preparing donors for oocyte donation; meeting with the recipient couple to address psychoeducational needs; facilitating the matching of donors and recipients; and adjusting both donor and recipient hormone levels in order to synchronize their menstrual cycles. The coordinator also acts as a clinical liaison between the patient and the medical team by relaying information and maintaining daily communication with the Assisted Reproductive Technology patient care representative, nurses, and physicians.

As a program administrator, the Donor Oocyte Program coordinator proposes program policies and procedures, manages financial issues, collects data and keeps outcome statistics. In addition, she develops educational material for the program and participates in public relations and community outreach education. She supervises the work of an administrative assistant who helps with correspondence, record keeping, and data collection. Frequent meetings are held with the Assisted Reproductive Technology director, the clinic manager and other departmental staff to monitor and facilitate program development and improvement.

EVALUATION OF RECIPIENTS

AGE LIMIT FOR DONOR OOCYTE RECIPIENTS

The UWMC Donor Oocyte Program has established an upper age limit of 50 years for patients receiving donor oocytes (there is no lower age limit for recipients). The age limit is based on the paucity of pregnancy outcome data for women over 50 and the well-established increase in maternal obstetric morbidity in women ≥35 years old. Age-related increases in perinatal and maternal mortality rates have also been reported. Factors contributing to this increased mortality may be related to the lower socioeconomic status, lack of access to contraception, and higher parity in the older age groups studied in prior published reports. A study of private obstetric patients revealed no increase in perinatal mortality in women ≥35 compared to women 20 to 34 years of age.[1]

Nonetheless, whether healthy older women who intentionally postpone pregnancy are subject to an increased mortality rate is currently not clear because of the low frequency of maternal deaths and only preliminary obstetric data from this population.[2] The incidence of chronic medical illness increases with age and may contribute to an increase in maternal morbidity. For this reason, recipient women in our program who are 45 years of age or older are required to have medical screening beyond a routine history and physical examination including the following:

1) mammogram
2) fasting and two-hour postprandial glucose
3) fasting lipoprotein profile
4) complete blood count
5) serum chemistries, including electrolytes, blood urea nitrogen, creatinine and hepatic enzymes
6) electrocardiogram
7) treadmill stress test

Women with medical risk factors identified by these tests are counseled regarding risks of pregnancy and referred for preconceptual counseling (perinatal consultation) if they desire to proceed. There are no strictly defined criteria for exclusion of recipients based on medical evaluation; patients are counseled and decisions made on an individual basis. However, the Donor Oocyte Program reserves the right to refuse to allow participation of a particular recipient if the physician(s) believe the medical risks are excessive. All DOP recipients over 40 years of age are counseled regarding the increased risk of gestational diabetes, hypertension, and cesarean section as well as the compounding of these risks by the high incidence of multiple gestation.

MEDICAL EVALUATION OF THE DOP RECIPIENT

The medical evaluation generally takes place over one or more clinic visits that occur at least two months before an anticipated active donation cycle. The evaluation of oocyte recipients at UWMC includes a medical history and physical examination with particular attention to specific risk factors for pregnancy, especially diabetes and hypertension. A uterine sounding to measure the depth of the endometrial cavity is performed in anticipation of embryo transfer at a later date. A hysterosalpingogram to evaluate the uterine cavity is recommended, particularly if the patient is nulliparous, has a history of infertility in the presence of ovarian function, or has risk factors for spontaneous abortion or abnormalities of the endometrial cavity (e.g., diethylstilbestrol exposure, recurrent abortion, fibroids, abnormal bleeding, or previous uterine instrumentation).

If either psychopathology or substance abuse is identified during routine medical history and physical examination or during the counseling session with the program coordinator, recipients are referred for psychiatric evaluation. It is recommended that patients with a history of addiction to drugs or alcohol have one year free of substance abuse prior to attempting conception to reduce the risk of relapse during pregnancy. Unless specific psychiatric disorders are suspected, no formal psychological testing is performed.

Prior to undergoing a donor oocyte IVF cycle, recipient women are asked to sign a written consent form acknowledging the medical risks and agreeing to accept donor oocytes and to maintain anonymity between donor and recipient.

COUNSELING

The recipient couple meets with the program coordinator for 45 to 60 minutes to discuss alternatives and are counseled with particular attention to psychosocial, ethical, and legal issues pertaining to oocyte donation. Included in this discussion are issues regarding disclosure of the donation to the child, maintenance of anonymity between donor and recipient (in cases of anonymous donation) and legal issues regarding maternity. The impact of pregnancy and childrearing on the marital relationship is also addressed. Generally, this discussion is directed toward informing recipients of these issues and providing an opportunity for discussion. The coordinator may also make recommendations or assist the couple in decision making based on information provided by the couple during this session. The program coordinator encourages the couple to employ various coping techniques during the cycle and to seek follow-up care regardless of cycle outcome.

EVALUATION OF THE DOP RECIPIENT MALE PARTNER

Male partners of recipient couples are asked to complete an extensive medical and genetic history to identify possible carrier status for genetic traits and their risk for transmitting genetic abnormalities. These men are also evaluated with a general medical and social history and swim-up semen analysis to identify possible subfertility. For men of unproven fertility or with two or more abnormal semen analyses, a sperm penetration assay (zona-free hamster egg sperm penetration test) may be recommended to help identify those at risk for fertilization failure. Patients with male infertility are not excluded from the program. However, when severe male infertility is present, sperm microinjection or donor sperm may be recommended and used for insemination.

SEROLOGIC TESTING

Serologic testing of donor recipient couples is routinely performed. They are tested for syphilis, hepatitis B and C, HIV I and II, blood type, and chlamydia within six months of an active cycle. If antichlamydial antibodies are detected in the serum of either partner, both are treated with a course of doxycycline for the possibility of active infection. Female recipients are also tested for antibodies to rubella and vaccinated prior to the cycle if nonimmune.

EVALUATION OF OOCYTE DONORS

DONOR RECRUITMENT (ANONYMOUS)

Healthy women aged 21 to 34 years with no significant genetic risk factors or history of infertility or pregnancy wastage are recruited from the general population. Advertising for oocyte donors is limited to advertisement in community publications and the posting of flyers around campus. As it turns out, most donors learn of the program by word of mouth. Phone or mail inquiries are answered with an information sheet and a written application, which includes a complete medical, social, and genetic history.

SCREENING, COUNSELING, AND CONSENT

Women with acceptable written applications are contacted and invited to attend an information class conducted by the program coordinator. In this class, the medical screening process, clinical procedures and mechanics of the donation cycle, risks and reimbursement are discussed. In addition, a video-tape is shown describing the basic process of IVF. A woman who has already participated as an oocyte donor is asked to attend the class to describe her experience and to answer questions.

Women who remain interested after the class are asked to schedule an appointment for a personal interview with the Donor Oocyte Program coor-dinator. The coordinator conducts a 45 minute interview with each donor applicant. During this interview the coordinator assesses the applicant's com-prehension and assimilation of the information previously presented in the donor class. Other essential elements of the interview include assessing (1) motivation for donation, (2) current life stressors, (3) coping skills and stability, and (4) strength of interpersonal relationships.

Women are questioned about their previous and current sexual practices and reproductive health, with attention to contraceptive practices and risk factors for sexually transmitted diseases. Potential personal, religious, and ethical concerns related to oocyte donation are explored with each donor candidate. Particular attention is paid to possible substance abuse, evidence suggestive of a personality disorder, other past or present psychopathology, or sexual abuse. Donors may be excluded from the program for any of the above-mentioned problems or issues.

The coordinator also emphasizes the importance of sexual monogamy or celibacy and the use of nonhormonal contraception in the absence of perma-nent sterilization. A review of the possible risks and side effects from ovula-tion induction medications and/or the sonographic egg retrieval is completed, and the donor's signature on the written consent form is witnessed. The interview is concluded with an explanation of the financial compensation offered by the recipient couple for the donor's time, effort, and discomfort. The information included in the donor profile is then approved by the donor to ensure both confidentiality and accuracy prior to putting the profile in the donor notebook (see section on matching, below).

Donor applicants are asked to keep a record of daily basal body tempera-ture for one cycle. A medical history and physical examination is performed (usually by a nurse practitioner or physician assistant), and the genetic history is reviewed by a genetic counselor. After this portion of the screening is completed, the written application, history and physical examination, pro-gram coordinator's and genetic counselor's comments, and basal body tem-perature chart are reviewed by the UWMC Assisted Reproductive Technology director for final approval.

SEROLOGIC TESTING

When a donor has been matched to a recipient couple, donor serologic testing is performed for syphilis, hepatitis B and C, and HIV I and II. Blood type and Rh status are also determined. Specific tests are performed such as hemoglobin electropheresis or screening for Tay-Sachs disease carrier status as indicated by risk associated with ethnic background.

KNOWN DONORS

Occasionally, patients request that a friend or relative serve as an oocyte donor. Known donors are screened as in the anonymous donor program; however, the program is more flexible with regard to the age and fertility status of the known donors (age limit 21–40). There is also more leniency exercised in relation to the genetic history of a known donor who is a relative, since the risks may be the same as if the female recipient were to have conceived using her own oocytes. When an older donor is selected, recipients are counseled regarding possible reduced pregnancy rate and increased risk of spontaneous abortion and chromosomal abnormalities. In counseling and obtaining informed consent from a known donor, particular attention is paid to psychosocial issues and motivation of the donor, with an effort to identify possible coercion.

REPEAT CYCLES

There is no well-established limit on the number of cycles in which a woman may serve as an oocyte donor, although a guideline to the *maximum* number of pregnancies would be the same as that recommended when donor sperm are used, that is, ten pregnancies per donor to reduce the possibility of future unintentional consanguineous marriages between unrelated offspring. However, due to limited data on long-term consequences of multiple egg-recovery procedures on subsequent fertility as well as possible unknown long-term effects of multiple cycles of aggressive ovulation induction in young women, we have not encouraged donors to undergo repeat cycles beyond three. Most of the UWMC Donor Oocyte Program donors donate one or two times. Donors are excluded from continuing in the program if previous cycles have not resulted in pregnancy in the presence of poor ovarian response to ovulation induction, poor oocyte or embryo quality, the occurrence of medical complications and/or noncompliance (e.g., lack of cooperation) in their previous cycles.

MATCHING DONORS AND RECIPIENTS

Matching of anonymous donors and recipients is accomplished in one of two ways. Couples can select their donor from the donor profiles listed in the anonymous donor notebook. The profiles contain information on ethnic background, physical traits, past fertility, academic interests, talents, motivation for donation, and general health information on the donor and her family. The medical/genetic history is complete through her grandparents' generation. All information in the profile is nonidentifying and approved by the donor before being put in the notebook. The second method of matching is for the program coordinator to select two possible donors based on a photograph of the recipient woman and a letter the couple has written briefly describing general characteristics they would prefer in a donor. Common requests are for donors who physically resemble the recipient woman, have a history of pregnancy, and have similar academic/social/athletic talents and interests. Occasionally couples will request donors who are specifically motivated by altruism or who are donating to improve their life situation (e.g., to pay for college tuition). The coordinator-facilitated matching is selected most often when the couple lives out of town. When a tentative match has been made, a phone appointment is arranged to present profile information on two donors to the couple. The couple is asked to choose one of the donors by the following day. Once the match has been made, the donor profile is taken out of the notebook and a copy is given to the couple. If a pregnancy occurs, it is suggested that the couple keep the profile in their family depository for important documents.

ACTIVE CYCLE

DONOR STIMULATION

Until the fall of 1994, ovarian stimulation had been achieved with a combination regimen of clomiphene citrate (CC) and human menopausal gonadotropins (hMG). This regimen was originally selected because of its relatively low cost and ease of administration. Our experience with this protocol had been excellent overall, with highly consistent ovarian responses requiring little deviation from the anticipated synchrony with the recipient's hormone replacement schedule. Cycle cancellation with this protocol was uncommon (<10%), and ovulation prior to egg recovery was rare (less than 1%).

However, it was noted that there was significant variability of oocyte quality and fertilization rates not generally experienced with the more standard ovulation induction protocol utilizing pituitary down-regulation with a gonadotropin-releasing hormone analogue (GnRHa). Therefore, we now utilize a stimulation protocol with nafarelin acetate beginning in the midluteal phase followed by gonadotropin stimulation beginning at any time after adequate ovarian suppression. This protocol generally results in recovery of more oocytes and eliminates the possibility of an LH surge prior to egg recovery. Embryo quality and pregnancy rates have also improved since this change in donor stimulation was implemented.

EGG RECOVERY AND INSEMINATION

Oocytes are usually recovered from the donor transvaginally under ultrasound guidance in an outpatient setting. Most donors receive only oral diazepam and intravenous fentanyl for sedation during the oocyte recovery procedure with oral promethazine as prophylaxis for nausea. This level of anesthetic treatment is referred to as conscious sedation. However, donors are offered the opportunity to have the procedure performed in the operating room with an anesthesiologist present to administer propofol for more complete anesthesia. The vast majority of donors do well in the clinic setting with conscious sedation. Oral doxycycline is given after the procedure as prophylaxis against infection. Donors are instructed to return to the clinic for a follow-up visit and ultrasound one week after the procedure to evaluate them for signs or symptoms of ovarian hyperstimulation syndrome or other complications.

Insemination is performed on the day of oocyte recovery with prepared sperm from the recipient's husband (or donor sperm when indicated). The standard sperm preparation consists of either a swim-up technique or a density gradient centrifugation. Men are scheduled for specimen collection after the donor has been discharged from the clinic to ensure anonymity.

EMBRYO TRANSFER AND CRYOPRESERVATION

Embryo transfer is scheduled approximately 48 hours after egg recovery. Up to four embryos are transcervically delivered to the fundal region of the uterine cavity. Embryo quality is graded by the embryologist and is taken into consideration when determining the number of embryos to transfer. Generally, the best quality embryos (subjectively determined) are selected for the fresh transfer. Until 1993, four embryos were routinely transferred; however, this number was reduced to three if there was good to excellent embryo quality because of the high percentage of multiple gestations, including many triplet and one quadruplet pregnancy.

All Donor Oocyte Program transfers are performed transcervically unless precluded by an anatomic abnormality in the recipient woman. Gamete intrafallopian transfer (GIFT) and zygote intrafallopian transfer (ZIFT) are not routinely performed in the Donor Oocyte Program because of the increased risk and cost to the recipient in the absence of well-established evidence of improved pregnancy rates. In fact, a comparative study failed to demonstrate an advantage of GIFT over IVF in a donor oocyte program.[3]

If more than three good quality embryos are available on the day of transfer, the remaining embryos are cryopreserved with the consent of the recipient couple. In some cases with more than eight pronuclear embryos available on the day prior to transfer, six are held out from which to select for the fresh transfer, and the remaining embryos are frozen at the pronuclear stage.

HORMONE REPLACEMENT THERAPY

Premenopausal recipients

Recipient patients with evidence of recent ovarian function (spontaneous menses within one year) are placed on daily subcutaneous leuprolide acetate

(LA) or intranasal nafarelin acetate to suppress endogenous gonadotropins and ovarian function. Suppressed recipients are maintained on low-dose estrogen replacement and LA until ovarian stimulation of the donor is initiated. At the initiation of the active donor cycle, the recipient's hormone replacement therapy (HRT) is then augmented. Our current regimen consists of oral micronized estradiol given in graduated doses throughout donor stimulation; oral estradiol along with intramuscular progesterone-in-oil is continued throughout the luteal phase. Each patient is given a calendar outlining the HRT regimen. This recipient HRT regimen is much more complex and at a higher dose than those used for standard replacement in postmenopausal women. Variations in the donor's response to ovarian stimulation can lead to alterations in the recipient's HRT schedule; therefore, recipients remain in contact with the IVF nurse or physician throughout the stimulation so that these alterations can be communicated to the patient as needed.

Postmenopausal recipients

Postmenopausal patients and those with ovarian failure receive a similar regimen of estradiol and progesterone replacement with the exception that the GnRha is not required. They are placed on cyclic HRT until the donor menses are expected; at that time, low-dose estradiol is continued until ovarian stimulation is begun and then the specific high-dose Donor Oocyte Program HRT calendar is followed. Withdrawal menses are scheduled to occur within 30 days of anticipated embryo transfer so that a given recipient has not had prolonged uterine stimulation by estrogen prior to initiating the accelerated HRT regimen. All recipients receive at least 14 days of estradiol from the onset of the last menses to progesterone initiation.

PREGNANCY MONITORING

Blood for assay of quantitative bhCG is obtained 13 days after embryo transfer. If positive, a repeat bhCG is done 48 to 72 hours later to confirm rising levels, and the luteal phase hormone replacement therapy is continued until eight completed weeks from embryo transfer. No routine monitoring of serum estradiol or progesterone levels is performed during early pregnancy. Transvaginal ultrasound is performed approximately five weeks after embryo transfer to confirm a viable intrauterine pregnancy and also to evaluate for extrauterine and multiple gestations. Patients with normal ultrasound findings are referred for obstetric care. The program coordinator contacts the patient within several weeks after her expected date of delivery to obtain data on pregnancy outcome.

COST

Anonymous oocyte donors are compensated by the recipient for their time and inconvenience in the amount of $1,500 per egg recovery. If the cycle is canceled after ovulation induction has been initiated but prior to egg recovery, recipients provide partial compensation at their discretion. The recipient is responsible for all charges related to the cycle, including donor screening, medications, monitoring costs, egg recovery and embryo transfer procedures, and laboratory charges. The total is about $9,000 per cycle, including donor compensation.

DONOR OOCYTE PROGRAM OUTCOME AT UWMC

Since the UWMC Donor Oocyte Program began in 1988, 222 treatment cycles (with either known or anonymous donors) have been initiated. Eighteen cycles (8%) were canceled prior to egg recovery due to poor ovarian response (8 cycles), development of a single dominant follicle (5 cycles), premature luteinization (3 cycles), or recipient medication error (2 cycles). A significant male factor (sperm concentration <20 million/ml and/or motility <40%) was present in 26 cycles (12%). Of the 204 cycles in which oocytes were obtained, embryo transfer did not occur in six cycles because of fertilization failure. Sixty-three clinical pregnancies have resulted, with an ongoing pregnancy rate of 30% per embryo transfer. The multiple pregnancy rate is 42%, and the spontaneous abortion rate is 9%. No oocyte donors have experienced medical complications requiring hospitalization in the UWMC Donor Oocyte Program. Occasionally, additional follow-up visits have been required to monitor for signs or symptoms of mild or moderate ovarian hyperstimulation syndrome.

With a growing number of women who delay childbearing until their later reproductive years and increasing public awareness of oocyte donation, the UWMC Donor Oocyte Program continues to grow. As the number of women conceiving through donor oocyte IVF increases, obstetric risks for women in and beyond the late 40s will become better defined. Also, the potential impact of psychosocial and legal ramifications of oocyte donation will become more apparent. The protocol outlined in this chapter will require ongoing evaluation as more data on the outcome of donor oocyte pregnancies become available.

NOTES

1. G. S. Berkowitz, M. L. Skovron, R. H. Lapinski, R. L. Berkowitz, "Delayed Childbearing and the Outcome of Pregnancy," *New England Journal of Medicine* 322 (1990): 659–64.

2. M. V. Sauer, R. J. Paulson, R. A. Lobo, "Pregnancy after Age 50: Application of Oocyte Donation to Women after Natural Menopause," *Lancet* 341 (1993): 321–23.

3. J. P. Balmaceda, V. Alam, D. Roszjtein, T. Ord, K. Snell, R. H. Asch, "Embryo Implantation Rates in Oocyte Donation: A Prospective Comparison of Tubal Versus Uterine Factors," *Fertility and Sterility* 57 (1992): 362–65.

TWO

OOCYTE DONATION PROGRAM AT MONTE-FIORE MEDICAL CENTER, ALBERT EINSTEIN

David H. Barad, M.D., and
Brian L. Cohen, M.D.

INTRODUCTION

Love, marriage, and children are among life's normal expectations. These expectations, however, are not always fulfilled. Approximately 12% of married couples in the United States are infertile and require help to realize their family goals. Relying on other people to help create a family is not a modern concept. In the Bible, Jacob and Sarah achieved their first child, Ishmael, by using Sarah's maid, Hagar (Gen. 16:1-4). Rachel's son Dan was given birth by her maid, Bilah (Gen. 30:3-6).

Oocyte donation is a procedure that contemporary women can use to achieve a pregnancy. The egg of a donor is substituted for an egg that the recipient cannot produce and is fertilized in the laboratory. The resulting preembryo is transferred to the recipient's womb. In about 30% of cases this leads to a pregnancy.

Hagar and Bilah acted as what we would now call surrogate mothers. Oocyte donation differs from surrogacy in several respects. The surrogate mother is lending her body for use by the infertile couple. She experiences pregnancy and exposes herself to its attendant risks. She develops bonding to the child through pregnancy and birth, and often feels grief on having to give the child up to the infertile couple.[1] Oocyte donation allows the recipient to be the gestational mother and spares the donor the emotional and physical risks of pregnancy. There seems to be greater justice in oocyte donation than in surrogacy in that with the former, those who will benefit from the procedure bear the risks of pregnancy. Oocyte donation also seems more natural, in that the mother who gives birth will raise the child.

In this chapter, we will describe our oocyte donor program, our screening procedures for oocyte donors and recipients, and our thoughts regarding issues that arise in relation to the use of anonymous or nonanonymous oocyte donors.

THE PROGRAM

Our oocyte donor program is located at the Fertility and Hormone Center, an ambulatory care facility developed by Montefiore Medical Center and the Albert Einstein College of Medicine. The program was founded late in 1987 following the development of our *in vitro* fertilization program, which had existed for two years and was responsible for several live births. Others had already reported successful pregnancies as a result of oocyte donation,[2] or embryo transfer.[3] We had as patients several young women with premature ovarian failure. Oocyte donation seemed to be a technique we could use to help them.

To assist us in formulating policies for our oocyte donation program we asked the dean of the Albert Einstein College of Medicine to appoint an ethics committee, which he did. The committee is chaired by an associate dean, and is composed of members of the Division of Reproductive Endocrinology, ethicists, lawyers, and psychologists. Since its creation, the group has met monthly and has provided valuable guidance to its clinical members. The committee has assisted in developing policies regarding oocyte donation, payment of donors, criteria for recipients, and psychiatric screening of donors and recipients. It has also discussed questions related to nonanonymous or anonymous donation of both oocytes and sperm.

OOCYTE DONORS

Why do women donate their eggs? When asked, most of our oocyte donors responded that they wanted "to help other women." Among women undergoing tubal ligation who were asked to be oocyte donors, we noted that those who agreed to participate were more likely to have had a voluntary abortion in the past. We can speculate that oocyte donation was an act of contrition for them. Or it may be that they placed less value on the products of their reproductive processes than women who did not choose to be donors. More than half of our donors have been unmarried and many of them do not plan to have children of their own. Oocyte donation may allow these women to fulfill their own urge to reproduce.

Potential donors may be subject to emotional and financial coercion. They may be unable to refuse friends and family members if asked to donate their eggs. Anonymous donors may find that the financial incentives offered by oocyte donor programs are irresistible. Some women who were proposed by recipients as nonanonymous oocyte donors were only casual acquaintances. One potential donor was approached in a shopping mall by her prospective recipient because the two women resembled each other physically. Another donor worked as an administrative assistant for the recipient. A casual acquaintance has less potential for emotional coercion than a donor known well by the recipient, but a greater chance for financial coercion. Like Hagar and Bilah, employees may not be able to deny assistance to their employers.

DONOR ELIGIBILITY

Healthy women age 35 years and younger are eligible to be anonymous oocyte donors. Our age limit for nonanonymous oocyte donors is 39 years. Married women who have had children are the most suitable donors, but single nulliparous women have also been accepted. We limit oocyte donors to ten successful pregnancies, the same limit advised by the American Fertility Society for donor sperm pregnancies in a single geographical area. In practice, we have not had to invoke this limit, as we have never used the same anonymous oocyte donor in more than one cycle of ovulation induction and oocyte retrieval. Nonanonymous oocyte donors have gone through as many as three cycles before their recipient became pregnant. One nonanonymous oocyte donor returned to help her recipient achieve a second pregnancy.

ANONYMOUS OOCYTE DONORS

When our program was initiated, our anonymous oocyte donors came from two sources; women who were undergoing *in vitro* fertilization (IVF) or women having laparoscopically guided bilateral tubal ligation. The development of embryo cryopreservation techniques eliminated excess oocytes derived from women having IVF as a source of donated oocytes.

Tubal ligation patients were approached only after they had consented to that procedure. In a 1988 study, we found that only 2.5% of 194 women undergoing laparoscopic tubal ligation were eligible to donate oocytes. Of these, 55% were disqualified because they were over the age of 35 and 16% because they were pregnant at the time of their tubal ligation. The remaining eligible women were not willing to participate.[4]

ADVERTISING FOR ANONYMOUS OOCYTE DONORS

Paid donors recruited by advertising are a third source of anonymous oocytes. With the development of embryo cryopreservation, we realized that

Radio Advertisement

A Westchester fertility center is seeking altruistic and compassionate women under 36 years of age who are willing to donate their eggs to women who are unable to have children because of a lack of eggs. Financial compensation is available. Call 914-693-8820 for more information.

Print Advertisement

If you are a woman under 36 years of age and would like to help a woman who cannot have children because she has no eggs of her own, you can help by donating eggs. This involves stimulation with fertility drugs, having several blood tests and ultrasound examinations, and undergoing a procedure to obtain the eggs. If you want to have a tubal ligation, it could be performed at the time the eggs are retrieved at no charge to you. Financial compensation is available. Please call The Fertility and Hormone Center at 914-693-8820 for more information.

Figure 1.

our former sources would no longer be as numerous. We would have to advertise for anonymous donors or allow more women to use nonanonymous oocyte donors if we were to continue our program.

In 1992, we began advertising (Figure 1) for anonymous oocyte donors on radio and in local newspapers. Twenty-four potential donors responded to our last advertisement. Most gave "wanting to help other women" as a reason for responding. Only three went beyond the screening phone call to make an initial visit. Several made appointments, but didn't keep them. Women who said they wanted to donate only for financial reasons were not encouraged to participate further in the program.

OOCYTE DONOR SCREENING

When a potential donor contacts the center by phone, she is given the information listed below (Figure 2). Information obtained from her includes: date of birth, race and ethnic background, number of pregnancies, number of children, date of last pregnancy, method of contraception being used, last grade completed in school, reason for considering donating eggs.

- 6–7 visits will be required for consultations and tests at no cost to you to determine if you can donate eggs.
- If you are accepted as a candidate to donate eggs, the treatment necessary to retrieve eggs will involve: taking fertility medication, having several blood tests and sonograms, and undergoing a procedure to obtain the eggs.
- If accepted into the program, the maximum reimbursement for your time and effort is $1,500.
- A limited number of donors are needed. If you are interested, I will ask you some information about yourself which will be reviewed by a doctor. We will contact you within two weeks to let you know if you are a candidate to donate eggs.
- Further information about the medical and financial issues can be discussed at the time of the appointment.
- All information is confidential.

Figure 2. Information given to potential oocyte donors who respond to our advertisement.

If she maintains her interest, an appointment is made with the donor oocyte program director, who obtains a complete medical and social history, takes a family history documenting common inherited diseases such as Tay-Sachs, cystic fibrosis, and sickle-cell disease, and performs a physical examination. The potential donor is given the opportunity to ask questions about the medical procedures involved. The risks of ovulation induction and ovum retrieval are discussed, including the possibility of ovarian hyperstimulation and its consequences. The hypothesized link between ovulation-inducing medications and ovarian cancer is also presented. The candidate is told that she will have to abstain from intercourse or use barrier contraception while taking medications or else risk becoming pregnant.

A large part of the second visit is devoted to discussing and analyzing the candidate's motivation for participation. At the third visit, she is evaluated by the psychiatric counselor. Conflicting feelings about children who may arise

Cultures:	GC, chlamydia, mycoplasma.
Blood tests:	FSH, estradiol, HIV, hepatitis screen, RPR, CMV, CBC, chemistry screen, blood type.

Figure 3. Donor screening.

out of the oocyte donation are evaluated. She is also assessed for her ability to comply with the rigors of ovulation induction and ovum retrieval. If the oocyte donor is married, her husband is expected to attend a session with the psychiatric counselor along with, in the case of nonanonymous donors, the recipient couple.

Information about the potential donor is presented at the weekly staff meeting, and if she is approved, she is asked to return for further testing (Figure 3). Following the results of these tests, the donor is instructed regarding medications, a recipient is matched, and the cycle is commenced.

FINANCIAL COMPENSATION TO DONORS

We are very concerned about the commercialization of reproductive technologies. We do not believe that human eggs should be treated as a commodity. Our policy for compensation of egg donors was approved by our ethics committee and was based on our medical school's published guidelines for compensation to subjects participating in clinical research.

When our program was initiated, we accepted the insurance of women undergoing tubal ligation who agreed to be oocyte donors as payment and offered no other financial incentive for participation. However, it became clear that frequent visits for monitoring during ovulation induction were a burden for these women. During our second year, we elected to cover these expenses, which were usually just a few hundred dollars. In order to maintain parity among different donors, we began to offer $1,000 as reimbursement for time and expenses.

Our present compensation for oocyte donors consists of a $700 honorarium plus $100 per visit with a maximum payment of $1,500. This is paid regardless of the number of oocytes retrieved or recipients involved. If more than one recipient benefits, the cost of the donor is distributed among the recipients. This has occurred on six occasions. One donor became angry when she learned that her oocytes had been used for two recipients. She demanded double reimbursement and has threatened to sue for additional compensation.

OOCYTE RECIPIENTS

In our program, candidates for receiving donor oocytes must fulfill medical and some social criteria. Recipients must be in good physical and mental health. There is no absolute age limitation. Women over the age of 43 are required to have a medical and perinatal consult early in the evaluation, and those over the age of 47 must have a cardiology evaluation.

Donated oocytes are a scarce resource. Consequently, we try to assign donated oocytes to recipients who will be most likely to have a successful pregnancy as a result of the procedure. Most potential recipients have experienced premature loss of ovarian function. Women who have menstrual cycles are evaluated for standard IVF before being considered as oocyte recipients. Those who are unable to produce oocytes in response to ovulation induction during the course of a standard IVF cycle can be accepted as recipients in the donor oocyte program. A third category of potential recipients are women with a genetic trait or disorder in whom pregnancy may result in a fetus with a lethal or debilitating inherited condition.

UNMARRIED RECIPIENTS

Our oocyte donation program does not require that potential recipients be married. We require that single women demonstrate that they have social support to help share responsibilities of childrearing and to care for the child if the mother should become ill. Such support could be from a partner, sibling, parent, or friend. If there is a partner, we require that he or she participate in the preparation and counseling prior to ovum donation. We ask, but do not require, that we meet other adults who may participate in childrearing. We urge single women to advise their parents of their plan to become pregnant, since the grandparents could become guardians by default. We have similar requirements for single women seeking donor sperm insemination.

We did not all embrace the concept of allowing unmarried single oocyte recipients access to donated oocytes. Some of us felt that oocyte donation to a single woman (who also requires sperm donation) was the same as adoption. However, the majority of members of the ethics committee noted that a woman who receives ovum donation experiences pregnancy and childbirth; this is a significant physiological and philosophical difference from adoption that some women value.

Financial security is an important part of child care. Ovum donation is one of the most expensive of the assisted reproductive technologies because we are managing two patients, the donor and the recipient. Both must go through extensive pre-cycle screening and preparation. The expenses of the donor cannot be charged either to her or the recipient's insurance carrier. Thus, more than any other assisted reproductive technology, most of the expense of these cycles are paid out of the recipient's pocket. It has been our experience that only people with considerable disposable income have sufficient funds to undertake this procedure. Most of the recipients will be able to give their children great financial security.

RISKS OF CYCLE

Risks for the recipients include those related to the procedure and those related to pregnancy itself. The medical preparation of an ovum recipient is dependent upon whether or not she is still menstruating. If premenopausal, the donor's stimulation can be programmed in parallel with the recipient's "natural" cycle. In this way, the recipient does not have to use any medications. One of the risks of a natural cycle embryo transfer, however, is that the recipient and donor may not cycle in tandem and embryos would be transferred when the endometrium is not ready to receive them. Among the risks of transfer itself are discomfort, perforation of the uterus, or infection. The latter two outcomes are exceedingly rare.

Suppression of the premenopausal recipient's menstrual cycle is an alternative to the natural cycle embryo transfer. In this case, recipients are made hypogonadal by administration of a GnRH agonist. Oocyte recipients who use GnRH agonist experience menopausal symptoms, including vaginal dryness and hot flushes. It is not known if there are any long-term risks of a short course of GnRH agonist.

Postmenopausal women and women who have used GnRH agonist to induce a hypogonadal state require estrogen and progesterone replacement. We developed a protocol using estradiol valerate to establish a proliferative endometrium. Patients receive 1 to 3 mg of estradiol valerate i.m. twice weekly. Nadir serum concentrations of estradiol are maintained at 400 to 600 pg/ml. After two weeks of therapy, the recipient is given 50 mg of progesterone in oil i.m. daily for four days together with progesterone vaginal suppositories 100 mg bid. Progesterone serum concentrations are maintained between 15 and 40 ng/ml. Levels achieved with this regimen mimic those of natural cycles and are generally an order of magnitude less than the estrogen levels obtained following ovulation induction with human menopausal gonadotropins. Women with a history of deep vein thrombosis have an increased risk of recurrent thrombosis or pulmonary embolism on high-dose estrogen replacement. It is unlikely that there are any other significant long-term risks of this type of estrogen replacement. Patients on this regimen for lengthy periods may not undergo adequate endometrial shedding and may be at risk for the development of endometrial hyperplasia or endometrial cancer. For this reason, women who are waiting for a donor are placed on an alternate estrogen replacement regimen until a donor has been located.

RISKS OF PREGNANCY

Premature menopausal patients

Risks of pregnancy for a healthy woman of normal reproductive age who has experienced premature ovarian failure and become pregnant following hormone replacement and embryo transfer are no greater than those of other women in her age group. There is no known increased risk to the woman or the fetus as a result of hormone replacement and embryo transfer once the pregnancy has been established. Women must remain on hormone replacement through the first trimester of pregnancy. Serum concentrations of estradiol and progesterone are maintained at those found in a normal pregnancy. After the first trimester, the placenta is capable of sustaining the pregnancy without exogenous hormonal supplementation. From then on the pregnancy proceeds as if the woman had conceived on her own without assisted reproduction.

Menopausal patients

These techniques may also be used to establish a pregnancy in women who are beyond the usual reproductive age. There is no established database to assess the risks of pregnancy for women in the later reproductive years. Oocyte donation from a young donor decreases the risk of genetic abnormalities, a risk usually associated with pregnancy in women over the age of 35. Other risks include spontaneous abortion, medical complications, fetal growth abnormalities, dysfunctional labor, cesarean section, and maternal-perinatal death. Maternal mortality and morbidity increase after the age of 40.[5]

Recently we have had several requests for ovum donation from patients older than the usual reproductive age. Our oldest patient to achieve a pregnancy was 50 years old at the time of her embryo transfer. One 57-year-old patient was evaluated cautiously because she was overweight and hypertensive and therefore might have had an extremely high probability of morbidity for herself and her child. Even if this patient were fit and healthy, we would have had reservations about including her as an oocyte recipient out of the belief that it would be unfair to the child to have aged parents who might be infirm or die before the child reached its majority. The validity of this point is challenged by reality. In the Bronx, where our medical school is based, there are many children who are raised by their grandparents. Is it worse to have older parents or not to be born at all?

SUCCESS RATES

Our clinical pregnancy rate per embryo transfer has remained between 25 and 35% for the past five years. Ovum recipients are told that they may have to go through more than one cycle to achieve a pregnancy. They have to be reminded of the possibility of failure more than once, since the spirit of hope and anticipation they bring to this endeavor seems to cloud any notion that they will not achieve a pregnancy.

RECIPIENT SCREENING

Recipients are screened at our center in a series of six steps. The objective is to evaluate relevant medical and psychological issues and provide the potential participants with appropriate information they need for their decision-making process. We try not to evaluate potential recipients for eligibility, but rather to empower them with the information to determine their own eligibility.

The first visit is with one of our reproductive endocrinologists. General information about the donor program is given. A history and physical of the potential recipient is performed to determine whether or not oocyte donation is indicated and to begin to determine her physical ability to support a pregnancy. If medical problems are discovered that could jeopardize the recipient's health or the success of a pregnancy the potential recipient is asked to obtain a medical consult. Use of an anonymous oocyte donor versus a nonanonymous oocyte donor and the length of time anticipated until an anonymous oocyte donor is available are also discussed. In addition, the recipient is told of the remaining screening visits.

The second visit is with the psychiatric counselor. The purpose of this visit is to allow the couple to explore their feelings about receiving another woman's oocytes. It also permits the couple to express any reservations they may have about the process and to ensure that both husband and wife freely consent to be recipients. The couple is asked to discuss plans for informing a potential child of his or her biological origins. The issue of secrecy is addressed. Our advice to potential couples is not to create a family secret, as we believe this makes it difficult to build a healthy family. If a couple decide that they prefer to maintain secrecy about the donation, however, we respect their wishes. The difference between secrecy and confidentiality is discussed. Their medical records will reflect all procedures that they have undergone. Information about their treatment will not be released without their consent.

Couples with a nonanonymous oocyte donor have an additional visit with the counselor together with the donor and her spouse. At that visit the potential for ambivalent relationships between the donor and the recipients' future child are discussed.

The counselor and primary physician present the case at the weekly staff meeting. The primary physician arranges a follow-up visit with the couple to address any issues raised at that meeting, review the reports of any medical or perinatal consults, and allow the couple to ask further questions. A series of laboratory tests is performed on both husband and wife (as appropriate) at

	Patients	Percent per Cycle	Percent per Transfer
Cycles initiated	56		
Transfers completed	49	(87.5)	
Clinical pregnancies	15	(26.7)	(30.6)
Deliveries	11	(19.6)	(22.4)
Twins	2		
Triplets	1		
Miscarriage	4		

Figure 4. Pregnancy rates following oocyte donation.

this time including: a semen analysis, Papanicolaou smear, HIV screen (after counseling and consent), hepatitis screen, RPR, rubella, CMV, a complete blood count, chem screen, and cervical cultures for GC, mycoplasma, and chlamydia. A recent evaluation of the uterine cavity by either hysteroscopy or hysterosalpingogram is also required.

A mock cycle is conducted whose primary purpose is to acquaint the recipient with the technique of hormone replacement that will be used during her actual transfer cycle. An endometrial biopsy is performed to determine the endometrial response to hormone replacement. This mock cycle allows the couple and our staff to develop confidence that medications will be administered properly during the transfer cycle. A third visit with the primary physician is scheduled at which results of the tests and the mock cycle are discussed. Consents for receiving ovum donation are reviewed and signed.

NONANONYMOUS OR ANONYMOUS DONORS

Seven years ago when our donor program was instituted we favored anonymous oocyte donation. This bias arose from our experience with anonymous sperm donation. We believed the issues of parenthood were less ambiguous when gamete donation was anonymous. In *The Fertility Fallacy,* Lynn Baker wrote, "One of the main reasons why people [don't arrange their own artificial inseminations] is that secrecy would be lost. In the current practice of artificial insemination, the paternity of the child is kept strictly secret from all concerned. Often the couple chooses an obstetrician who doesn't know how the baby was conceived, to avoid the necessity for formal adoption and to place the husband's name on the birth certificate."[6] Secrecy is still a major part of sperm donation. A 1989 survey of sperm donors found that most favor strict anonymity.[7] We felt that oocyte donation would best be dealt with in a similar manner. Others shared our bias. Rene Frydman et al. described a protocol to satisfy the "ethical" issues raised by oocyte donation.[8] What were these ethical issues? They said, " . . . assuring anonymous donation of oocytes would limit the risk of possible tension in the future between the participating parties. . . . "

Our feelings favoring anonymous donation may have been partly formed by the Baby M trial, in which custody of a child born to a surrogate mother was awarded to the genetic father. We realized that oocyte donation differed from surrogacy: in surrogacy, the gestational mother and genetic mother are the same, whereas in oocyte donation, they are different. The court's decision seemed to support the genetic definition of parenthood over the gestational. This put our oocyte recipients at risk, since they would not be the genetic mothers of the children to whom they gave birth. Anonymous oocyte donation would help protect them from a legal challenge to their maternity.

Over time our philosophy changed. Our present view of motherhood is closer to that of A. D. Hard who, in discussing the first reported case of donor insemination, said, " . . . the mother is the complete builder of the child. It is her blood that gives it material for its body and her nerve energy which is divided to supply its vital force."[9] In this paradigm, the gestational mother is not a passive vessel, but an active force in the creation of a new life. Motherhood brings much more than genetics to reproduction.

Until gamete donation became a reality, people had the luxury of choosing the father or mother of their children for what they perceived to be desirable characteristics. Anonymous donation takes away the choice of all but the most rudimentary characteristics in a child's genetic parent. This additional loss of control is a major burden for infertile couples who are already dealing with a loss of control of basic biological functions.

Oocyte donation by a nonanonymous donor allows the parents to participate in selection of the child's genes in a way that is very different from selection based on a list of donor characteristics. It also frees the child and family from the "secret" of its conception. Schaffer and Diamond[10] have stated that "It is the political, moral, and ethical position . . . that people are entitled to know who are or are not the biological parents of children." In coming to this conclusion they rely greatly on Mahlstedt and Greenfeld,[11] who wrote, "The reality in the use of donor gametes is that there are more than two 'parents' involved in the conception. Though this reality may be kept secret from others, it cannot be changed nor denied by the couple nor, in some cases, by the [nonanonymous] donor."

In practice, we learned that many of our fears about nonanonymous donation were unfounded. On several occasions, we were able to help a candidate excuse herself as a donor if she felt she had been emotionally coerced to participate. Interviews with oocyte donors who were friends or relatives of our oocyte recipients have convinced us that donors view their relationship to the child as similar to that of an aunt. Most of our recipients who have had a child with the help of a nonanonymous oocyte donor still see the donor, although a few feel threatened by her.

We now believe that a nonanonymous oocyte donor, if available, is preferable to one who is anonymous. A known donor is less likely than an anonymous donor to participate in the program for purposes of financial gain and more likely to be acting out of beneficence toward the recipient who is her friend or relation. We believe that continued emphasis on anonymous oocyte donation will lead to the inevitable definition of human oocytes and embryos as commodities to be bought and sold, as has occurred with human sperm. Although use of a nonanonymous oocyte donor increases the obligations of all of the participants, we believe it serves the purpose of family building, decreases secrecy, and protects against commercialization.

CONCLUSION

Oocyte donation is an act of beneficence, especially in the case of a nonanonymous donor. Unlike the birthmother of an adoptive child whose pregnancy may be the result of accident or ignorance, the child of oocyte donation results from carefully orchestrated planning. These two factors, beneficence and planning, may allow the donor to be incorporated into the child's life in a way that an adopted child's birthmother cannot.

Since biblical times men and women have sought ways to help the infertile couple. The proposed solutions have often met with social criticism. One modern critic of assisted reproduction has said that "making babies in laboratories—even 'perfect' babies—means a degradation of parenthood."[12] Babies are not made in the laboratory. Even the most sophisticated of technologies does not "make" a baby, any more than the surgeon welds tissue together. He uses suture to attach tissues atraumatically and reconstruct natural relationships. If he has done his job well, the tissues will join. Assisted reproductive technology allows physicians to facilitate reproduction in much the same way. We atraumatically bring the components needed for reproduction into contact with each other. If we do our job well, nature will take its course, resulting in fertilization, pregnancy, and hopefully, a child.

NOTES

1. Lori B. Andrews, *New Conceptions* (New York: St. Martin's Press, 1984), pp. 221–23.

2. Zev Rosenwaks, "Donor Eggs: Their Application in Modern Reproductive Technologies," *Fertility and Sterility* 47 (1987): 895–909.

3. Maria Bustillo et al., "Non-Surgical Ovum Transfer as a Treatment in Infertile Women," *Journal of the American Medical Association* 251 (1984): 1171–73.

4. Michael Feinman, David Barad, Ivan Szigetvari, and Steven G. Kaali, "Availability of Donated Oocytes from an Ambulatory Sterilization Program," *Journal of Reproductive Medicine* 34 (1989): 441–43.

5. Christopher O'Reilly-Green and Wayne R. Cohen, "Pregnancy in Women Age 40 and Older," in *Perimenopausal Health Care,* ed. David H. Barad, *Obstetrics and Gynecological Clinics of North America* 20 (1993): 313.

6. Lynn S. Baker, *The Fertility Fallacy* (Philadelphia: Saunders Press, 1981), p. 209.

7. Mark V. Sauer et al., "Attitudinal Survey of Sperm Donors to an Artificial Insemination Clinic," *Journal of Reproductive Medicine* 34 (1989): 362–64.

8. Rene Frydman et al., "A Protocol for Satisfying the Ethical Issues Raised by Oocyte Donation: The Free, Anonymous, and Fertile Donors," *Fertility and Sterility* 34 (1990): 666–72.

9. A. D. Hard, "Artificial Impregnation," *Medical World* 27 (1909): 163.

10. Judith A. Schaffer and Ronny Diamond, "Infertility: Private Pain and Secret Stigma," in *Secrets in Families and Family Therapy*, ed. Evan Imber-Black (New York: Norton, 1993), p. 109.

11. P. Mahlstedt and D. Greenfeld, "Assisted Reproductive Technology with Donor Gametes: The Need for Patient Preparation," *Fertility and Sterility* 52 (1989): 908–14.

12. Ethics Committee, American Fertility Society, "Ethics and the New Reproductive Technologies," *Fertility and Sterility* 53, Suppl. 2 (1990): S17.

THREE

OOCYTE DONATION SERVICE AT IVF AMERICA-BOSTON

Patricia M. McShane, M.D.

BEFORE WE SET UP THE PROGRAM

Although pregnancy rates for assisted reproductive technologies have increased steadily over the last ten years, two groups of patients have had historically poor outcomes—men with severe male factor infertility and women with frank ovarian failure (lack of menstrual periods before the age 40) or diminished ovarian reserve. Advances in IVF laboratory practices, such as microinjection of sperm, have closed the gap dramatically in recent years for men with very diminished sperm function. Oocyte donation has been utilized with increasing success since the mid-1980s for young women with frank ovarian failure, and pregnancy rates are consistently high for this therapy.

More recently, treatment of "perimenopausal" women, who are not yet in menopause and yet manifest reduced responsiveness to stimulatory drugs, has been initiated. It appears that chronological age is a factor affecting the outcome of infertility treatment; several reports have documented dropping IVF success rates in women beyond 37 years of age.[1] The blood level of follicle stimulating hormone (FSH) is another indicator of ovarian "age,"[2] which may be distinct from the chronological age of the woman. This level tends to rise in all women in late reproductive years prior to onset of definite menopause. Thus, it appears that both chronological age and FSH level are independent risk factors for poor outcomes with assisted reproductive technology. It was believed that uterine responsiveness was also a significant factor in this lack of success, since morphologically normal embryos of many older women have been transferred on several occasions without initiating pregnancy.[3]

Many IVF programs used to make 40 years of age their cut off point for treatment. Other programs that did accept older women counseled them strongly regarding the poor pregnancy rate and increased miscarriage rates for older women that were documented in numerous national registries.[4] Therefore, it was with great optimism that the assisted reproductive technology community greeted early reports of a high success rate with donor oocytes in women over 40 years of age, regardless of prior hormonal response or FSH level. Once the proper levels of steroid replacement therapy were recognized, pregnancy rates for these women appeared to mirror those of younger, frankly menopausal women.[5] A new door was opened to couples who had deferred pregnancy until later in their reproductive lives or had suffered longstanding infertility and were in their fifth decade.

It was upon this background that IVF America set up our donor oocyte service in 1991. Prior to performing our first oocyte donation, we talked extensively with staff at other programs who had been active in this field; several of our clinicians and psychologists visited other programs. We were well aware of the controversial nature of some of our decisions, and therefore embarked upon this service with a set of guidelines that have remained in effect during the first four years.

INDICATIONS FOR THERAPY

The following are the medical indications for donor oocyte that we use:

1. Premature ovarian failure (menopause), whether natural, surgical or secondary to chemotherapy
2. Incipient ovarian failure
3. Age greater than 40 years, regardless of ovarian status, if unsuccessful with IVF
4. Poor response to controlled ovarian hyperstimulation at maximum doses
5. Consistently poor embryo quality at IVF
6. Multiple failed IVF cycles
7. Failed fertilization with normal sperm and at least two attempts
8. Risk of transmission of genetic disease through female partner oocytes

Frequently, use of donor oocytes is discretionary—that is, persistence in therapy with the woman's own oocytes is possible, but is not likely to result in a pregnancy. Therefore, the clinical staff counsels patients at length about their treatment options, including moving to alternative forms of family building such as adoption.

The upper age limit of the donor recipient was, and continues to be, a broadly debated topic. Our major concern in setting guidelines was the well-being of the potential offspring; we wanted to ensure as far as possible that the children would have healthy parents to raise them to adulthood. We consulted actuarial tables and chose 45 years of age as the cutoff. We allow women up to age 50 to cycle if their partner is significantly younger, however, reasoning that the child is likely to have at least one healthy parent at age 21.

We have been advised by legal counsel that requiring couples to be married is discriminatory and in violation of federal and state statutes. Therefore, this is not a requirement in our program for any service. On rare occasions, we have discussed donor oocyte with single women. Since these women would be using donor sperm and donor oocyte, transferring donor embryos would appear to be preferable to oocyte donation; it is certainly much less expensive and does not involve a third party in a minor operative procedure. The ethical concerns when simultaneous donor oocyte and donor sperm are used are different from those when either technology alone is used, since we are using assisted reproductive technology to create a potential new life with a genetic connection to neither parent. However, donor embryo service is not widely available because of the paucity of available cryopreserved embryos.

Women, especially those over age 40, are counseled and screened regarding possible medical contraindications to pregnancy. If there is significant concern about a medical issue, we ask for consultation with an internist or a perinatologist prior to initiating pregnancy. Potential recipient couples are given our current statistics regarding the clinical outcomes of both anonymous and known donor oocyte services prior to their consultation.

OOCYTE RECIPIENT SCREENING

Recipient couples are screened according to the American Society of Reproductive Medicine (ASRM) guidelines for Gamete Donation for infectious diseases prior to receiving donated oocytes. All couples in our assisted reproductive technology program fill out a short form entitled "Genetic History" to ascertain risks for common genetic disorders. If appropriate, the husband is screened for such conditions as thalassemia or sickle-cell disease. At the time of consultation, couples meet with a physician, psychologist, and financial coordinator. The physician's role in the consultation is to explain the medical procedures, the limitations of genetic and infectious disease screening for the donor, the limitations of the phenotypic (physical appearance) matching with the donor, and general issues pertaining to policies and procedures of the program. Couples are counseled to consult an attorney regarding legal issues and the possibility of having a contract with the donor, even maintaining confidentiality through an escrow attorney.

The psychologist reviews the psychological and emotional implications of oocyte donation for the couple, whether they are using a known or anonymous donor. When known donors participate, the psychologist first meets with the donor and her partner (if applicable) (see "Oocyte Donor Screening") and later with the recipient and her partner; she or he then meets with all three (or four) parties together. Of particular concern are the historical and future social relationships between the couples, family background if they are related, issues regarding cryopreservation and disposition of any cryopreserved embryos in the future, and any reservations that any party may have regarding the donation. Whether and how to disclose to the child is also discussed.

OOCYTE DONOR SCREENING

For anonymous donation, the donor must be between the ages of 21 and 35. Both anonymous and known donors and their sexual partners, if any, undergo the infectious disease screening test as per the ASRM guidelines. Anonymous donors complete an extensive genetic questionnaire and undergo any appropriate testing that might be indicated. Donors with known genetic disease (e.g., asthma, diabetes) are excluded prior to meeting with the clinic staff. Those with a strong family history of a life-threatening disorder in early life (e.g., premature coronary artery disease) are handled individually and often excluded. Donors are counseled regarding the need for monogamy and sexual abstinence at times during the donation treatment cycle. Those who are unwilling or unable to comply are excluded.

Donors with questionable obstetrical history are asked about this in detail. Those who are thought to have any gynecological or obstetrical issues of relevance may undergo further testing; some are excluded. Donors undergo the Minnesota Multiphasic Personality Inventory (MMPI); those who manifest psychopathology or substance abuse problems are rejected.

DONOR COUNSELING

Oocyte donors, whether anonymous or known to the recipient, are seen in consultation by a physician, psychologist, and nurse prior to inclusion in the program. The physician visit serves to emphasize the medical risks of controlled ovarian hyperstimulation and oocyte retrieval. The need for absolute adherence to monogamy and need for sexual abstinence at times during the treatment cycle are reinforced. The importance of an accurate personal and family medical history is emphasized. The unknown late psychological implications of being an oocyte donor are also mentioned. Lastly, the donor is thanked for her generous act!

When the psychologist meets with the donor, she or he emphasizes the potential for long-term unknown medical or emotional complications as a result of oocyte donation. If the donor is known to the recipient, the nature of their relationship is assessed with a special note of any guilt or sense of obligation. The major concern of the psychologist is to ascertain whether the donor feels any untoward external or internal pressure to proceed with the donation against her wishes or better judgment. If a donor opts not to proceed at that point, the psychologist will discuss with the donor how to tell the potential recipient. If the potential donor does not wish to tell her sister or a close friend the true reason for the refusal to donate, the clinical team will assist by finding another reason for not proceeding.

During the consultation, the issues of payment are discussed in more detail. For anonymous donation, the donor is compensated $1,500 if she undergoes a complete treatment cycle (controlled ovarian hyperstimulation and oocyte retrieval).[6] If the cycle is cancelled prior to retrieval, there is a pro rata share of the compensation given for the inconvenience and time lost from work for the injections and monitoring, communications with the clinical team, etc.

WHAT WE HAVE LEARNED THUS FAR

Our anecdotal experience to date is that oocyte donation is a viable option for a small but not insignificant percentage of the couples who are medically eligible. Most couples confronted with poor response to medication or lack of success over age 40 will choose to move on to adoption or accept child-free living. It is only a minority who actively pursue donor oocyte services. Many couples have ethical reservations about third-party parenting and would use assisted reproduction only if they could become pregnant with their own gametes. Other people treasure the experience of gestational parenting and are not particularly concerned regarding the genetic aspects of oocyte donation. Many couples are profoundly concerned regarding the possibility of infectious disease transmission; for others, the potential risk of genetic diseases and the lack of subsequent genetic information is deeply disturbing.

Many couples would utilize donor oocytes from a close relative if they had one, but are unwilling to use anonymous donors. Others who have a sister or friend who has repeatedly offered to donate do not desire to accept the donation. They may feel that it is "too much to ask another person," or know, on some level, that it would complicate their relationship and jeopardize the upbringing of the child.

Because the institutional review board and board of trustees of Waltham Weston Hospital & Medical Center were concerned regarding potential legal risks of introducing anonymous donors to recipients, even if no names were used, the service is offered only for those who accept total anonymity. For this reason, we have not to date allowed couples to advertise for their own donor. However, we are constantly struggling to recruit donors and are entertaining the possibility of allowing couples to advertise, but then "swapping" donors with another couple in order to help our waiting list. There is currently a wait of approximately one year for an anonymous donation. One concern has been that this arrangement makes possible financial abuses. We are concerned that excessive rewards might provide a disincentive to donors to give accurate information regarding their risk behaviors, medical and family histories. Excessive compensation would also be potentially coercive.

Our experience to date is that most anonymous donors have a strong sense of pride regarding reproduction and their reproductive history. Most have a young child or children, and many have had close friends or family members who have experienced infertility and wish to provide an alternative for another person. Some donors are financially comfortable, but many are in marginal financial circumstances. We have specifically sought not to recruit among students, although this could be easily done logistically.

Another contentious issue within our program has been the possibility of reducing cycle fees for assisted reproductive technology patients who are willing to donate some of their oocytes. In our Massachusetts-based program, this is seldom an issue insofar as we currently enjoy a mandate for insurance coverage for most couples. In other IVF America programs, this is being done on a limited basis. Since the advent of efficient cryopreservation, reduction in the number of oocytes inseminated would seem to compromise the chance of pregnancy for the woman considering subsequent transfer cycles with thawed embryos. On the other hand, many couples would not be able to try IVF or GIFT at all were it not for the price reduction afforded by donation of some of the oocytes.

NOTES

1. Society for Assisted Reproductive Technology, The American Fertility Society, "Assisted Reproductive Technology in the United States and Canada: 1991 Results from the Assisted Reproductive Technology Generated from the American Fertility Society Registry," *Fertility and Sterility* 59 (1993): 956–62; French In Vitro National, "French National IVF Registry: Analysis of 1986 to 1990 Data," *Fertility and Sterility* 59 (1993): 587–95; S. L. Tan, P. Royston, S. Campbell, H. S. Jacobs, J. Betts, M. Bridgett, G. E. Edwards, "Cumulative Conception and Livebirth Rates after In-vitro Fertilisation," *The Lancet* 339 (1992): 1390–94.

2. J. P. Toner, C. B. Philput, G. S. Jones, S. J. Muasher, "Basal Follicle-Stimulating Hormone Level Is a Better Predictor of In vitro Fertilization Performance than Age," *Fertility and Sterility* 55 (1991): 784–90.

3. D. R. Meldrum, "Female Reproductive Aging—Ovarian and Uterine Factors," *Fertility and Sterility* 59 (1993): 1–5.

4. Society for Assisted Reproductive Technology, "Assisted Reproductive Technology," pp. 956–62; French In Vitro National, "French National IVF Registry," pp. 587–95; Tan et al., "Cumulative Conception and Livebirth Rates after In-vitro Fertilisation," pp. 1390–94.

5. D. Navot, P. A. Bergh, M. A. Williams, G. J. Garrisi, I. Guzman, B. Sandler, L. Grunfeld, "Poor Oocyte Quality Rather than Implantation Failure as a Cause of Age-Related Decline in Female Fertility," *The Lancet* 337 (1991): 1375–77.

6. M. M. Seibel, A. Kiessling, "Compensating Egg Donors: Equal Pay For Equal Time?" [Letter to the Editor]. *The New England Journal of Medicine* 328 (1993): 737.

FOUR

OOCYTE DONATION PRO-GRAM AT HUNTINGTON REPRODUCTIVE CENTER

QUALITY CONTROL ISSUES

Paulo D. Serafini, M.D.,
Jeffrey R. Nelson, D.O.,
Shelley B. Smith, M.A., M.F.C.C.,
Ana Richardson, R.N., B.S.N., and
Joel Batzofin, M.D.

INTRODUCTION

The unveiling of the DNA molecule, the rapid progress of molecular biology and genetics, and the development of human *in vitro* fertilization (IVF) and related assisted reproductive treatments, have astounded the world in the past few decades. These advances, however, have introduced a myriad of social, ethical, moral, legal, and religious issues involving several disciplines.[1] In this study, we address some aspects of the psychological, medico-scientific, and laboratory quality control issues related to the highly successful assisted conception treatment that uses eggs from a woman donor.

INDICATIONS FOR OOCYTE DONATION

Women with either primary or secondary ovarian failure (cessation of ovarian function) are the primary candidates for assisted procreation treatments using an oocyte donor.[2] Oocyte donation has also become an accepted modality of treatment for women who exhibit serious genetic abnormalities (autosomal dominant, sex-linked, and autosomal recessive traits).[3] The documentation of repeated failures to retrieve eggs (the so-called empty follicle syndrome) or the presence of abnormally shaped eggs with poor fertilization *in vitro* qualify women for this assisted procreation modality.

Patients with normal oocytes and spermatozoa who experience repeated lack of fertilization *in vitro* could also be considered candidates for oocyte donation.[4] In a small number of women, egg retrieval may be contraindicated for medical reasons or because the ovaries are anatomically inaccessible (e.g., ovaries shifted away from the pelvis for radiation therapy).[5] Repeated failure to respond to ovarian stimulation regimes that might establish a viable pregnancy after several trials of IVF treatment, as well as advanced maternal age, have become acceptable indications for the use of donated oocytes.[6]

Several couples have recently requested assisted procreation with oocyte donation alone or with both oocyte and sperm donation because the woman is approaching the age of 40 and has not become pregnant after several assisted reproductive treatments. Intriguingly, this scenario is increasing because the alternative of adoption has certain negative potentials to some, and adoption has become more difficult for those of advanced parental age. Therefore, some find attractive the selection of an oocyte donor and a sperm donor followed by the creation of an embryo with subsequent transfer and recipient gestation.

The possibility of controlling present indications, the establishment of an acceptable number of patients' own cycle failures, advanced maternal age, and the desire for a healthy child must be carefully weighed before using oocyte donation. There appears to be a trend among infertility specialists to employ oocyte donation for recipients over 50 and even 60 years of age.[7] While there is no doubt that the technology supports such a medical odyssey, the ultimate goals of initiating pregnancy at an advanced age are not clear. Even though the life span of women has increased significantly in the last century, there is uncertainty about the physical ability of older women to rear a child, especially since oocyte donation treatments carry a high probability of multiple pregnancies. The concerns regarding fairness to the child weigh heavily. On the other hand, ending a patient's hope to gestate and establish a family is equally heartbreaking.

OOCYTE VERSUS SPERM DONATION

The introduction of third-party gametes via donor sperm can be traced back to the nineteenth century.[8] More recently, fairly strict guidelines for sperm donation have been developed by the American Fertility Society.[9] The medical questionnaires and screening procedures adopted by sperm banks have been introduced into oocyte donation practices.[10] However, there are major differences between oocyte donation and sperm donation with respect to recruitment, motivation, number of collections, method of obtaining gametes, potential medical hazards to the donor from the collection procedures, and psychological screening.

The method of retrieving sperm gametes (masturbation) is very easy when compared to oocyte retrieval via an ultrasound-guided transvaginal ovarian puncture and needle aspiration of follicles under drug analgesia and/or anesthesia. With the use of prophylactic antibiotic therapy, an associated ascending infection process in the oocyte donor is extremely rare, but it does occur. A pelvic infection following an egg retrieval could culminate in infertility and sterility.

A more contemporary concern is the risk of ovarian cancer in patients exposed to several cycles of ovulation induction.[11] At present, the scientific evidence for this appears clouded because of methodological flaws in the original study.[12] Nevertheless, infertility specialists should use caution and limit the maximum number of hormonal stimulations of oocyte donors. We have adopted a maximum of four to six cycles of ovarian stimulation in patients without ovarian cancer risk factors, acknowledging that this number is totally arbitrary. It may also be prudent to counsel oocyte donors regarding the advisability of pregnancy soon after the series of ovarian stimulation cycles, since the authors of the collaborative ovarian cancer study found that pregnancy reduces the risks of this malignancy.[13] Consideration could also be given to recommending the use of oral contraceptives when oocyte donors complete the series of egg retrievals, since oral contraceptives hormonally simulate gestation and are known to reduce the risks of ovarian cancer.

Finally, oocyte donors should also be advised about the risk of ovarian hyperstimulation, a syndrome induced by the ovulatory drugs, that could represent a life-threatening situation for them.[14] Further, if an oocyte donor experiences an unprotected sexual encounter around the time of egg retrieval and the infertility specialist fails to retrieve all eggs, the donor may face the possibility of a pregnancy. Therefore, caution should be exercised to avoid overstimulating the donor; barrier contraception should be advised if any sexual activity is engaged in around the time of egg retrieval.

MEDICAL AND PSYCHOLOGICAL SCREENING

The disastrous potential for transmission of genetically linked disorders, sexually and infectious transmitted diseases, and psychosocial aberrations make medical and psychological screening of couples and third parties entering into oocyte donation programs imperative.[15] Preconception assessment of the egg donor and her sexual partner, as well as the recipient couple, should be comprehensive and follow the minimum requirements set by the guidelines of the American Fertility Society.[16] This approach will protect oocyte recipients from major medico-obstetrical disasters and decrease the probability of serious genetic, infectious, and other offspring disorders.[17] However, one must bear in mind that contemporary standards for medical and psychological screening are continuously being redefined in view of new technological advances.

At Huntington Reproductive Center, the approach to both anonymous and nonanonymous donors includes an initial history and physical exam, baseline blood count, chemistry, ABO-Rh and antibody screening tests.[18] Oocyte donors must be of legal age and ideally should be under the age of 35. Proven fertility, while desirable, is not required, since several investigators have established healthy progeny from donors who have not previously been pregnant.[19] Donors should be in good general health and not suffer from any multifactorial congenital disorders such as cleft palate, spina bifida, congenital heart defects, hip dislocation, albinism, hypercholesterolemia, juvenile diabetes mellitus, epilepsy, hypertension, psychosis, sickle cell anemia, and so on.[20] Finally, highly efficient screening should be performed for genetically inherited diseases. Inborn errors of metabolism such as Tay-Sachs and Gaucher's disease should be considered in Eastern European Jewish donors when the recipient's husband is from the same ethnic background.[21] Cystic fibrosis, a common disease among European descendants, should be considered when there is an historical risk.[22] Information on the lifestyles of donors and their partners also needs to be closely examined in order to lower the medical risk to the recipients and offspring.

In addition to these congenital and genetic disorders, socially and sexually transmitted diseases should be assessed including infections caused by Chlamydia trachomatis; Mycoplasma hominis; Ureaplasma urealyticum; Neisseria gonorrhea; syphilis; toxoplasmosis; cytomegalovirus (CMV); herpes; hepatitis A,B,C, and possible D and E; rubella; and immune deficiency virus disorder. Since substance abuse carries major sociolegal implications, as well as an increased risk of multiorgan fetal anomalies, routine drug screening should be a mandatory component of the initial donor evaluation. A positive screening dictates counseling, and exclusion of the donor from the program.

Due to the lack of qualified psychological staff and often because of the desire to save time and expense, many egg donation programs adopt the sperm donor minimalist approach to psychological screening.[23] However, this may not adequately protect those involved from severe mental-psychological impairments. Psychological screening of donors and recipients, contrary to the established minimal standards for sperm donors, should incorporate counseling and formal testing. The tests should include the Minnesota Multiphasic Personality Inventory, and possibly both a Thematic Apperception Test (TAT) and a Wechsler Adult Intelligence Scale.[24] The inclusion of additional tests such as psychiatric assessment through the life events checklist, Perceived Stress Scale (PSS), and the Hopkins Symptom Checklist-90 (SCL-90) among others, may provide additional insights.[25] These precautions will aid psychologists in detecting underlying pathologies and will work toward the best interest of the donors, while providing reassurance to the egg recipients. Bartlett reported that one donor in their nonanonymous oocyte donation program, had a younger male sibling with an autistic-like condition, and that she desired to donate her own oocytes as a "test" for that condition.[26] A high level of quality control will prevent prospective egg donors with similar motivations from participating in oocyte donation programs and exposing unborn humans to catastrophic outcomes.

The health profile of the recipient couple should be evaluated in a similarly careful manner. Cardiovascular and obstetrical assessment and a recent mammogram appear mandatory for women over the age of 40. Preferably, a recipient should be under age 45. However, individual considerations must be taken into account with all prospective patients.[27] Documentation of a normal uterine cavity by hysterosalpingo-graphic exam and/or by hysteroscopic evaluation seems prudent to make sure that the small risk of multiple pregnancies can be safely accommodated and to avoid treatment failure, including early and late obstetrical complications.[28]

The recipient's spouse should be evaluated with a semen analysis, semen culture with sensitivity to antibiotics, and possibly the "hamster egg penetration test."[29] We do not exclude patients who need sperm microsurgical techniques to benefit from the oocyte donation program, although the couple is fully informed of the lower likelihood of success. On the other hand, an improved oocyte quality enhances sperm penetration capacity and final treatment outcome.

Finally, the recipient couple must be counseled about the increased likelihood of twins and higher-order pregnancies experienced among oocyte recipients. These pregnancies carry a relative increased risk for severe handicap of 1.7 for twins and 2.9 for triplets when compared to singletons.[30] Preterm labor, hospitalizations during pregnancy, the necessity of using neonatal intensive care facilities, an increased number of surgical deliveries, and associated rearing difficulties are among some of the immense hardships created by multiple pregnancies. The psychological ability of recipient couples to deal with the risks and realities associated with multiple births must be carefully addressed.

An important question regarding the screening of recipients concerns the reproductive center's ability to say "no" to couples who desperately want a child. Unresolved issues that couples may have and anger they may feel about their lack of fertility should be addressed before they enter the oocyte donation program. Psychological unpreparedness may require further education, counseling, and perhaps psychotherapy before potential recipients are accepted into the program. Clearly, most people, when faced with their own infertility and loss, will hope for a donor who is attractive to them on as many levels as possible. A process of transference takes place and the couple may begin projecting their fantasies and feelings for the child they are attempting to create onto the oocyte donor. Problems can develop if the couple is attempting to create a "super baby" to regain the great loss of control brought about by infertility.

Above and beyond the medical and psychological concerns, the commitment required of the oocyte donor in terms of compliance with the treatment regimen, frequency and timing of clinic appointments, and flexibility in her work schedule so that she can be available on short notice, should be explained. In the course of the screening process, expert legal counsel to develop comprehensive contracts outlining commitments, obligations, rights, and unknowns are mandatory. These documents should be independent of those that cover donor compensation for time and expenses. Knowledge of country or state legal statutes is important before such treatments are initiated. In the United States, courts are likely to recognize an agreement that excludes the oocyte donor from all rearing rights for offspring born to the recipient who gestates.[31] Provisions regarding possible intrafamilial problems, as well as other potential difficulties that could lead to violation of the agreement, should be carefully spelled out.

ANONYMOUS VERSUS NONANONYMOUS

Is there any advantage to using anonymous donors? We will briefly discuss issues related to anonymity that we have encountered in performing hundreds of oocyte donation cycles.

Intrafamilial donations maintain some genetic tie with the offspring, reduce costs, allow the choice of a person with a known background, facilitate custody decisions in the event of the recipient's death, and are considered an ethically more acceptable form of assisted procreation by some commentators.[32] Conversely, maintenance of genetic ties may be detrimental in cases of unrecognized autosomal recessive traits within a clan. A known background does not assure certain offspring characteristics or behavior, nor does it guarantee that the donor's participation is a gesture of love. In addition, one must seriously consider the possibility of unintentional coercion of a friend or family member by the infertile couple. We have unfortunately observed on a few occasions, usually by the tail end of the treatment, that the donor did not want to be involved in such activities but could not refuse her own sister or mother (marrying a stepfather). Indeed, these situations may be very incestuous and lead to various maladjustments within the family, as well as confusion for the child later during the process of forming an identity.

The use of donated oocytes harvested from an infertile patient undergoing an assisted reproductive treatment cycle may not be the most attractive alternative since she may have an infertility problem that she might be passing on.[33] This practice gives complete control of the treatment of an especially vulnerable patient to the physician, and such power can be subject to misuse. Furthermore, how can one choose the eggs that will be used in attempts to achieve pregnancies in both donor-patients and recipients? Programs using this approach may need much more strict quality control and treatment guidelines.

An anonymous donor, while initially more costly, may represent a more acceptable alternative than known or intrafamilial donors. This alternative accommodates a search for healthy donors, reduces risks of inbreeding, and reduces inconveniences and obligations on the part of donors, since they are also receiving a return for their generosity. Legal issues are also more easily handled when anonymous donors are used.

SUCCESS AND REPORTS

Reports of pregnancy and delivery rates vary greatly due to differences in clinics, physician expertise, laboratory efficiencies, patient selection, inclusion of male factor infertility, the wide spectrum of donors, recipient age, variable ovarian responses to hormonal stimulation, primary infertility factors, inadequate workup of recipients, the number of procedures carried out on the same patient, and the lack of cumulative reports. The lack of a statistical formula that could correct all variables, along with the lack of uniformity in providing success rates among centers, undermines attempts to report treatment outcomes. It is also important to realize that the total number of treated individuals is still relatively small and that technology and training are progressing at an ever increasing pace. Of equal importance is the fact that government organizations and special interest groups have inconsistently and deficiently reported their statistics. Consequently, potential consumers have only general, noncomparable information about the success rates of various clinics, and, in turn, about their individual likelihood of success.[34]

Because of such problems, investigators have suggested that evaluation of the effectiveness of a treatment should include the number of couples beginning treatment, the number completing each step of the IVF-donor oocyte process, the number of either fresh or frozen embryos transferred, and the number of clinical pregnancies and liveborns.[35] The authors also believe that whether oocytes are provided by other infertility patients or by fertile donors will skew results. A valuable source of information for prospective patients would be the analysis of the United States IVF Registry reports from the years 1988 to 1991.[36] Although this analysis overlooks several of the concerns mentioned above, it summarizes the results from over 200 clinics.

Since oocyte quality appears to play a central role in the establishment of a healthy pregnancy, we analyzed the results of IVF-embryo transfer in women under the age of 40 and compared these with those obtained with frozen-thawed embryo transfer procedures, as well as those obtained with the recipients of donated oocytes. Due to the inconsistency of yearly reports, we could only compare the results of clinical and delivery rates per embryo transfer procedure. Table 1 depicts the results of the four-year U.S. IVF Registry reporting analysis. Using the chi-square analysis to evaluate treatment outcomes, it became apparent that IVF-oocyte donation results are much superior to those associated with cryopreservation. However, one must understand that the report did not provide information about the age of the women who received frozen embryos. Investigators from Clamart, France,[37] have reported higher implantation rates from transfers of cryopreserved embryos originating from donated oocytes (33%) than from regular IVF treatment (9%). Interestingly, these results compare favorably with the four-year data on cryopreservation and oocyte donation, not taking into account that oocyte donation embryos reported by the Clamart group were previously frozen.

Table 1: Combined 4 years (1988–1991) assisted reproductive treatment results from the IVF Registry in the U.S. regarding oocyte donation, *in vitro* fertilization in women younger than 40 years and cryopreservation.[38]

	OD	IVF<40	CRYO
# ET	2,065	22,136	10,664
# CLIN PREG	648 (31.4)*	5,363 (24.2)*	1,316 (12.3)*
# DELIVERIES	503 (24.4)*	4,295 (19.4)	967 (9.1)*

OD = oocyte donation; IVF = *in vitro* fertilization;
CRYO = cryopreserved embryos; ET = embryo transfer;
CLIN PREG = clinical pregnancies; ( ) percent per ET;
*P<0.0001 (significance level)
= number

It is also very important to note that a center may have difficulty providing realistic pregnancy rates to prospective patients since many anonymous donors may produce over two dozen oocytes of which most fertilize; the resulting embryos are cryostored for future use. The calculation of pregnancy rates becomes difficult if the recipient becomes pregnant during the synchronized fresh cycle, and subsequently during a frozen embryo transfer attempt. These calculations become even more complicated when the recipient becomes pregnant in the fresh cycle and after two consecutive frozen cycles, as the authors have observed in a few cases. These examples make it apparent that reports of success with oocyte donation should also take into account cumulative pregnancy rates.

Finally, some centers may choose relatives, other infertile patients, or designated anonymous donors. The 1991 IVF Registry report accounts for results obtained among 819 anonymous oocyte donor cycles compared to 288 known egg donor treatments.[39] Delivery rates per egg retrieval of 26% and 23%, respectively were reported. Unfortunately, the report does not consider how the donors were selected. Future studies need to be carefully and prospectively designed to unequivocally answer these questions. Control of treatment quality will rest on the above considerations.

Data on the method of embryo transfer are also critical in determining success rates.[40] This can be broken down into two aspects: (a) the recipient's endometrial preparation and (b) the route of embryo transfer. Various successful protocols for uterine preparation have been described since the initial report of a term pregnancy in a woman without functioning ovaries.[41] In a landmark study, New Jersey Medical School researchers demonstrated a threefold higher pregnancy rate among patients prepared with a combination of estrogen and progesterone than those following natural ovulation.[42] Furthermore, reproductive endocrinologists from Mount Sinai Medical Center found that hormonal manipulation provided a great deal of flexibility to accommodate for a fresh, synchronized embryo transfer and a lesser chance of spontaneous abortion (miscarriage) in the recipients receiving the hormones for an extended period of time.[43] Several other investigators have found similar results. Therefore, hormonal manipulation appears to be the treatment of choice for recipients.[44]

Several investigators have reported that either zygote (day 1 embryo or pronucleus oocyte) or embryo tubal transfer render higher pregnancy rates than transcervical, intrauterine transfers among infertile patients.[45] While this hypothesis has been recently questioned because of the lack of consistent superiority among different infertility centers, some groups have performed tubal transfer for recipients of donated oocytes.[46] In the authors' experience, there has been no advantage in performing a laparoscopy or a minilaparotomy for transfer of embryos in patients who receive exogenous estrogen and progesterone endometrial preparations.[47] These results essentially negate surgical transfer as an option for recipients undergoing endometrial preparation. However, considerations must be incorporated in the individual decision-making process for women with a nonaccessible uterine cavity or an acute cervical herpetic infection. In addition, surgical transfers may be valuable in recipients during cycles of spontaneous ovulation or human menopausal gonadotropin endometrial preparation.

Finally, as noted earlier, the current practice of transferring multiple embryos per cycle to increase the implantation or pregnancy success rate results in twin and multiple pregnancies at a higher rate than is normal for women in the general population. The corresponding increase in medical problems for the woman during pregnancy and for the infants in the neonatal period, and increased rearing problems over the longer term, must be addressed prudently. Until scientists can determine *in vitro* which embryo will become a baby, it is essential to limit the number of embryos transferred despite a small reduction in pregnancy rates during that cycle attempt.

CONCLUSION

In summary, oocyte donation is a wonderful assisted procreation treatment alternative for many couples. This option allows each parent to have a true biological tie to the offspring, genetic on the part of the father and gestational on the part of the mother. Issues of quality control require careful monitoring in order to enhance the family unit, reduce problems, and avoid unscrupulous use of genetic breeding and selection.

ACKNOWLEDGMENTS

The authors are grateful to Professor Alan DeCherney, M.D. for his encouragement, intellectual and scientific motivation, to Mrs. Gayle Norbryhn, R.N., NAACOG, for the initial establishment of Huntington Reproductive Center Oocyte Donation Program and to Mrs. Jeana Lago for typing this manuscript.

NOTES

1. Luther M. Talbert, "Oocyte Donation," *Current Opinion in Obstetrics and Gynecology* 4 (1992): 732–35; Ethics Committee, American Fertility Society, "Ethical Considerations of the New Reproductive Technologies," *Fertility and Sterility* 46, Suppl. 1 (1986): 1S–94S; Joseph G. Schenker, "Religious Views Regarding Treatment of Infertility by Assisted Reproductive Technologies," *Journal of Assisted Reproduction and Genetics* 9 (1992): 3–8; John A. Robertson, "Ethical and Legal Issues in Human Egg Donation," *Fertility and Sterility* 52 (1989): 353–63; David Wasserman, Robert Wachbroit, "The Technology, Law, and Ethics of *In Vitro* Fertilization, Gamete Donation, and Surrogate Motherhood," *Clinical Laboratory Medicine* 12 (1992): 429–48.

2. Talbert, "Oocyte Donation," pp. 732–35; Ethics Committee, American Fertility Society, "Ethical Considerations," pp. 1S–94S; Ethics Committee, American Fertility Society, "Guidelines for Gamete Donation," *Fertility and Sterility,* 59 (1993): 1S–9S; P. Lutjen, A. Trounson, J. Leeton, J. Findlay, C. Wood, P. Renous, "The Establishment and Maintenance of Pregnancy Using *In Vitro* Fertilization and Embryo Donation in a Patient with Primary Ovarian Failure," *Nature* 307 (1984): 174; H. I. Abdalla, R. J. Baber, A. Kirkland, T. Leonard, J. W. W. Studd, "Pregnancy in Women with Premature Ovarian Failure Using Tubal and Intrauterine Transfer of Cryopreserved Zygotes," *British Journal of Obstetrics and Gynaecology* 96 (1989): 1071–75; Mark V. Sauer, Richard J. Paulson, "Human Oocyte and Preembryo Donation: An Evolving Method for the Treatment of Infertility," *American Journal of Obstetrics and Gynecology* 163 (1990): 1421–24; G. Pados, M. Camus, L. Van Waesberghe, I. Liebaers, A. Van Steirteghem, D. Devroey, "Oocyte and Embryo Donation: Evaluation of 412 Consecutive Trials," *Human Reproduction* 7 (1992): 1111–17.

3. Talbert, "Oocyte Donation," pp. 732–35; Ethics Committee, American Fertility Society, "Guidelines for Gamete Donation," pp. 1S–9S; P. Lutjen, "The Establishment and Maintenance of Pregnancy," p. 174; Abdalla, "Pregnancy in Women with Premature Ovarian Failure," pp. 1071–75; Sauer, "Human Oocyte and Preembryo Donation," pp. 1421–24; Pados, "Oocyte and Embryo Donation," pp. 1111–17.

4. Abdalla, "Pregnancy in Women with Premature Ovarian Failure," pp. 1071–75.

5. Ibid.

6. Talbert, "Oocyte Donation," pp. 732–35; Ethics Committee, American Fertility Society, "Ethical Considerations," pp. 1S-94S; Ethics Committee, American Fertility Society, "Guidelines for Gamete Donation," *Fertility and Sterility,* 59 (1993): 1S-9S; Abdalla, "Pregnancy in Women with Premature Ovarian Failure," pp. 1071–75; Sauer, "Human Oocyte and Preembryo Donation," pp. 1421–1424; Pados, "Oocyte and Embryo Donation," pp. 1111–17; Mark V. Sauer, Richard J. Paulson, "Demographic Differences between Younger and Older Recipients Seeking Oocyte Donation," *Journal of Assisted Reproduction and Genetics* 9 (1992): 400–402; Randy S. Morris, Mark V. Sauer, "Oocyte Donation in the 1990s and Beyond," *Assisted Reproduction Reviews* 3 (1993): 211–17; Ryzszard J. Chetkowski, Thomas E. Nass, "Use of Donated Eggs Sharply Reduces Cost of IVF in Women Over 40," *Obstetrics and Gynecology News,* Dec. 15, 1993, p. 9.

7. Sauer, "Demographic Differences," pp. 400–402; Morris, "Oocyte Donation in the 1990s," pp. 211–17; Chetkowski, "Use of Donated Eggs," p. 9.

8. Ethics Committee, American Fertility Society, "New Guidelines for the Use of Semen Donor Insemination: 1990," *Fertility and Sterility,* 53, Suppl. 1 (1990): 1S-13S.

9. Ibid.

10. Ethics Committee, American Fertility Society, "Guidelines for Gamete Donation," pp. 1S-9S.

11. Alice S. Whittemore, Robin Harris, Jacqueline Itnyre, and the Collaborative Ovarian Cancer Group, "Characteristics Relating to Ovarian Cancer Risk: Collaborative Analysis of 12 US Case-control Studies," *American Journal of Epidemiology* 136 (1992): 1212–20; Robert Spirtas, Steven C. Kaufman, Nancy J. Alexander, "Fertility Drugs and Ovarian Cancer: Red Alert or Red Herring?" *Fertility and Sterility* 59 (1993): 291-93.

12. Ibid.

13. Whittemore, "Characteristics Relating to Ovarian Cancer Risk," pp. 1212–20.

14. Paul A. Bergh, Daniel Navot, "Ovarian Hyperstimulation Syndrome: A Review of Pathophysiology," *Journal of Assisted Reproduction and Genetics* 9 (1992): 429–38.

15. Ethics Committee, American Fertility Society, "Guidelines for Gamete Donation," pp. 1S-9S; Paulo Serafini, "Screening of Donors and Surrogates," *Proceedings of the VI Annual In Vitro Fertilization and Embryo Transfer—A Comprehensive Update* 6 (1993): 328-51.

16. Ethics Committee, American Fertility Society, "Guidelines for Gamete Donation," pp. 1S-9S.

17. Ethics Committee, American Fertility Society, "Guidelines for Gamete Donation," pp. 1S-9S; Serafini, "Screening of Donors and Surrogates," pp. 328-51.

18. Serafini, "Screening of Donors and Surrogates," pp. 328-51.

19. Jose P. Balmaceda, Veronica Alam, Daniel Roszjtein, Teri Ord, Kellie Snell, Ricardo H. Asch, "Embryo Implantation Rates in Oocyte Donation: A Prospective Comparison of Tubal versus Uterine Transfers," *Fertility and Sterility* 57 (1992): 362-65.

20. Ethics Committee, American Fertility Society, "Guidelines for Gamete Donation," pp. 1S-9S.

21. Ethics Committee, American Fertility Society, "Guidelines for Gamete Donation," pp. 1S-9S; Serafini, "Screening of Donors and Surrogates," pp. 328-51.

22. Ibid.

23. Talbert, "Oocyte Donation," pp. 732–35.

24. H. J. Brand, "Complexity of Motivation for Artificial Insemination by Donor," *Psychiatry Report* 60 (1987): 951–55; L. R. Schover, J. Reiss, R. L. Collins, J. Blankstein, G. Kanoti, M. M. Quigley, "The Psychological Evaluation of Oocyte Donors," *Journal of Psychosomatic Obstetrics and Gynecology* 2 (1990): 299–309; Jacqueline A. Bartlett, "Psychiatric Issues in Non-Anonymous Oocyte Donation—Motivations and Expectations of Women Donors and Recipients," *Psychosomatics* 32 (1991): 433–37; A. Kirkland, M. Power, G. Burton, R. Baber, J. Studd, H. Abdalla, "Comparisons of Attitudes of Donors and Recipients to Oocyte Donation," *Human Reproduction* 7 (1992): 355–57; David Pettee, Louis N. Weckstein, "A Survey of Parental Attitudes toward Oocyte Donation," *Human Reproduction* 8 (1993): 1963–65; Mary Lisa Sanschagrin, Elaine B. Humber, Carol Cumming Speirs, Sydney Duder, "A Survey of Quebec Pediatricians' Attitudes toward Donor Insemination," *Clinical Pediatrics* 4 (1993): 226–30; Roberta Lessor, Nancyann Cervantes, Nadine O'Connor, Jose Balmaceda, Ricardo H. Asch, "An Analysis of Social and Psychological Characteristics of Women Volunteering to Become Oocyte Donors," *Fertility and Sterility* 59 (1993): 65–71.

25. Schover, "The Psychological Evaluation of Oocyte Donors," pp. 299–309.

26. Bartlett, "Psychiatric Issues in Nonanonymous Oocyte Donation," 433–37.

27. Sauer, "Demographic Differences," pp. 400–402; Morris, "Oocyte Donation in the 1990s," pp. 211–17; Chetkowski, "Use of Donated Eggs," p. 9.

28. Dominique Cornet, Jean-Marie Antoine, S. Casanova, U. Uzan, Jacqueline Mandelbaum, Michelle Plachot, Jacques Salat-Baroux, "Obstetric Evolution of Pregnancies Obtained from Donated Oocytes," *Fetal Diagnosis and Therapy* 7 (1992): 31–35.

29. Morris, "Oocyte Donation in the 1990s," pp. 211–17; Serafini, "Screening of Donors and Surrogates," pp. 328–51.

30. Louis Keith, Jose A. Lopez-Zeno, Barbara Luke, "Triplet and Higher Order Pregnancies," *Contemporary OB/GYN* June 1993, pp. 36–50.

31. Robertson, "Ethical and Legal Issues," pp. 353–63.

32. Ethics Committee, American Fertility Society, "Ethical Considerations of the New Reproductive Technologies," pp. 1S–94S; Sauer, "Human Oocyte and Preembryo Donation," pp. 1421–24; Kirkland, "Comparisons of Attitudes," pp. 355–57; Rene Frydman, Helen Letur-Konirsch, Dominique de Ziegler, Monique Bydlowski, Anne Raoul-Duval, Jacqueline Selva, "A Protocol for Satisfying the Ethical Issues Raised by Oocyte Donation: Free, Anonymous, and Fertile Donors," *Fertility and Sterility* 53 (1990): 666–72.

33. Serafini, "Screening of Donors and Surrogates," pp. 328–51; Jerome H. Check, Kosrow Nowroozi, Jeffrey Chase, Ahmad Nazari, Carolyn Braithwaite, "Comparison of Pregnancy Rates Following *In Vitro* Fertilization-Embryo Transfer between the Donors and the Recipients in a Donor Oocyte Program," *Journal of Assisted Reproduction and Genetics* 9 (1992): 248–50; Daniel Navot, Paul A. Bergh, Maryanne Williams, G. John Garrisi, Ida Guzman, Benjamin Sandler, Janis Fox, Patricia Schreiner-Engel, Glen E. Hoffman, Lawrence Grunfeld, "An Insight into Early Reproductive Processes through the *In Vivo* Model of Ovum Donation," *Journal of Clinical Endocrinology and Metabolism* 72 (1991): 408–14.

34. Pados, "Oocyte and Embryo Donation," pp. 111–17; Richard J. Paulson,

Mark V. Sauer, Rogerio A. Lobo, "Embryo Implantation after Human *In Vitro* Fertilization: Importance of Endometrial Receptivity," *Fertility and Sterility* 53 (1990): 870–74; F. Zegers-Hochschild, E. Fernandez, C. Fabres, A. Mackenna, J. Prado, L. Roblero, T. Lopez, E. Altieri, A. Guadarrama, F. Escudero, "Pregnancy Rate in an Oocyte Donation Program," *Journal of Assisted Reproduction and Genetics* 9 (1992): 350–52; Society for Assisted Reproductive Technology, The American Fertility Society, "*In Vitro* Fertilization-Embryo Transfer in the United States: 1988 Results from the IVF-ET Registry," *Fertility and Sterility* 53 (1990): 13–20; Society for Assisted Reproductive Technology, The American Fertility Society, "*In Vitro* Fertilization-Embryo Transfer (IVF-ET) in the United States: 1989 Results from the IVF Registry," *Fertility and Sterility* 55 (1991): 14–23; Society for Assisted Reproductive Technology, The American Fertility Society, "*In Vitro* Fertilization-Embryo Transfer (IVF-ET) in the United States: 1990 Results from the IVF-ET Registry," *Fertility and Sterility* 57 (1992): 15–24; Society for Assisted Reproductive Technology, The American Fertility Society, "Assisted Reproductive Technology in the United States and Canada: 1991 Results from the Society for Assisted Reproductive Technology Generated from the American Fertility Society Registry," *Fertility and Sterility* 59 (1993): 956–62.

35. Lynne S. Wilcox, Herbert B. Peterson, Florence P. Haseltine, Mary C. Martin, "Defining and Interpreting Pregnancy Success Rates for *In Vitro* Fertilization," *Fertility and Sterility* 60 (1993): 18–25.

36. Society for Assisted Reproductive Technology, The American Fertility Society, "*In Vitro* Fertilization-Embryo Transfer in the United States: 1988 Results," pp. 13–20; "*In Vitro* Fertilization-Embryo Transfer (IVF-ET) in the United States: 1989 Results," pp. 14–23; "*In Vitro* Fertilization-Embryo Transfer (IVF-ET) in the United States: 1990 Results," pp. 15–24; "Assisted Reproductive Technology in the United States and Canada: 1991 Results," pp. 956–62.

37. Dominique de Ziegler, Rene Frydman, "Different Implantation Rates after Transfers of Cryopreserved Embryos Originating from Donated Oocytes or from Regular *In Vitro* Fertilization," *Fertility and Sterility* 54 (1990): 682–88.

38. Society for Assisted Reproductive Technology, The American Fertility Society, "*In Vitro* Fertilization-Embryo Transfer in the United States: 1988 Results," pp. 13–20; "*In Vitro* Fertilization-Embryo Transfer (IVF-ET) in the United States: 1989 Results," pp. 14–23; "*In Vitro* Fertilization-Embryo Transfer (IVF-ET) in the United States: 1990 Results," pp. 15–24; "Assisted Reproductive Technology in the United States and Canada: 1991 Results," pp. 956–62.

39. "Assisted Reproductive Technology in the United States and Canada: 1991 Results," pp. 956–62.

40. Talbert, "Oocyte Donation," pp. 732–35; Abdalla, "Pregnancy in Women with Premature Ovarian Failure," pp. 1071–75; Pados, "Oocyte and Embryo Donation," pp. 1111–17; Balmaceda, "Embryo Implantation Rates," pp. 362–65; Zegers-Hochslchild, "Pregnancy Rate in an Oocyte Donation Program," pp. 350–52; P. Devroey, C. Staessen, M. Camus, E. de Grauwe, A. Wisanto, A. C. Van Steieghem, "Zygote Intrafallopian Transfer as a Successful Treatment for Unexplained Infertility," *Fertility and Sterility* 52 (1989): 246–49.

41. Talbert, "Oocyte Donation," pp. 732–35; P. Lutjen, "The Establishment and Maintenance of Pregnancy," p. 174; Sauer, "Human Oocyte and Preembryo Donation," pp. 1421–24; Navot, "An Insight into Early Reproductive Processes," pp. 408–

14; Paulson, "Embryo Implantation after Human *In Vitro* Fertilization," pp. 870–74; Cecilia L. Schmidt, Dominique de Ziegler, Carol L. Gagliardi, Richard W. Mellon, Frances H. Taney, Mary J. Kuhar, Jose M. Colon, Gerson Weiss, "Transfer of Cryopreserved-Thawed Embryos: The Natural Cycle versus Controlled Preparation of the Endometrium with Gonadotropin-Releasing Hormone Agonist and Exogenous Estradiol and Progesterone (GEEP)," *Fertility and Sterility* 52 (1989): 609–16.

42. Schmidt, "Transfer of Cryopreserved-Thawed Embryos," pp. 609–16.

43. Navot, "An Insight into Early Reproductive Processes," pp. 408–14.

44. Talbert, "Oocyte Donation," pp. 732–35; P. Lutjen, "The Establishment and Maintenance of Pregnancy," p. 174; Sauer, "Human Oocyte and Preembryo Donation," pp. 1421–24; Navot, "An Insight into Early Reproductive Processes," pp. 408–14; Paulson, "Embryo Implantation after Human *In Vitro* Fertilization," pp. 870–74; Cecilia L. Schmidt, Dominique de Ziegler, Carol L. Gagliardi, Richard W. Mellon, Frances H. Taney, Mary J. Kuhar, Jose M. Colon, Gerson Weiss, "Transfer of Cryopreserved-Thawed Embryos: The Natural Cycle versus Controlled Preparation of the Endometrium with Gonadotropin-Releasing Hormone Agonist and Exogenous Estradiol and Progesterone (GEEP)," *Fertility and Sterility* 52 (1989): 609–16.

45. Abdalla, "Pregnancy in Women with Premature Ovarian Failure," pp. 1071–75; Balmaceda, "Embryo Implantation Rates," pp. 362–65; Devroey, "Zygote Intrafallopian Transfer," pp. 246–49; Y. L. Yovich, D. G. Blackedge, P. A. Richardson, P. L. Matson, S. R. Turner, R. Draper, "Pregnancies Following Pronuclear Stage Tubal Transfer," *Fertility and Sterility* 48 (1987): 851–57.

46. Balmaceda, "Embryo Implantation Rates," pp. 362–65.

47. Ibid.

PART B

Ethical and Policy Issues
Raised by Egg Donation

FIVE

NEW REPRODUCTIVE TECHNOLOGIES AND THE FAMILY

Thomas H. Murray, Ph.D.

My wife and I have been discussing whether to get a bread machine. We both love the smell and taste of fresh-baked bread. But our lives are so busy, rarely do either of us have the time to make bread. I can't say that the nation's journalists have been particularly interested in our quandary. Instead, they are terribly interested in such matters as the cloning of human embryos in a laboratory.

What do my wife's and my deliberations whether to buy a bread machine have to do with cloning human embryos? They both involve decisions whether to incorporate some new entity into a family's life. But, you may protest, surely you are not equating a piece of machinery with—and this of course is the ultimate point of cloning human embryos—something that could become a baby? To be honest, I'm a little reluctant to make that equation—but some of my bioethics colleagues seem to find it less troubling. Norman Fost, for example, is quoted in the *New York Times* as saying he begins "with a presumption of privacy and liberty, that people should be able to live their lives the way they want and to make babies the way they want."[1]

Fost is by no means alone in his effort to portray questions about cloning human embryos, along with other means of creating babies, in terms like privacy, liberty, and individual preferences—and their intimate conceptual relations, property and contract. In this way of thinking about human reproduction, if people desire to obtain a child, they have a right to pursue that goal, just as they have a right to fulfill their desire for fresh bread by trying to buy a bread machine. We may want to put boundaries on the pursuit of babies that are more strict than those we place on the pursuit of bread machines. In neither case do we think it is permissible to walk into a place where the desired items lie (respectively, a newborn nursery and an appliance store), slip one under our coat and walk out with it. At a minimum, we insist on a mutually voluntary transfer. We may also want to forbid the sale of used versions of the one type (say, three-year-old children) while feeling completely comfortable with a market in used versions of the other (that is, three-year-old bread machines).

By now, this discussion will strike some readers as utterly bizarre. That is only because it is. Our sense that something is out of joint here arises because we are tempted to apply the same conceptual scheme to two very different entities. Babies are not bread machines, although both can smell very good in the morning (though the baby may need a change and bath first). Nor is the relationship of one who supplies the genetic material or who gestates a baby to that infant the same as that of one who manufactures or retails a bread machine to that appliance.

In the realm of commerce, moral relationships are relatively simple. There are owners and property and prospective buyers. The property itself has no intrinsic moral significance. Its "worth" is measured fully by the price agreed by buyer and seller. The relationship of buyer and seller is governed by contract—an agreement that specifies in precise detail what each party expects from the other. The relationship between buyer and seller is merely instrumental to the exchange of goods: I give you, the store owner, $150; you give me this bread machine. In the realm of parents and children, of family, the new additions—that is, children—have a richer moral status than mere property. The relationships among the various parties who may be involved in providing babies—suppliers of gametes, gestational services, and those who wish to rear the children—are more complex as well, to say nothing of the relationships between each of those parties and the children they create. Indeed, it could be said that the main point of having a child is to initiate the relationships that will develop between that child, its siblings, and the adults in its life.

We should not accuse people who champion liberty, privacy, property, and contract in the sphere of new reproductive technologies of wanting to treat children as nothing more than property. To the contrary, proponents of strong individual rights in reproductive technology frequently acknowledge the great moral importance of children. Indeed, they might argue that the liberty to pursue parenthood is even more important than the liberty to pursue more prosaic commercial transactions.

The problem as I see it is this: We recognize that thinking of children as property, and of family life as essentially a series of commercial transactions, is a grievous distortion. We know of cultures that have treated children as a form of property; indeed, there are practices in our society that appear to be surviving remnants of that idea. It is also possible to analyze family relationships in economic terms. That may be a useful heuristic for understanding how family arrangements interact with the larger world of markets. But it remains a fiction, not an insightful description of how successful families function, or more importantly, why people live in families.

One of the most important things that happen in families—indeed, many take it to be the single most important defining feature of families—is procreating and raising children. New reproductive technologies are a challenge to our notions of family because they expose what has been at the core of the family to the vicissitudes of the market. At the heart of our often vague concerns about the impact of new reproductive technologies, such as those about the purchase of human eggs, is our sense that they threaten somehow what is valuable about families. To understand whether those apprehensions are well-based or mistaken, we need to have a better idea of what families are, what important values are served by families, and the scope and limits of moral relationships among parents and children.

As the champions of reproductive liberty proclaim, the freedom to pursue parenthood is one of the most important expressions of individual liberty. Acquiring the child is usually as far as they take the story. My experience as a parent—shared I believe with countless other contemporary parents—is that having a child has profound consequences for one's liberty. The responsibility of caring for an infant, then a child, then a young adult, is among the most constraining experiences a parent can have. Unless they have arranged for someone else to do it for them, the parents of an infant are not free to sleep late on weekends (or sleep through the night, for that matter). They are not free to leave their young child home alone while they go to a movie or a meal. Many of the freedoms they experienced prior to having a child are altered radically.

What I have just said takes one notion of liberty—the capacity to do what one wishes—and portrays having children as a diminishment of that sort of liberty. I believe this is only being honest. The kind of liberation I have in mind here is certainly not the liberty of the marketplace. It is not the liberty of conspicuous consumption—to stand out from the crowd by my acquisitions—nor is it the liberty of consumer conformity—to avoid disapproval by making certain I look like every other member of my group. It is, rather, the sort of liberation that comes from knowing what genuinely matters, what carries real meaning into my life. This is not just some sort of intellectualized self-persuasion, either, like trying to convince yourself that what tastes bad really is good for you. The experience of knowing what matters *feels* liberating.

Contemporary Americans overwhelmingly identify their family as the primary source of meaning in their lives.[2] In a culture that celebrates autonomy and individualism, this may seem surprising. Our freedom is, in one respect, the liberty to seek or create meaning in our lives; it does not itself provide that meaning. We are deeply sociable creatures who find much of what gives our life meaning and purpose in our enduring, intimate relationships.

Erik Erikson, in his interpretation of development through the human life cycle, described a period in adult life during which individuals must develop the capacity for generativity, or fall into a kind of stagnation. We must learn to care for persons and projects outside of ourselves, or we are prone to sink into a narrow preoccupation with our own needs and worries.[3] Liberty, in the sense of freedom from intimate, intricate moral ties with other persons, turns out—if Erikson is correct—to be antithetical to liberty in the sense of a full development of our humanity, or what he calls a ripening of the vital virtues. Making a family, in the sense of having children—not just genetically, but the experience of responding to their needs and guiding their development—is surely the most common way, but by no means the only way, to meet the challenge of generativity.

Defining "family" is not a trivial matter. The paradigm of a nuclear family remains a woman, a man, and their biological offspring. But if we limited our notion of family only to groups that strictly adhered to this model, death, divorce, adoption, foster care, remarriage, single parenthood, and some of the new reproductive technologies would disqualify most of us who live with or have raised children. We need a more encompassing definition, one that reflects what we value in family life.

Carol Levine, in an insightful and compassionate essay on AIDS and the family, suggests three characteristics of human relationships that seem to capture well what we mean when we describe the relationships that typify family. First, the intention, if not always the reality, is that the relationships are permanent, lifelong. Second, the relationships embody a commitment to mutual support—economic, social, and emotional. Third, family bonds have an intimacy that distinguishes them from other attachments. Levine offers a working definition of family that seems a good starting point for this study: "Family members are individuals who by birth, adoption, marriage, or declared commitment share deep, personal connections and are mutually entitled to receive and obligated to provide support of various kinds to the extent possible, especially in times of need."[4] This notion of family serves two purposes: It emphasizes what distinguishes family bonds from other, less central, human relationships; and it highlights the problem with the punitively narrow concept of family deployed in the rhetoric of "family values."

"FAMILY VALUES" AND THE VALUES FAMILIES SERVE

As we turn toward a consideration of the impact of new reproductive technologies on the family, we will need to talk about the values characteristic of family life, and the larger social values served by having families. The phrase "family values," however, has become a political slogan, a shorthand for a lengthy catalogue of political views, ranging from affirmations that families are important, through condemnations of homosexuality, to approval of narrowly limited roles for women and prayer in schools.

"Family values" in contemporary American political discourse has become synonymous with the views of a narrow portion of the political right. Both right and left in American politics share the blame for the sorry recent history of discussions of values and the family. The right has shamelessly promoted its particular roster of positions as *the* only, exclusive, and legitimate values associated with family life and at the same time has implied that those who disagree have *no* values, or at least none worth mentioning. The left, for its part, has done virtually nothing to challenge the right's claim to a monopoly on values. This inaction is due in part to a greater tolerance for diversity, but also, I believe, to the suspicion that to affirm any set of substantive values is inherently oppressive. The characteristic view seems to be that we should throw all questions back to what each individual would freely choose, on the assumption that this would be wholly liberating. Individuals, that is, should be free to do anything—except talk seriously about what among the things they would *not* always freely choose might be good for themselves and others. Other than an espousal of liberty and justice, and a defense of diversity, the left was reluctant to talk about values. I believe one of the great failures of American political life in the 1970s and 1980s was the reluctance to engage in a balanced discussion of values. The only way I know to reinvigorate the political and moral debate is to call us back to the reasons why people make families—to the crucial values served by families. But to do that requires first taking a closer look at the way the debate over the ethics of new reproductive technologies typically has been framed.

The public debate over the ethics of new reproductive technologies has tended to be framed in a manner that reinforces a highly individualistic, rights-oriented understanding of moral relationships within families. Some of the practices associated with new reproductive technologies, for example, the purchase of eggs from young women, have tended to insert commercialism into the heart of family relationships. I want to look at some of the aspects of new reproductive technologies that people find most uncomfortable. That discomfort, however widely shared, is not proof that the practices giving rise to the discomfort are immoral. It could be due to misunderstanding, or superstition, or what some authors dismiss as merely "symbolic harm."[5] But I want to take seriously the possibility that the discomfort people feel at a practice such as commercial surrogacy has legitimate moral concerns at its root. Intellectuals too swiftly reject such concerns. The impulse to rejection is the harder to resist when the culture's ideology supports certain values that exclude, or are incongruous with, the sources of misgiving—when the language of rights, property, consent, and contract disguises what is morally significant about families.

JUSTICE AND FAMILY LIFE

The reasons why people form families, what people hope to find in family life, are different in significant respects from the reasons why people enter the public spheres of commerce and politics. Likewise, the ethics that govern family life are distinctive, in many ways, from the ethics that govern commerce and politics. It would be easy to overemphasize the distinction between the sphere of the family and the spheres of the market and politics, but family life intersects with these other spheres in countless ways. It would also be a mistake to collapse the distinction, to see family life as essentially the same as life in these other spheres. To do so would ignore that families serve very important values, values not served at all well by the marketplace or the public forum.

For one thing, well-functioning families are the locus for the development of emotionally and physically healthy children. Families are also a principal place for the emotional and moral development and maturation of adults. Families provide the setting for nurturing relationships characterized at their best by love, loyalty, and a healthy measure of forgiveness.

Of course, not even in the best of families do all things go well. And many families are riven by anger, cruelty, and bitterness. When we think about families we must avoid the temptation to romanticize the family—to picture only one type of family as the ideal, to deny the ambivalence that infuses even the best of family relationships.

On the other hand, neither should we demonize the family. Families are not the primary sources of evil in the world, and even in many troubled families, good things can happen. Children can experience love, learn that at least some people are trustworthy, develop a sense of their own worth and efficacy. We need to be realistic about the many difficulties families encounter or cause, about the rich varieties of ways in which people make families. But we must not allow cynicism, which is occasionally justified, to blind us to what is valuable in families.

Values that are fundamental in shaping our relationships in other spheres may play a different role in the family. Take justice, for example. In our relations with strangers in the public sphere and in the marketplace, justice is a crucial value. Perhaps the highest moral compliment we can pay to a social institution is to say that in this institution justice prevails. In the sphere of politics, we may not need to love one another, but we do need to treat each other justly.

The emphasis is different within families. Certainly, justice remains an important virtue in family life. And I believe that we learn our first and most memorable lessons about justice as members of families. Most parents are familiar with the procedure for fairly distributing the last piece of pie between two children: You have one cut it, and the other gets first pick. Within families, attentiveness to justice is necessary to prevent the wounds that family members habitually inflict on each other from becoming persistent, suppurating sores that drain the individual's moral and emotional strength, and ultimately sicken the family. Justice is a kind of maintenance value in family life. If you don't keep it fresh and vigorous, then you will find it impossible to achieve the values you sought when you entered your family. Families poisoned with injustice are poor soil for the growth of enduring love and loyalty and intimacy.

Insisting, though, that justice be the predominant value in family life is, I think, a mistake. It's a very understandable mistake, when we consider how readily injustice can seep into our lives as spouse, parent, or offspring, and how pernicious such injustice can be. The mistake is in forgetting why we make families. We enter families not to seek justice but to seek other values— love, learning to care for other people, enjoying the mutual affection and interdependence of parent and child. Without justice, those other values are lost. Justice is not the reason we make families, but it is crucial to any chance we have for achieving those values.

FAMILIES AND THE CONCEPT OF "RIGHTS"

The concept of rights is a blunt and crude instrument with which to understand the ethics of life within families. Suppose you knocked on the doors of all of the houses in your neighborhood with young children in them, and asked the parents in each why they fed their children. I expect that they would usually mention two sorts of reasons: that children need to be fed to be healthy and grow; and that making certain one's child is well nourished is just one of those things that a good parent does. One answer I do not expect to hear from these parents is that they feed their children because their children have a right to be fed.

Does this mean that these parents believe that their own children, or other parents' children, have no right to be fed? Hardly that. There are times when it seems appropriate—indeed necessary—to assert that a child's right is being ignored. If parents persistently fail to feed their child, then the agencies of the state may intervene. But the state's intervention becomes necessary only because of a grave breakdown within the family, a failure, for whatever reason, to provide one of the essential elements of child nurture.

Talk about "rights" seems to be most clear and to work best when it is doing one of two things. First, we invoke rights when we want to erect boundaries against interference by others. The other party may be the government, an institution or corporation, or individuals. This sort of claim against interference by others is often called a "negative right" — for example, the right to be left alone or the right to privacy. Second, we sometimes use the language of rights to state a positive claim—a claim *to* something, such as a claim to be fed by you. One way of thinking is to presume that all cases in which you have a duty to provide me with certain goods or services are best expressed in terms of rights. But there are many circumstances in which the language of rights seems awkward and second best—when talking about why parents feed their children, for example. Perhaps it is more useful to see claims about positive rights as fallbacks—efforts to obtain something that could not be better assured by ties of affection, loyalty, or by moral duties deeply ingrained into complex social practices—like parenting.

Understanding the moral intricacies of family relationships through a concept such as rights is like opening a beautifully carved front door with an ax. It is undeniably effective; it is justified only by an emergency such as a fire; it thrusts the state into the middle of family life; and it can leave a heavy toll of destruction in its path. A fireman's ax, of course, is not the preferred way of opening your front door. It does violence to your house. Similarly, asserting that someone's rights are being violated within a family is typically a way of justifying state intervention into that family's life. It may be necessary; it is probably wise to limit it to occasions when great harm would otherwise be caused; and it certainly inflicts its own kind of violence on that family.

The language of rights is a language most at home in the spheres of public life, government and commerce. I have a right to keep you from trespassing on my land; I have rights of free speech and freedom from governmental interference into my political and religious activities; I have a right to go to court to ask that you fulfill the terms of the contract we both signed. In these spheres, the concept of a right is powerful, and important, and in many instances represents a great moral and political advance. The concept of human rights, as it gains increasing international momentum, is a growing bulwark against oppression by governments of any political stripe that succumb to the temptation to exercise their considerable power against their own citizens.

The language of rights is also a common and comfortable way of talking about our legal relationships with one another. There again it serves important purposes. But even outside the sphere of the family, rights talk captures only a small part of what is important in our moral relationships with one another. We do many things out of friendship, or kindness, or sympathy, or solidarity—not principally or even partly because you have a "right" to our friendship, or kindness, or sympathy, or solidarity. Because the decision whether to make a family, especially whether to have children, is perhaps the most profoundly important life decision most individuals face, it should be no surprise that we are inclined to the language of rights in thinking about the ethics of such choices. But perhaps a moral concept most helpful for understanding our moral relationships with the state, and with strangers in the marketplace, is not as helpful in understanding family life—especially a language that carries with it powerful connotations of property, and that elevates choice to a position of near-supreme moral importance.

WHAT DOES IT MEAN TO
HAVE AN "ILL-FITTING" ETHIC?

Talking of rights as a way of understanding family relationships is not like talking about a "purple idea" or a "repentant toaster." Unless the adjectives are being used merely as bizarre metaphors, a person who utters such non-sense is committing what the philosopher Gilbert Ryle called a category mistake. It is not, however, a category mistake to insist that the ethics of family relationships are best understood through concepts such as rights or justice. It is more like being slightly off-center, for it misses something very important about families. It is a bit like wearing a tuxedo to a beach party. You might at first think the person in the tuxedo had a wry sense of humor; but when you realized that he was completely serious, that he honestly thought this is what to wear to the beach, you might, at best, feel a little sorry for him. Obviously, he did not understand what beach parties were all about.

Both kinds of mistakes—category mistakes and missing the point—are errors in meaning. In a category mistake, one fails to grasp the meaning of a concept. The result is a linguistic absurdity. On the other hand, when we try to analyze family ethics with a concept like rights, there is a misfit between the moral concept and the meaning of the social institution and the practices that accompany it. Meaning here signifies the point of the institution and prac-tices, their place in human affairs, the relationships they call forth, the values they support and exemplify. A mistake here results in a moral, not a linguistic, absurdity. Trying to understand families primarily through concepts such as rights and justice is not incoherent, but it misses the point of why people make families, the sorts of human relationships people strive to create within families, and the values families serve.

THE VALUES SERVED BY FAMILIES

Love. Loyalty. Affection. Forgiveness. Trust. Care. Nurturing. Maturation. This is at best a partial list of the values families serve. But I believe that it will be a recognizable list to most of my cultural compatriots in late-twentieth-century America. For that matter, it should not have seemed strange to a literate American in the mid-1800s. The ideal of companionate marriage and the view that children are creatures to be nurtured and loved, rather than little demons to be broken, were already a part of American popular culture nearly 150 years ago. Nor would it surprise me to learn that many of these values were present in families made by people in far distant times and cultures. John Boswell's study of child abandonment in ancient Rome and medieval Europe suggests that some parents in those times and places were at least as fond of their children as contemporary Americans fancy themselves to be.[6] A study of eighteenth-century families in the Chesapeake region of Virginia and Maryland likewise found abundant evidence for great affection between parents and children—and great grief when, as often happened, the child died.[7] Thomas Jefferson, probably the best-known resident of that place and time, wrote to his daughter about his hope that his granddaughter "will make us all, and long, happy as the center of our common love."[8]

At their best, families are institutions that support human flourishing—of the adults in the family, as well as the children. Families, although they constitute a distinctive sphere of human life, do not and cannot exist in isolation. Just as children need families and many adults need children, so do families need supportive social institutions and communities. Without a web of support in the wider culture, individual families may collapse under the weight of external blows and the inevitable injuries that even the best of families inflict on themselves.

Within families, the relationships among the various members of the family are centrally important. The values we think of as crucial to family life tend either to be found only in the context of relationships—love, loyalty, affection, trust, care—or, given our social natures, to depend utterly on good, enduring relationships—identity, self-confidence, maturation. The centrality of relationships in the values important to families points up another contrast with the spheres of the market and of politics.

In the market, relationships are secondary to the purpose of the market—the fair and efficient exchange of goods and services. In a market transaction, I deal with you not because I prize the intrinsic value of our relationship, but because you have something I want, and vice versa. The relationship is merely instrumental to the exchange of goods. On the other hand, in the realm of the family, the relationship is prior and primary and brings about the exchange of goods or gifts to build and sustain the relationship.

NEW REPRODUCTIVE TECHNOLOGIES
AND THE VALUES SERVED BY FAMILIES

Certain values at the core of new reproductive technologies are at odds with the values most central to creating and sustaining the relationships that are at the heart of family life. The new reproductive technologies emphasize values such as control, choice, and contract. This constellation of values leads readily to the view that commercialization in reproduction is acceptable, even desirable.

Commercial surrogacy illustrates these values. The paid surrogate may be contractually obliged to watch her diet, take vitamins, avoid liquor and alcohol, and of course, get regular prenatal care. The contracting couple, in this way, seek to control her behavior. The interest in control can manifest itself in another way, when the contracting couple insist on prenatal diagnosis. The importance of choice emerges clearly when the payors reject a baby born with impairments. The surrogate may also want to exercise her own choice, rejecting the same child. Honoring choice in this case may serve the interests of the adults involved; it does not seem to serve the child.

Control is linked closely to choice. John Robertson, in a defense of cloning human embryos, argues that couples wishing to "adopt" (his word) an embryo which is a clone of already living children should have the option of knowing as much as possible about those children. He says: "the right of adoptive parents to receive as full information as possible about the children whom they seek to adopt is increasingly recognized. There is no reason why the same principle should not apply to embryo 'adoptions.' Even though the couple seeking the embryos will be choosing embryos on the basis of expected characteristics, such a choice is neither invalid nor immoral. . . . "[9] A couple, that is, may exercise quality control through choice.

The emphasis here on control and choice does not fit at all well with our understanding of families. Good families are characterized more by acceptance than control. Furthermore, families are the preeminent realm of unchosen obligations. We may choose our spouses (although a powerful argument could be made that for most of us this choice bears scarce resemblance to the model of rational, autonomous, considered decision making). We may choose to have a child, but—unless we are "adopting" one of Robertson's cloned embryos—we do not in any informed way choose to have this *particular* child, with its interests, moods, and manners. And as offspring, we certainly did not choose our parents. Yet I think most of us would agree that we do have moral obligations to our parents, our spouses, and our children. An interesting problem for an ethics founded on autonomous choice as the fundamental requirement for moral obligation is this: How do you explain the enormously powerful web of moral obligations that supports family life, despite the only partly chosen or wholly unchosen nature of those relationships?

Many of the new reproductive practices require enlisting third parties. Women sell their eggs, men sell their sperm, and women may gestate their own or someone else's fetus. Justifying the involvement of third parties usually builds on the values of choice and control, and invokes the concept of liberty. The question immediately arises, Why would any third party agree to participate in another couple's effort to have a child? For many people the answer is obvious: money. Robertson states the case bluntly: "If collaborative reproduction is viewed positively, reproduction contracts become the instruments of reproductive freedom."[10] He acknowledges the implication of this view: "Legal liberty allows persons to treat each other as means to reproductive ends, with their negotiating ability and other resources determining the fate of future offspring. The extracorporeal embryo becomes subject to the vagaries of a market that drives people to buy or sell reproductive factors and services. Yet such freedom also allows people to determine and satisfy their welfare more efficaciously than by government prescription. In liberal society, the invisible hand of procreative preference must be allowed to flourish, despite the qualms of those who think it debases our humanity."[11] Freedom equals the right to make a contract, to welcome, in a memorable paraphrase of Adam Smith, "the invisible hand of procreative preference." The price we pay for that freedom, including markets for human eggs, sperm, and embryos, is the necessary cost of liberty, or so Robertson argues.

With admirable tenacity, John Robertson leads us down the reproductive path paved by the values of the market—individual liberty, choice, personal preference, contract, and commercialization. We are now in a position to see where we have arrived—and what beautiful, perhaps fragile, shoots have been bulldozed in the rush to build this particular highway.

Having someone else's baby for pay is a good example of the problem. How does a paid surrogate childbearer explain to her other children what has happened? Does she say: "Mommy loves her children so much that she wants to give another woman a chance to have her own children to love"? Does she add: "Oh, by the way, it also lets us buy groceries / pay off the mortgage / go to Disney World / finish the third floor"? What do her children think about their own security? Their relationship with their parents? What have they learned about the nature of the parent-child relationship? Have they learned that it is subject to the same harsh rules of supply and demand as any other commodity? Will such doubts make them more secure, contribute to their emotional development? Are children more likely to flourish in a culture where making children is governed by the same rules that govern the making of automobiles or VCRs? Or is their flourishing more assured in a culture where making children, and matching children with nurturing adults, is treated as a sphere separate from the marketplace? A sphere governed by the ethics of gift and relationship, not contract and commerce?

My claim is not that a market in children or gametes violates some abstract principle in the noumenal realm. It is that, given the sort of creatures we humans are, our patterns of psychosocial development, our needs at different stages of our lives, the set of social institutions and practices we have developed—given these facts—some values, institutions, and practices support our mutual flourishing better than others. The values of the marketplace are ill suited for nurturing the values, institutions, and practices that support the flourishing of children and adults within families.

Debates over the ethics of new reproductive technologies shine a stark light on one common but peculiar tendency in modern thought: the habit, at least since Descartes, of elevating a single, isolated aspect of our humanity—our reason—above everything else that characterizes us. The capacity to reason is important to be sure, but why not give equal stress to other morally relevant characteristics of humans, for example, our capacity for love, our concern for others, for self-sacrifice? The explanation for this modern elevation of rationality above all else may have more to do with the historical circumstances of modernity than anything defensible by sound reasoning.[12] Isolated, disembodied, autonomous reason is, so far as we know it, a fiction. It may be a useful fiction for thinking about certain kinds of problems. But it seems to be a particularly inept framework for understanding families—the contexts in which we irreducibly social, inevitably embodied creatures actually develop and live.

A market in gametes, or even in offspring, might not be a moral and social problem for some other sorts of creatures for whom rationality is preeminent. But such a market is a threat for us humans who need affection, trust, and above all intimate and enduring relationships in order to flourish.

AT THE HEART OF OUR CONCERNS

The ever growing array of reproductive alternatives are not equally troubling. Artificially inseminating a woman with her husband's sperm, for example, strikes most people as eminently acceptable. (The Roman Catholic Church is an exception to this general chorus of approval.) For a variety of reasons, a man might produce some normal sperm, but not be able to place enough of them in a good position to reach an ovum ready for fertilization. Using another man's sperm is more complicated morally. The usual practice in the United States, known as artificial insemination by donor, or AID, is a misnomer. The "donor" is usually paid for his sperm, making him a sperm vendor. I think this is a more serious error than a minor semantic quibble. Calling the supplier of sperm a donor invokes the realm of gifts, not sales, and with it the sphere of family and friendship. In commercial sperm banks, the vendors are actually anonymous strangers, paid for their "product" and then sent away, with presumably no more interest in what happens to it subsequently than a seller of office supplies has with what happens to his or her post-it notes.

In fact, there is evidence that at least some men who sold sperm discover later that they have a great deal of interest in what has happened to it. I take this as evidence that in human reproduction, the market is a poor description of what transpires when gametes are transferred from one party to another. Because the market fails as a description, it is unlikely to be a faithful guide to ethical understanding as well.

If what I am arguing about the dangers of the values of the market intruding upon the sphere of the family is correct, then AIV—artificial insemination by vendor—should make us uneasy. Not because of any sexual squeamishness, but because commerce in this realm may threaten what is genuinely valuable within it. Using gametes provided by another man raises other morally relevant difficulties.[13] Even if, as seems likely, those are outweighed by the good of creating new parent-child relationships, we should still worry about the impact of commercializing the practice. Men who provide sperm should indeed be donors, not vendors.

Would such a change create a shortage of sperm? There is reason to believe that it would not. First, in at least one country, an adequate number of men volunteer to be genuine, unpaid donors. Second, in the United States it used to be assumed that you could only obtain an adequate supply of whole blood by paying individuals for it, or by offering them some other advantage. That assumption was false. People give blood because they are convinced other persons need it, and they do not have to undergo great inconvenience in order to make a donation.[14] Although like any change it would unsettle those accustomed to business as usual, the United States should see if it could move from its current dependence on vendors to relying on genuine sperm donors.

Whatever moral difficulties we find in a market for sperm, they are magnified in the market for ova. There are fewer healthy ova available for treating infertility than there are women who want them. Getting healthy ova to use in IVF and related procedures is a much more elaborate and invasive procedure than the one used to obtain sperm. The woman who will be the source of these eggs typically takes hormones that stimulate her ovaries to ripen multiple eggs, which must then be removed by aspiration or laparoscopy.

Why would a woman go through such an ordeal? In many instances, the woman is a genuine donor, providing an egg for a relative or a friend. In other cases, the woman receives money. Compensating the supplier is fine, according to the American Fertility Society's report "Guidelines for Gamete Donation: 1993." The Guidelines say in VI. A. that "Donors should be compensated for the direct and indirect expenses associated with their participation, their inconvenience and time, and to some degree, for the risk and discomfort undertaken."[15] One proposal calculates that with all the interviewing, testing, examinations, the procedure itself, and a full day to recover, an egg donation takes 56 hours of a woman's time. Assuming that men are paid $25 an hour for sperm, the authors of this proposal conclude that a woman should "receive $1,400 for her time alone, exclusive of any compensation for travel, risk, or inconvenience."[16] They ask, "Since it is standard to compensate men for sperm donation, shouldn't the policy be equal pay for equal time?"[17] A survey of infertility programs found that women who were paid for their ova received an average of $1,548, with a range from $750 to $3,500.[18]

"Equal pay for equal work" sums it up well. Despite the repeated reference to "donors" of both ovum and sperm, paying individuals for their biological products makes them vendors, not donors. And it places the interactions between the parties squarely in the marketplace. If you believe that markets, the values markets exemplify, and the relationships that typify market interactions, celebrate human freedom, and that such freedom is the preeminent good, then none of this should bother you. If, however, you regard families as a sphere distinct from the marketplace, a sphere whose place in human flourishing requires that it be kept free of destructive incursions by the values of the market, paying gamete providers should trouble you.

WHAT DIFFERENCE DOES IT MAKE?

If we did set aside the moral framework of contract and market in favor of one more in tune with what we value about families, how would we regard alternative methods of reproduction? The most significant alteration in our understanding of the ethics of reproductive alternatives would be a shift in how we frame the moral question. The currently fashionable way to think about such matters is to place individual liberty and choice on one side of the balance, and the harms caused on the other side. John Robertson uses this strategy frequently and skillfully. His analysis of surrogacy provides a typical example.[19] Robertson emphasizes the voluntary nature of the agreement between the paying couple and the paid surrogate. He looks at potential harms to the couple and the surrogate as implausible, not that different from other things we already tolerate, and in any event a consequence of their own free choice.

The child who would be the consequence of the surrogacy contract is a more difficult story. But not that much more difficult. The prospect of harms to such children could be dismissed as implausible or unproven, or not so different from other practices we tolerate anyway, especially adoption. The parallel with harms to the adults involved in surrogacy ends there. Robertson, like other defenders of commercial surrogacy, cannot use the child's fictional "consent" to justify any harms that might come to it. But he has another strategy. The child, he argues, benefits because "but for the surrogacy contract, this child would not exist at all . . . even if the child does suffer identity problems, as adopted children often do . . . this child has benefited, or at least has not been wronged, for without the surrogate arrangement, she would not have been born at all."[20]

Try now to imagine some novel method of bringing children into this world which such a way of framing the issues would condemn, as long as the adults participating did so freely. Cloning human embryos? No problem. Cloning embryos, freezing some, and thawing them out later for implantation in someone else? Still, no problem. Implanting an aborted fetus's ovary, with its millions of yet-unripe eggs, into a woman's body, so that she might become pregnant with that fetus's ova? It is difficult to see how anyone who frames the argument as Robertson and other enthusiasts do could make a strong objection to the practice. Who is harmed? Certainly not the woman who wanted the abortion and gave her consent to using the fetal ovaries. Not the recipient woman or her spouse, who want this supply of healthy ova. And for any children born from these eggs, how could anyone claim that they would have been better off never existing?

Would it matter if the reason the woman desired the fetal ovary was because of her own infertility, or because she is 35 and wanted to avoid the increased risk of birth defects that comes from older eggs? Or that she and her spouse wanted children with blue eyes, or some other genetically linked characteristics? I doubt that Robertson or most other supporters of reproductive alternatives would embrace such bizarre practices. But, on the other hand, it is hard to see how, given the way they structure the ethical balancing, they could argue persuasively against them. You would have to demonstrate harms of such magnitude and certainty to individuals who have not, by their own choice, accepted the risk of such harms, that they overwhelm the enormously powerful presumption in favor of liberty.

What of healthy fertile women who want to have their own genetic children, but don't want to go through pregnancy? Robertson believes that "surrogacy for convenience . . . may turn out to be more acceptable if it proves to be an effective way for women to combine work and reproduction. . . . As long as surrogate interests are protected, an optimal situation for all might result from surrogacy for convenience, if one accepts the change in the concept of mother that it would appear to entail."[21] This is precisely the inexorable moral logic of the marketplace. It is a logic that sweeps everything before it, deterred only by convincing evidence of serious, direct harm to those who have not consented by virtue of their own participation. As for the children thus created, we would have to prove that they would have been better off never being born. An awesome, perhaps insurmountable burden of proof.

If framing the ethics of new reproductive technologies in terms like markets, liberty, and contract is unsatisfactory, what is the alternative? We could instead ask if these novel means of creating children support or interfere with the values that characterize family and parenthood. Would they, on balance, create not just individual parent-child relationships, but the kind of relationships that foster mutuality, loyalty, and love; relationships that endure, that survive the inevitable occasions when the relationship is causing a great deal more pain than pleasure? Beyond individual relationships, would they help build social attitudes and institutions that support the flourishing of children and adults within families?

I am suspicious of practices such as paying gamete suppliers or surrogate childbearers, practices that thrust the values of the market into the heart of the family. It would be ridiculous to argue that all children born of such arrangements are irreparably damaged, or their relationships with their rearing parents warped. But I do not think it is silly to worry about the net effect such practices have on our intimate relationships more generally, and on parent-child relationships in particular. Unreflective ideological commitments can and do lead entire cultures astray, away from what they genuinely and deeply value. The attitudes and institutions that provide the absolutely necessary cultural support for what we value can be eroded, so gradually that we scarcely notice.

The intimate conceptual and moral connections between the moral discourse of reproductive autonomy and the cultural sphere of the market makes commercialization in reproduction a potent threat to what we value about families. John Robertson and I actually agree about the enormous importance children can play in the lives of adults. And we both want to promote social practices that match children with adults. But where he regards contract and commercialization as "the instruments of reproductive freedom," I view them as, at best, threats and, at worst, inimical to the values families are meant to promote. They should be our culture's last resort, if we allow resort to them at all. Cultural meanings are shared creations, and their protection, or change, a shared project.

In order to protect the few against the tyranny of the majority, the law may have to permit some practices in the name of liberty that we believe are unwise. But our moral vision must not be trimmed to meet the requirements of the law. If commercializing reproductive practices threatens cultural meanings and institutions, then our respect for political liberty does not require us to declare that such practices are ethically acceptable. Preserving what we value about families is more important than whatever good might be derived from reproductive commerce.

Nor does our commitment to political liberty demand that we permit or facilitate reproductive commercialization. Some commentators argue that procreative liberty is a fundamental constitutional right. Under our constitution, the government must have a compelling purpose in order to justify interfering with such a right. But other experts disagree with the claim that our reproductive rights are so broad as to encompass practices such as gestation for pay. Alex Capron and Margaret Radin conclude that the "claim that the right to privacy protects surrogacy may be more plausible for noncommercial than for commercial surrogacy; even if the Constitution should be understood as including a right to bear a child for someone else, it should not be interpreted as including a right to be paid for it."[22] They argue that there is no obstacle in the Constitution to prevent a community through its government from banning commercial surrogacy agencies, brokers, or advertising.

A woman who is willing to bear her sister's or best friend's child out of loyalty and affection is acting in harmony with the values we prize in families. I would urge caution on the part of everyone involved, but I see what she is doing as an act of generosity, an extraordinary gift. Despite the outward physiological similarity between surrogacy-for-love and surrogacy-for-pay, the meanings of the two acts could not be more different. The former builds on one relationship of affection in order to create new affectionate relationships. The latter transmutes the creation of a child into a commercial transaction—a sort of reverse alchemy, turning gold into dross.

I began this chapter with the vague uneasiness many people feel about some of the new reproductive alternatives, wondering if the qualms were the product of mere habit and superstition, or if they sprung from well-founded concerns. I looked at the terms in which the public debate has been conducted, and found them severely wanting because they disguise or devalue what is morally significant about families. Finally, I wanted to see if we could recast that debate on terms more faithful to what we value about families and the relationships families make possible, and whether that recasting could help us make moral sense out of the proliferation of new ways to make children. Our concerns, I believe, were very well founded. The commercialization of reproduction is indeed a threat to what we value about families. The purchase of human ova, along with other reproductive alternatives, needs to be examined in the light of those same values.

NOTES

1. Gina Kolata, "Cloning Human Embryos: Debate Erupts over Ethics," *New York Times*, October 27, 1993, pp. A1, B7.

2. B. Berger and P. L. Berger, *The War over the Family: Capturing the Middle Ground* (New York: Anchor/Doubleday, 1983).

3. Erik H. Erikson, *Insight and Responsibility* (New York: W. W. Norton, 1964).

4. Carol Levine, "AIDS and Changing Concepts of the Family," in *A Disease of Society: Cultural and Institutional Responses to AIDS*, ed. Dorothy Nelkin, David P. Willis, and Scott V. Paris (New York: Cambridge University Press, 1991), p. 48.

5. See any of the articles about reproduction by the distinguished legal scholar John A. Robertson, e.g., "Embryos, Families and Procreative Liberty: The Legal Structure of the New Reproduction," *Southern California Law Review* 59/5 (1986): 939–1041.

6. John Boswell, *The Kindness of Strangers: The Abandonment of Children in Western Europe from Late Antiquity to the Renaissance* (New York: Pantheon, 1988).

7. Daniel Blake Smith, "Autonomy and Affection: Parents and Children in Chesapeake Families," in *The American Family in Social-Historical Perspective* (Third edition), ed. Michael Gordon (New York: St. Martin's Press, 1983), pp. 209–28.

8. Letter from Thomas Jefferson to Mary Jefferson Randolph, May 31, 1791, in Sarah N. Randolph, *The Domestic Life of Thomas Jefferson* (New York, 1939), p. 202. Cited in Smith, op. cit., p. 217.

9. John A. Robertson, "The Question of Human Cloning," *Hastings Center Report* 24/2 (1994): 6–14.

10. Robertson, 1986, p. 1031.

11. Ibid., 1040.

12. Stephen Toulmin, *Cosmopolis: The Hidden Agenda of Modernity* (New York: Free Press, 1990).

13. Paul Lauritzen, *Pursuing Parenthood* (Bloomington: Indiana University Press, 1993).

14. Alvin W. Drake, Stan N. Finkelstein, and Harvey M. Sapolsky, *The American Blood Supply* (Cambridge: MIT Press, 1982).

15. American Fertility Society, "Guidelines for Gamete Donation: 1993," *Fertility and Sterility*, Suppl. 1, 59 (1993): 5S-9S, p. 6S.

16. Machelle M. Seibel and Ann Kiessling, "Compensating Egg Donors: Equal Pay for Equal Time?" *New England Journal of Medicine* 328 (1993): 737.

17. Ibid.

18. Andrea Mechanick Braverman, "Survey Results on the Current Practice of Ovum Donation," *Fertility and Sterility* 59 (1993): 1216–20.

19. John A. Robertson, "Surrogate Mothers: Not So Novel After All," *Hastings Center Report* 13 (1983): 130–36.

20. Ibid., p. 131.

21. Ibid.

22. Alexander M. Capron and Margaret J. Radin, "Choosing Family Law over Contract Law as a Paradigm for Surrogate Motherhood," *Law, Medicine & Health Care* 16/1–2 (1988): 34–43, p. 40.

SIX

MORAL CONCERNS ABOUT INSTITUTIONAL- IZED GAMETE DONATION

Lisa Sowle Cahill, Ph.D.

GAMETE DONATION AS INFERTILITY THERAPY

Sperm and oocyte donation programs are generally seen as offering therapies to alleviate a medical condition, and as doing so in a spirit of compassion for those who suffer from reproductive dysfunction. The justification of gamete donation is usually formulated in terms of cost-benefit ratios, in which the lack of demonstrable physical or social harm to donors, families, and offspring is a central consideration, and also in terms of the informed consent of the participating parties.

A CRITICAL MORAL PERSPECTIVE

Because of moral pluralism in our culture, our respect for differences, and the value we ascribe to tolerance, we tend to approach disagreements over moral practices in terms of procedural solutions, rather than substantive ones. Procedures that support the equality and self-determination of every individual are no doubt extremely important. Yet certain areas of moral concern can be neglected by a criterion that emphasizes individuality, liberty, and autonomy. These include the nature of human parenthood as ideally grounded in biological kinship relations, as well as in chosen social commitments; the contextualization of choice by inevitable and universal aspects of "the human condition" (e.g., health and illness, aging, diminishment of some of our youthful powers, death, our interdependence within communities and families); the relation of individual choices to the common good, especially when these choices become social practices; and the moral role of policy in a culture in which legality is often equated with unobjectionability.

I believe it would be well to ask some second questions about a society that sets up large, profitable, and science-driven programs in which donors and recipients are encouraged to dissociate genetic from social parenthood, biological partnership in conceiving from social partnership in rearing, and to see medicine and technology as "desperate" but inevitable and "necessary" solutions to problems which have social as well as medical origins. A fundamental concern about oocyte donation that also pertains to other forms of reproductive technology is the degree of pressure on clients, especially women, to "choose" this means of resolving infertility.

GAMETE DONATION, CHOICE, AND A LARGER HORIZON OF VALUES

Although some programs have age-based cutoffs (which are primarily for medical rather than for social reasons, and are applied earlier and more strictly to donors than recipients), few if any other limits are placed on the free choice of participants.[1] The age of recipients of oocytes, once considered a medical, if not a social, factor, is increasingly being extended. An appendix to the 1993 report on gamete donation of the American Fertility Society (AFS) recommends only that donors over 40 be thoroughly evaluated for psychological and physical counterindications.[2] Mark Sauer, a practitioner in a clinic which was among the first to implant oocytes in postmenopausal women,[3] commented to the press, "They have a purpose again."[4]

Do older women lose purpose without fertility? A professor of philosophy and women's studies, Susan Sherwin (of Dalhousie University, Nova Scotia) has a different perspective. "An enormous industry has grown up in recent years to postpone or prevent menopause through hormone replacement therapy; now reproductive life can also be prolonged. . . . There are questions of what we value in women."[5] That older men beget children without public concern says little about the suitability of persons at the far end of the life cycle to parent infants. Such men often have young wives to mother their children—and usually a divorced wife their own age.

Questions about the fundamental human values which come into play in sexuality, parenthood, and gender relations receive little sustained attention in discussions of gamete donation, except for freedom of choice and risk of measurable harm. John Robertson, a lawyer, addresses the ethics of oocyte donation primarily in the categories of consent and of "risk" to participants and offspring. Moral considerations which "do not depend on the actual effects of the practices in question" are categorized as "deontologic views" which "are not universally shared."[6] The term "deontologic," whose Greek root means "duty," is evidently meant to denote positivistic or authoritarian positions unsupportable by publicly accessible argumentation. Such views are associated with religious teachings, especially of the Roman Catholic Church.[7] What counts are quantifiable data about bad consequences. In the absence of hard data the freely chosen life plans of individuals should not be curtailed.

Similarly, the reproductive technology guidelines of the American Fertility Society Ethics Committee identifies the "common thread running through . . . possible constraints on the moral right to reproduce" as "a concern about harm. . . . " Absent harm, couples have "a liberty right to reproduce" that includes the right to enlist third parties.[8]

Yet philosophical questions can be raised about the ultimacy of liberty and choice, and the adequacy of cost-benefit ratios as a reasonable guide. Charles Taylor[9] identifies a prevalent cultural "ethics of authenticity" to one's own original and freely chosen ideals. Yet, he warns, if choice is its own rationale, morality is trivialized. Although the modern ideal of self-creating and sincere selfhood undergirds democratic societies with their values of equality and respect, this ideal can slide into subjectivism, self-centeredness, and finally nihilism (as with many "deconstructionist" philosophers).

Moreover, the ethic of authenticity coalesces in dangerous ways with another cultural attitude, a scientistic rationalism focused on finding the most efficient means to the self's chosen projects. This "instrumental reason" is often expressed technologically. And it operates on a delusory model of the detached human subject, which, even when predicting costs and benefits, is hardly free from its "messy embedding in our bodily constitution, our dialogical situation, our emotions, and our traditional life forms."[10] Technological instruments in the hands of a disembodied reason, thinks Taylor, tend to slide toward dominance and hence to subvert the very goal (beneficence) toward which they were originally directed. Taylor is convinced that we can and must discuss the larger order of values in public. Otherwise, public life will degenerate into advocacy politics (or remain there), with judicial decisions creating winners and losers in matters that should be subjected to public debate and the growth of consensus.[11]

PUBLIC CONSIDERATION OF VALUES

Interestingly, the American Fertility Society policy report on reproductive technologies, which ultimately limits consent by few, if any, criteria other than good medical prognosis and absence of risk, begins on a footing not far from Taylor. In laying out the basis for ethical evaluation, the guidelines observe that many factors, such as religious authority, personal experience, immediate utility, vocational commitments, autonomy, and what is legally required, may weigh in favor of a moral conclusion by a given individual or group. Yet such appeals come together insofar as they illuminate a more fundamental moral criterion, "the human person integrally and adequately considered."[12] The welfare of the human person is not derived from quantitative studies alone, but "calls for an inductive approach, based on experience and reflection."[13]

The phrase "human person integrally and adequately considered" reveals the hand of committee member Richard A. McCormick, a Catholic theologian. It is based on *The Pastoral Constitution on the Church in the Modern World* (.51, .59, .61, .64), a document of the Second Vatican Council of the Roman Catholic Church.[14] Note that the AFS report does not advance respect for persons fully considered under the aegis of religious authority, but as the expression of a fundamental moral insight that can be shared, even in a pluralistic society. An insight that originates within a religious group is not thereby disqualified from the public conversation, where it may find a more "universal" resonance. A humanistic, and not merely tribal, basis for debate of the fundamental values at stake in reproductive practices was acknowledged when the committee as a whole accepted McCormick's basic criterion and inductive approach as part of its general considerations. McCormick himself concluded that the use of donors "is not for the good of persons integrally and adequately considered. It involves risks to basic dimensions of our flourishing," such as the unity of marriage.[15] This is especially true when the institutionalization of gamete donation is considered. The point is not that McCormick's analysis is necessarily correct, but that his concerns can be discussed publicly.

The fact that McCormick is a Roman Catholic may account for some of his moral sensibilities, but it does not relativize their significance. All contenders in the policy arena will necessarily come from some background or perspective that is not universally shared. No theologian, lawyer, medical practitioner, or philosopher can claim to occupy a neutral space free from shaping moral influences. Social consensus is built by testing every consideration in the public forum on the basis of its ability to persuade and its confirmation by the moral experience of others.

Human beings share experiences which are in some form universal and fundamental to human societies. Among these are sex, parenthood, and gender relations. Although common ground in human moral experience is often denied in the interests of resisting (rightly) the constraints of hegemonic definitions of human "nature," some moral commonality is required and presumed by the very existence of cross-traditional and cross-cultural debates about women's status, human rights, war and peace, trade agreements, and global ecology, as well as issues of reproduction and population.

The confidence Westerners place in informed consent as a moral guarantee is itself a verification of this point. Even if we could never demonstrate empirically that human beings would be harmed or worse off if they were sustained in a state of drug-induced euphoria while a central planning system supplied their every need, we would still say that a life devoid of freedom is not humanly fulfilling or worthwhile, and that the deprivation of freedom would be a great evil. In making this judgment, we rely on a general but nonetheless real consensus about some of the things that make a meaningful human life. Taking such shared values from the level of general affirmation to that of concrete practice is never simple, easy, or free of conflict. This, however, does not nullify our ability—or our responsibility—to expand the public ground on which such values and their implications can be discussed.

A WIDER MORAL VIEW:
KINSHIP AND THE FAMILY

The deep and broad sociality of being a parent and having children is neglected when we use the term "reproduction" to denote a medicalized view of acts of conception. The term "parenthood" carries with it a richer connotative load of relational meaning. To speak of parenthood is to envision a child, and to set both parent and child within a series of relationships to past and future generations, as well as to a co-parent, to possible siblings, aunts, uncles, and cousins, and to a larger community. Whether such a community supports those family relationships or fails to do so, it shapes the way in which they are institutionalized and experienced.

Although we often call the rearing parent of the child of a gamete donor that child's "social" parent, this terminology tends to make the biological and social meanings of parenthood independent variables. The division of biological and social roles neglects the ways in which social relationships are built on material, embodied ones. It reduces sociality to voluntarily, even contractually, undertaken relationships among individuals. In a full moral picture of the human experience of parenthood, however, biological relation as intergenerational kinship has a high profile. Kinship, in turn, is a shaping component of the networks of relationships and the worldviews that define all human societies, however variously expressed. Moreover, our moral bonds to our kin are not defined by voluntary agreement alone. When we consider our responsibility to a family member, the fact that he or she is related to us by blood or genes counts. Biological relationship is, cross-culturally, the *foundation* of the social meaning of family. Even marriage, which is itself not a blood relation, is consummated biologically through sexual union and the procreation of offspring who are the genetic combination of both parents. In this way, a new nexus of kinship is formed.

Biology, however, is not an *absolute* criterion for defining the family as a social network. Virtually all cultures include in their understanding of "family" relationships which, while not biologically based, are *analogous* to biological ones. The adoption of family members, especially children, and the creation of stepfamilies are examples. Sociologists also describe "fictive kinship," by which friends assume the role of family members. "Since family is supposed to be more reliable than friendship, 'going for brothers,' 'for sisters,' 'for cousins,' increases the commitment of a relationship, and makes people ideally more responsible for one another."[16]

Moreover, biological relationships may be separated from their prima facie social meaning in exceptional situations. Children are given for adoption when the biological parents are not able or willing to realize the social aspects of parenthood. Parental (social) rights may also be legally terminated when biological parents do not adequately fulfill their social responsibilities to the child. In some circumstances, the social elaboration of a biological kin relationship is deliberately repudiated because of a history of mistreatment or ill will.

Based on his extensive studies of the natives of Yap in the West Caroline Islands, David M. Schneider describes some of the cross-cultural variability of the parent-child relation and its flexibility within a given society. His intent is to dismantle the whole category of kinship, and he therefore opens his book with the bombastic claim, "there is no such thing as kinship."[17] Yet his study proves, to the contrary, that the relation of mother to child provides a primal base for social relations,[18] and that parent-child roles that are biologically rooted serve as a paradigm case even when their social dimensions are transferred to those who are not kin.

Schneider discovered in his work among the Yapese that there exists a relationship of authority and dependence between two people who are termed, respectively, *citamangen* (male) or *citiningen* (female), and *fak*. A woman is a *citiningen* to her child, while her husband is the child's *citamangen*.[19] However, these roles can be assumed by others who behave in ways analogous to the parent-child relation. When the parents become old and dependent, they may call their own children *citiningen* and *citamangen*. If a man's son fails to care for him, another man may take that role, and become *fak* to the old man. If a woman leaves her husband in divorce, she may not take her children with her, and the father's next wife or sister will become the children's *citiningen*. The father may also "throw away" children who do not live up to expectations. Schneider shows, not that kinship does not exist, but that anthropologists should not approach it with too many preconceptions about the ways in which kinship systems define social organization or about the level of social importance that kinship will assume. Nonetheless, intergenerational connection is everywhere the basis of some form of recognition.

A more traditional anthropologist, assuming exactly the sort of privileged meaning of kinship against which Schneider rails, is still, I think, right when he generalizes that in many or even most societies historically,

relationships to ancestors and kin have been the key relationships in the social structure; they have been the pivots on which most interaction, most claims and obligations, most loyalties and sentiments, turned. There would have been nothing whimsical or nostalgic about genealogical knowledge for a Chinese scholar, a Roman citizen, a South Sea Islander, a Zulu warrior or a Saxon thane; it would have been essential knowledge because it would have defined many of his most significant rights, duties and sentiments.[20]

The family in industrialized societies has become functionally reduced to the nuclear unit. Even that is nearing collapse due to unprecedented divorce rates, out-of-wedlock births, and abandonment of families by fathers. We find a variety of nontraditional families springing up that are analogous to the more cross-culturally standard version oriented around a heterosexual, pro-creative couple. Nonetheless the basic human sense of the parent-child rela-tion, which is in a fundamental way shaped around the biological substruc-ture of the typical case, is still substantially in place. The assumption in our own culture that a paradigm for the parental relationship is the social collabo-ration of two mutually committed biological parents in nurturing and educat-ing the child they have created is attested by the very persistence with which infertile couples search out an alleviation of their condition, moving to gamete donation as an admitted last resort. The real parental relation of the donor to the child is also recognized tacitly in the sort of preparation and counseling that are offered to oocyte donors and recipients, and especially in the wall of separation that receiving families sometimes feel it necessary to erect between the donor and themselves.[21] A biological parent is, after all, a parent.

As James Lindemann Nelson has written, the family is ideally based in "nature," not contractual relationships. As he sees it, "genetic connections" are important "as a part of our interest in perceiving the connections between our lives and the lives of others—connections which add depth and richness to the continuing story in which we participate, and which can therefore be referred to as narrative connections." Such connections give "cohesiveness and quality to our lives," and make us "feel both situated and recognized as individuals."[22] One adoptee remarked, "there's a primal need to find your roots," despite one's love and loyalty to an adoptive family. "I was feeling like the center of a wheel with two spokes missing. . . . Then those two spokes were put in place, and all of a sudden the wobble was gone."[23] Certainly persons can get along and enjoy fulfilling lives even when their social families are not reinforcements of their biological ones. But the issue is how to define the humanly and morally preferable linkage between the natural and the social aspects of family, and then how to promote and encourage that ideal, without necessarily excluding all exceptions.

The human experiences of parent-child and of family are not best served and enhanced by social institutions that treat their genetic and social dimen-sions as coming together only in occasional, accidental, or fortuitous ways, or as related only when individuals happen to make that choice. The humanly experienced value of family is realized most fully when family is the social elaboration of biological kinship. The unity of kinship and social roles ought to be advanced as a guiding ideal even if not always accessible as a practical reality.

FROM IDEAL TO APPLICATIONS

The question before us, then, is not whether it is ever justified to separate the biological from the social dimensions of parenthood. Indeed, it is evident that, of these two ideally united dimensions, the social is the more important for human beings, even if the biological is more fundamental. Biology may provide a cross-cultural basis for forms of social recognition, but it is the social relations of commitment and care which most distinguish the human family from other species. What we regard as the highest forms of human relations—love, friendship, marriage, intellectual inquiry, political life—are defined more by intentional commitment to others than by the material or bodily associations which are nevertheless their preconditions. So, too, in parenthood. Our social notion of parenthood flows from our experience of human interactions around biological reproduction. But it is in intentional commitment to and love for one's children that one's procreative actions are fulfilled. In human terms, the social realm is the genuinely moral and interpersonal realm, even if human society is grounded in material, including bodily, conditions.

The open moral question is twofold. First, what are the criteria for determining the legitimate, if exceptional, separation of the ideally united biological and social aspects of parenthood? Second, how, especially as a matter of social practice, can we respect and affirm the biological dimension of parenthood as a morally important guide to reproductive decisions, even as we sometimes permit it to be set aside in favor of (nonbiological) social parenthood? These two queries are the flip sides of one another. The boundaries within which exceptions are permitted will be established, in part, by the practices we think necessary to uphold the importance of kinship as an integral meaning of human parenthood—even if kinship is superseded in certain cases by the importance of the personal relationship of parent and child.

My own suggestion is that separation is generally justified only in order to prefer the social to the biological, not the other way around, when the motivating factor is the best interests of the child, and when the circumstances requiring the separation are preexisting and now beyond human control. I would also stipulate that, *all other things being equal*, it is better to transfer parental responsibility for a child to an adult or family who shares some biological kinship relation with the child. (This final stipulation must still meet the criterion of the best interests of the child.)

At the practical level, these four criteria work to permit adoption and stepparenting, but not gamete donation. They put in a negative light reproductive arrangements in which adults freely elect to conceive a child who is never intended to enjoy the unity of kinship and social identity. These criteria place the donor who sees procreation as merely a biological act with no personal consequences in a more negative light than the recipient couple who want "desperately" to parent a child and who would create one biologically if that were possible. The criteria make it possible to see oocyte donation, in which the infertile woman gestates the child, as less a departure than sperm donation from the ideal in which a couple with a shared biological relation to the child also parent him or her together.[24] Finally, these criteria work to reject the removal of a child from adoptive parents who have established a social parenting relationship with that child, even when this is proposed to honor the tie of biological parents who have no similar realized social relation with the child.

Because human beings are often forced to act in devastating circumstances for which there is no morally unambiguous resolution, I am reluctant to propose an absolute rule against any and all gamete donation. One can imagine too readily, for instance, a bride in a culture which so prizes female fertility and male heirs, and which makes women's worth so highly dependent on this, that the access of women to an anonymous gamete donor could be a matter of life and death. However, I want to place that option at the margins of our notions of moral value and responsibility in the sphere of human parenthood.

The desire to beget or bear a child is understandable and worthy, but not an absolute that must always be fulfilled. Neither men's nor women's identity should be so focused on biological fertility or on its simulation (through secret use of a donor) that they will stop at the use of virtually no technology or reproductive scenario in order to have a biologically related child. We are well on the way to establishing wide-scale social practices, such as high-tech and costly infertility programs, which take it as unproblematic to move incrementally toward a freely elected and instrumental separation of genetic from social parenthood for rearing parents, donors, and the resulting child. This is to move the exceptional anomaly into the center of what we take to make up the human child-parent-family relationship. It sunders values that humans experience deeply and cross-culturally as interrelated. It provides symbolic reinforcement of other present and future modes of separation, such as the slim social attachment many impregnating men feel to their mates and off-spring.

Noting that a sperm donor is as much a father biologically as one who achieves that status through heterosexual intercourse, Daniel Callahan expresses incredulity that "with hardly any public debate at all, the practice — indeed institution — of artificial insemination by an anonymous donor so easily slipped in. What could society have been thinking about?"[25] While he finds the urge to have a child understandable, he is unsympathetic to "an acceptance of the systematic downgrading of fatherhood brought about by the introduction of anonymous sperm donors." Even more perturbing is the possibility that "fatherhood had already sunken to such a low state, and male irresponsibility was already so accepted, that no one saw a problem."[26] Taking female donors into account, we pose the question from a different perspective. Does motherhood already involve such objectification and reproductive servitude of women, and such internalization by women of the demands of a patriarchal society, that we find it unremarkable that some women despair of purpose outside of their ability to achieve pregnancy? That others dissociate their connection to their children from their own personal and social identity?

FEMINIST CRITIQUES OF "CHOICE" IN REPRODUCTION

The radical feminist critique allows us to look below the surface of free and informed consent and to recognize that powerful social forces always shape choice and define the options that we discern as available to us. A morality of private choice is ultimately self-delusory. Many feminists, influenced by the work of Michel Foucault and other "postmodern" philosophers, urge us to recognize that our freedom can be coopted by "discourses" of power and knowledge, preeminently medical discourses, which structure our perceptions of ourselves and our world.

An ethicist who with his wife endured a taxing series of infertility therapies before attempting donor insemination, verifies that "the tyranny of available technologies" constitutes "a form of coercion."[27] After each unsuccessful attempt, the patient asks, "How can I not try the next technique?" Moreover, the pressure to advance to additional treatments carries with it relational problems for the couple, insofar as one who refuses to go any further may be blamed for denying the spouse the opportunity to procreate.

The trajectory toward the use of reproductive technologies is often given momentum by a rhetoric of "desperation" surrounding the couples and their need to bear a child. One IVF client, who quite understandably wanted to help assuage her parents' grief over the recent death of her brother, is portrayed as giving the goal of a birth nearly ultimate importance. She is repeatedly characterized as "desperate." We hear of prayers for the baby she "so desperately desired," she tells us how she "so desperately wanted to give my parents a grandchild," and we learn that during a phone-line wait for the doctor, she "despaired."[28] In an essay entitled "Deconstructing 'Desperateness,'" anthropologist Sarah Franklin recounts headlined and emotionally overloaded stories of infertility from the British press. She concludes that the media are contributing to a mythology in which parenthood is a precondition of adulthood and social approval, and in which the only real solution to childlessness lies in the capabilities of medical science.[29] The story of the desperate infertile couple is both an adventure story and a romance, in which a successful "fight against the odds" may end in "a dream come true." It is an epic story of medical heroism in the face of human suffering and the forward march of scientific progress. It is a story of winners and losers, of happy endings for some and hopelessness for others.[30]

The personal consequences of living this story cry out in the words of one woman who was obviously not only at the point of desperation, but also emotionally dependent on the medical profession. "After more than four years of infertility, I am pregnant. . . . The last three months have been a black hole of terror. The overwhelming fatigue and constant nausea were bad enough, but the fear of miscarriage nearly drove me crazy. . . . I live from one obstetrical appointment to the next."[31]

Even those who win the happy endings do so at an enormous emotional and financial cost. Many of the veterans speak of profound personal humiliation, as the intimacy of their sexual and procreative capacities is invaded, and their person is objectified into a set of body parts and reproductive processes. Gena Corea makes a disconcerting comparison of artificial insemination, IVF, embryo transfer, and sex determination in cows and in women. One veterinarian who worked for a company that transferred fertilized eggs from donor to host cattle "gently soothed a cow while he was hurting her, saying, 'I'm sorry, honey.' " One of the farmers with whom this man worked described the operation as "making babies." He herded cows into confining equipment by shouting, hitting them on the side, twisting their tails, and finally urging, "What's the matter with you woman? Step up!"[32]

Janice Raymond finds a disturbing sexualization of the technically de-sexualized procedures of reproductive medicine, which compounds the experience of the woman as object and victim. Even if sexual banter and phallic references among physicians are more rare than some critics report, teams which prod and inspect a prone woman, feet in stirrups, genitals exposed, all the while discussing ways in which she can be made pregnant, reduce her to a state of sexual humiliation. Raymond recounts attending a world IVF conference on reproductive technologies in Paris in 1991, at which part of the entertainment for the "appreciative male medical audience" was a "can-can" in which women's bodies were exposed in a display of thrusting pelvises and buttocks.[33] In such an atmosphere, it is difficult to dismiss the argument that infertility medicine is inherently coercive, especially for women. One may hope that as more women enter this specialty, its dehumanizing effects on women will be diluted. I believe that specialists who practice oocyte donation and other infertility therapies usually do so with honorable intentions and a Hippocratic commitment to relieve human suffering and "do no harm."

But a liberal philosophy and politics of choice do not adequately address the fact that women are presented from birth with images of mothering as crucial to their identity. Pregnancy and childbearing are depicted as the culmination both of their sexuality and of their relationships of intimacy, and fertility as a sign of youthfulness, desirability, and worth. Men are taught to see virility and sexual potency as confirmed in the ability to "father" a child (i.e., to inseminate a woman), and both men and women are led to see the sexual and reproductive services of women as men's natural right and due. Hence the "desperation" that surrounds the failure to realize the socially requisite roles of wife and mother, and the insidious power of a highly technological medical establishment which holds out promise of a reversal of fortune.[34] The fault does not lie only with the doctors, however. Their petitioners, as well as a larger public whose attitudes are represented by a laissez-faire policy, have a responsibility to consider carefully the human values at stake in family and parenthood, as well as our trust that technology will provide a way around intractable human difficulties.

THE ADOPTION OPTION

The desire to conceive and birth a child "naturally" is not only understandable and appropriate, but is prevalent cross-culturally, both among married couples and many singles. The disappointment of this desire is a heavy burden, and it is valid to attempt to relieve that burden by remedying possible physiologic causes. The moral question concerns the proper limits of recourse to medical therapy. That question must be answered partly in terms of nonmedical alternatives.

One social answer to infertility is adoption. Adoption allows an infertile couple to nurture a child without requiring a reproductive alliance of one member of the couple with a third party. Adoption preserves a symmetrical relation of parents to child. It allows them to accept the limits of their fertility (and perhaps age), while recognizing that other, creative ways of satisfying their generative impulses and their desire to share the rewards of childrearing can be found. This is not to say that the need to parent is itself so strong that infertile persons cannot deal with this limitation through nonparental forms of relationship, service, and fulfillment. But, given the availability and need of parentless children worldwide, adoption is a viable way to channel one's parental aspirations.

I have a personal interest in adoption because three of my five children are adopted from Thailand, and adoption has been a tremendously rewarding experience for our family. The adoption of a child in need of loving parents can be an opportunity for adults who strongly desire a child to transform their own needs and frustrations into compassion and care for another. Parties to adoption can recognize that the sundering of the biological and social relationships of birthparents to children often arises from social injustices, and that the causes behind the availability of children for adoption should be addressed in their own right. Moreover, adopted children, adoptive parents, and birthparents will all need to come to terms with their "loss" of a unified biosocial child-parent relation. Regret can be expressed for this loss, which is a subsequent necessity that the birthparents did not plan when the child was conceived. Yet adoption can transform a reproductive "failure" on the one side, and a disrupted birthing situation on the other, into a constructive reconformation of family relationships. The matching of adults' needs and children's needs is an equation in which a double negative can become a positive accomplishment.

Elizabeth Bartholet, an advocate for adoption as a resolution of infertility, makes the case that adoption laws, health insurance policies, and the medicalized infertility scenario conspire to make it easier for parents to seek high-tech therapies than to parent already-existing children. Bartholet writes of her own experiences with fertility specialists. Those who are financially able are led ineluctably "down the treatment path," by a doctor whose advice "is inevitably biased toward the treatment option." Few doctors see it as "their job to explore with patients why they are considering medical treatment, whether continued treatment efforts are worth it, or when enough is enough."[35]

Bartholet also addresses the argument that adoption is exploitative, since it takes advantage of the misfortune of birthparents, contributes to its social causes, and even constitutes a form of "trafficking" in babies.[36] Kidnappings may occasionally occur, as may coercion of birthparents—especially impoverished birthmothers—and improper payments to parents or to intermediaries are not as rare as one might wish. Moreover, it is true that the demand of relatively well-off Western couples for healthy white infants indicates that need fulfillment (a need for a specified kind of "acceptable" child) often dominates in the adoption situation over outreach to homeless children. Abuses and distortions of the adoption relationship must be identified and abolished, not tolerated.

Nevertheless, adopted children are not most accurately seen as "products" who are "marketed" to the middle class, or "exported" from Third World countries. As Bartholet insists, mistreatment of children and oppression of birthparents must be kept in perspective. Even if all abuses were eliminated, and long-standing and worldwide injustices, such as poverty and the subordination of women, began to be substantially addressed, it is difficult to imagine that the numbers of children in need of families would be drastically reduced in the near future. Moreover, in many cultures, biological kinship is seen as so indispensable to a parental attitude toward children, that adoption of those who are not related by blood is virtually inconceivable. Adopted "slum children" are suspected of having "bad blood," and their true origin is often hidden in secrecy. (This extreme is the opposite of the voluntaristic view of parenthood that we find in North America.) "International adoption clearly represents an extraordinarily positive option for the homeless children of the world, compared to all other realistic options."[37] To denigrate legitimately formed adoptive families in order to promote a position that is either for or against reproductive technologies,[38] to focus solely on the well-founded resentment by poorer countries of Western colonialism and the indignity many of these countries experience in not being able to care for their own children, is to reduce needy children who deserve families to pawns in political battles.

To counter charges of adoption racketeering and exploitation, it should also be recognized that many international adoption agencies (and the parents who have adopted through them) make contributions, both financial and social, to improve the situation of children in their birth countries. These include social services for families who are under duress and in danger of disruption; education for children of poor families, including girls; financial support for birthmothers who desire to keep their children; foster family programs; educational and social programs for institutionalized children; care for handicapped children and a chance to be adopted (almost nil within the country for most); advocacy for in-country adoption; and the reuniting of birth families where possible. These organizations typically provide counseling and support for adoptive families, including programs which reinforce the ethnic and racial identity of adopted children. While problems and difficulties undoubtedly exist in the practice of adoption, and while it will not be a satisfying solution for all couples experiencing infertility, it is one viable avenue to relieve the suffering that infertility unquestionably can bring.

POLICY AND MORALITY

It is a truism that Americans tend to equate law with morality. The legalization or legal facilitation of an activity is likely to short-circuit further public discussion (and personal consideration) of whether that activity is worthwhile or objectionable in itself or in certain circumstances. Conversely, illegality makes a negative moral statement in the minds of many. Contrast public attitudes to abortion and to the use of marijuana, in view of the fact that the former is, from almost any credible standpoint, a more serious moral decision.

Institutionalized gamete donation, especially when or if it is facilitated by policies which provide it financial support, or specify and protect the rights of the parties to it, makes a public statement. The message is that the separation of biological from social parenthood, and the equation of family relations with voluntarily assumed contracts, are morally unproblematic. Oocyte donation reinforces the view that women must become pregnant in order to be fulfilled as women, and that this goal is important enough to justify extreme measures, including subjecting oneself to serious emotional and physical stress, and having one's spouse conceive with a third party. Gamete donation as a personal "choice" also conveys the priority of privacy and liberty over sociality and the common good, and the validity of personal risk and harm as compasses of moral reasoning. It reinforces our expectation that technology will resolve complex human problems, and reposes in the medical profession a confidence and a set of expectations that it neither should receive nor should want.

Institutionalized gamete donation is thus morally questionable as a social practice for a number of reasons that go far beyond the concerns we might have in an isolated case. However well established sperm donation has already become, we need to take another look at what it represents, and the arrival of oocyte donation gives us that opportunity. This is not a matter of some marginal religious objection, but of our ability to think and act morally as a society and to use reason in a transformative as well as an instrumental way.[39] We need to consider, not just protections of the decision-making process and efficient means to freely elected ends, but the substantive values whose realization we encourage by means of the policies we set.

Outlawing and attempting to eradicate well-entrenched practices is not the only way to advance their moral reconsideration; nor is it usually the most prudent and effective way. Laws and policies often do not command compliance unless they are met by at least an approximate social consensus in their favor. But policy can have a role in shaping consensus if it proceeds by relatively moderate measures, and if it encourages and comes out of broad and civil public discussion. Policy-making bodies can express the importance of ongoing moral scrutiny of gamete donation in a variety of ways. Some examples of restraints on the practice (here more suggestions than proposals) are refusing to let donors totally off the hook and out of the picture, as by making identifying information available to the adult child; declining to make gamete donation a research funding priority; denying insurance coverage to these technologies; setting an age limit for recipients as well as donors; and discouraging or denying oocyte donation to single women.

Positively, policy could support other options, especially adoption, and could encourage more thoughtful and extended counseling about alternatives. Counseling should be offered by persons with no vested interest in the success of gamete donation as a socially approved and supported practice. This might include the opportunity to share experiences with other individuals or couples who have taken a variety of routes in coping with infertility. Counseling and opportunities for reconsideration should continue throughout the infertility treatment process.

NOTES

1. Mark V. Sauer and Richard J. Paulson, "Understanding the Current Status of Oocyte Donation in the United States: What's Really Going on out There?" *Fertility and Sterility* 58 (1992): 17.

2. American Fertility Society, "Guidelines for Gamete Donation: 1993," *Fertility and Sterility* 59, Supplement 1 (1993): 7S.

3. See Mark V. Sauer et al., "Reversing the Natural Decline in Human Fertility: An Extended Clinical Trial of Oocyte Donation to Women of Advanced Reproductive

Age," *Journal of the American Medical Association* 268 (1992): 1275–79. An editorial in the same issue identifies oocyte donation as "the most appropriate treatment" for women over 40, and calls its development "truly exciting" (Martin M. Quigley, "The New Frontier of Reproductive Age," 1321). Quigley's title speaks volumes about the individualist, conquest-oriented, and entrepreneurial attitudes toward women's bodies of which many feminists have been critical. See, for instance, Emily Martin, *The Woman in the Body: A Cultural Analysis of Reproduction* (Boston: Beacon Press, 1989).

4. Susan Chira, "Of a Certain Age, and in a Family Way," *New York Times*, Sunday, January 2, 1994, p. 5.

5. Gina Kolata, "Reproductive Revolution Is Jolting Old Views," *New York Times*, January 11, 1994, p. C12. Germaine Greer is reported to have remarked, "The problem is that nobody seems to know what is pathological behavior anymore. . . . These women are going to have a terrible time when they finally meet the Grim Reaper. They're really out of touch with reality, and most women are not" (in Chira, "Of a Certain Age," p. 5).

6. John A. Robertson, "Ethical and Legal Issues in Human Egg Donation," *Fertility and Sterility* 52 (1989): 354.

7. Ibid., p. 360.

8. Ethics Committee of the American Fertility Society, "Ethical Considerations of the New Reproductive Technologies," *Fertility and Sterility*, 53/6, Supplement 2 (1990): 24S.

9. Charles Taylor, *The Ethics of Authenticity* (Cambridge, MA, and London: Harvard University Press, 1993).

10. Ibid., p. 102.

11. Ibid., pp. 114–16.

12. AFS, "Ethical Considerations," p. 1S.

13. Ibid.

14. See Walter M. Abbot, S. J., ed., *The Documents of Vatican II* (New York: America Press, 1966).

15. "Appendix A," in AFS, "Ethical Considerations," p. 87S.

16. Rayna Rapp, "Family and Class in Contemporary America: Notes Toward an Understanding of Ideology," in Barrie Thorne and Marilyn Yalon, eds., *Rethinking the Family: Some Feminist Questions* (White Plains, NY: Longman, 1982), p. 178.

17. Ibid., p. vii.

18. Ibid., pp. 121, 123. The father's biological relation to the child is more difficult to recognize and may be explained in a variety of ways. When Schneider worked on Yap in the 1940s, the inhabitants thought that pregnancy was caused by spirits who looked with approval on a wife's conduct in her husband's social group (defined partly by kinship and partly by landowning). But 20 years later, coitus as well as spirit approval was understood to be necessary to pregnancy. The view was that the man planted a seed which grew in the woman as in a garden (ibid., p. 28).

19. David M. Schneider, *A Critique of the Study of Kinship* (Ann Arbor: University of Michigan Press, 1984), p. 30.

20. Robin Fox, *Kinship and Marriage: An Anthropological Perspective* (Harmondsworth, Middlesex, England; Ringwood, Victoria, Australia; Baltimore, MD: Penguin Books, 1967).

21. See Patricia P. Mahlstedt and Dorothy Greenfeld, "Assisted Reproductive Technology with Donor Gametes: The Need for Patient Preparation," *Fertility and Sterility* 52/6 (1989): 908–14.

22. James Lindemann Nelson, "Genetic Narratives: Biology, Stories, and the Definition of the Family," *Health Matrix: Journal of Law-Medicine* 2/1 (1992): 79, 82.

23. Susan Chira, "Years after Adoption, Adults Find Past, and New Hurdles," *New York Times*, August 30, 1993, p. B6.

24. The rationale for ovum donation to single women is weak insofar as it would involve the cooperation of two strangers in the conception of a child for whom neither would ever function as the social parent, in order that the recipient could experience nine months of gestation and obtain a child who was not genetically related either to herself or to any domestic partner.

25. Daniel Callahan, "Bioethics and Fatherhood," *Utah Law Review* 735/3 (1992): 739.

26. Ibid., p. 741.

27. Paul Lauritzen, "What Price Parenthood?" *Hastings Center Report* (1990): p. 41. The article preceded the choice to pursue donor insemination. A subsequent book defending that choice is *Pursuing Parenthood: Ethical Issues in Assisted Reproduction* (Bloomington and Indianapolis: Indiana University Press, 1993).

28. Cindy Loose, "A Holiday Comes to Life: Mom's Celebration Was 4 years in Making," *Washington Post*, May 9, 1993, pp. A1, A22–23.

29. Sarah Franklin, " 'Deconstructing Desperateness': The Social Construction of Infertility in Popular Representations of New Reproductive Technologies," in Maureen McNeil, Ian Varcoe, and Steven Yearly, eds., *The New Reproductive Technologies* (London: Macmillan, 1990), pp. 200–29.

30. Ibid., pp. 203–204.

31. Kirsten Kozolanka, "Giving Up: The Choice That Isn't," in *Infertility: Women Speak Out about Their Experiences of Reproductive Medicine*, ed. Renate Klein (London: Pandora, 1989), p. 128; as quoted in Janice G. Raymond, *Women as Wombs: Reproductive Technologies and the Battle over Women's Freedom* (New York: Harper Collins, 1993), p. 87.

32. Gena Corea, *The Mother Machine: Reproductive Technologies from Artificial Insemination to Artificial Wombs* (New York: Harper & Row, 1985), pp. 62, 64, 65.

33. Raymond, *Women as Wombs*, p. xxxi.

34. "Increasingly, more and more control is taken away from an individual's body and concentrated in the hands of 'experts'—the rapidly—and internationally—growing brigade of 'technodocs': doctors, scientists, pharmaceutical representatives (most of them male, white, and of Euro-American origin) who fiercely compete with one another on this 'new frontier' of scientific discovery and monetary profits" (Renate Duelli Klein, "What's 'New' about the 'New' Reproductive Technologies?" in Gena Corea et al., eds., *Man-Made Women: How New Reproductive Technologies Affect Women* [Bloomington and Indianapolis: Indiana University Press, 1987], p. 65.)

35. Elizabeth Bartholet, *Family Bonds: Adoption and the Politics of Parenting* (Boston and New York: Houghton Mifflin, 1993), p. 30.

36. Bartholet cites an organization which has been critical of international adoption, Defense for Children International, as acknowledging that abuses are numerically rare. Trafficking cases undoubtedly "constitute only a tiny proportion of the displacements of children for adoption purposes" (Marie-Francoise Lucker-Bubel,

Inter-Country Adoption and Trafficking in Children: An Initial Assessment [Geneva: Defense for Children International, 1990], p. 2, as cited in Bartholet, *Family Bonds*, p. 248).

37. Ibid., p. 156.

38. Janice G. Raymond argues against reproductive technologies, seeing "trafficking" in women's reproductive body parts as of a piece with the market in children and with the sexual prostitution or enslavement of women (*Women as Wombs: Reproductive Technologies and the Battle over Women's Freedom* [New York: Harper Collins, 1993]). Paul Lauritzen does not totally reject adoption, but argues that donor therapies are preferable because the institution of adoption is exploitative (*Pursuing Parenthood*, pp. 115, 120, 125).

39. Nelson, "Genetic Narratives," p. 75.

SEVEN

PARENTS ANONYMOUS
Cynthia B. Cohen, Ph.D., J.D.

How much care do parents owe to their children? Ought they to provide them with the best possible life? Or need they only offer them a minimally decent one, free from severe physical and mental abuse? These questions, which have been debated with special force for the last two decades, presume that parents owe their children *something* in the way of care. Yet this presumption is dismissed in the case of women and men who donate gametes to others. Egg and sperm donors provide the very biological material that allows children to come into the world—yet they assume no parental responsibility for these children once born. Indeed, most donors are strangers to these offspring, and have no idea of where and how they are. Do gamete donors owe anything to these biological children? Ought they to offer them care and concern? Or have they an obligation to disappear into the shadows after they have donated, never to be seen again?

CONFLICTS IN ATTITUDES TOWARD
GAMETE DONOR ANONYMITY

These questions have been thrust to the fore by the striking growth of reproductive technologies that require the biological assistance of third parties. Sperm donation, which has been employed for over 100 years,[1] has rapidly increased in use over the last three decades. Usually it has been carried out anonymously in the belief that this contributes to the welfare of all involved.[2] Oocyte or egg donation, a procedure analogous to sperm donation, was introduced much more recently, in 1984.[3] At that time, infertility specialists planned to keep egg donors anonymous, just as they had sperm donors.[4] However, they could not find many women willing to experience the risks and inconvenience of having eggs extracted from their ovaries to be given to strangers.[5] Only women with close personal ties to recipients, such as sisters, cousins, friends, and even mothers, were willing to undergo the procedure. Therefore, when oocyte donation was first introduced, donors usually were known by recipients.[6]

All of this is changing today.[7] Calls are increasingly heard for openness about the identity and background of sperm donors.[8] Recent surveys indicate that many sperm donors are receptive to being known by those who receive their gametes and the children born of them.[9] When a law was passed in Sweden in 1985 abolishing anonymity for sperm donors, the number of donors initially decreased, but rose to its previous level a few months later.[10] Donors, who were now more often older and married, were willing to be open about their contribution to the creation of a child.[11]

This trend away from donor anonymity in sperm donation is taking place, in part, because of changes in social attitudes toward adoption.[12] Although sperm donation and adoption differ in significant respects, both involve rearing a child who is not genetically linked to at least one parent. For this reason, sperm donation has been conceptualized by some as "semi-adoption."[13] As greater openness about the origins of adoptees has developed, sperm donation has begun to move along a parallel path.[14]

Paradoxically, oocyte donation appears to be moving in the opposite direction. With the advent of a less intrusive means of collecting eggs, ultrasound-guided transvaginal follicular aspiration,[15] the risks and inconvenience to oocyte donors have lessened. This has made it possible to attract greater numbers of stranger donors. As the use of oocyte donation has increased, there has been a reversion to the old presumption in favor of gamete donor anonymity. By 1991, out of 1,107 donors who provided eggs for donation in the United States, only 288, roughly one-quarter, were known.[16] The move toward openness in sperm donation has not yet overtaken oocyte donation because the latter is a new procedure still absorbing the old norm in favor of donor anonymity. Moveover, oocyte donation seems less like adoption and more like ordinary reproduction than sperm donation. In oocyte donation, both rearing parents have a biological stake in the child: The man contributes the sperm and the woman her gestational capacities. The woman and her partner can view the child as a result of both their efforts and contributions. This gives them reason to bracket the involvement of a donor after a pregnancy has been initiated, and this, in turn, strengthens their impetus to use anonymous donors who can be forgotten after donation has occurred.

This conflict in attitudes toward donor anonymity in sperm and oocyte donation suggests that no firm picture of the appropriate role of the gamete donor has emerged. I propose that this is due to the disparate views of the very nature of gamete donation presumed by those who take opposing positions about donor anonymity. To test this contention, I will briefly examine the major arguments advanced for and against gamete donor anonymity to sift out the views of the moral meaning of gamete donation they presuppose. I will go on to argue that a broader, more coherent moral conception of gamete donation and of the role of the gamete donor is needed if we are to reach a justified conclusion about whether those providing gametes should remain anonymous or be known.

ARGUMENTS OF THOSE WHO FAVOR THE USE OF ANONYMOUS GAMETE DONORS

Anonymity and secrecy are logically distinct concepts. Anonymity has to do with keeping the identity of the donor hidden. Secrecy has to do with keeping the origins of the child hidden. The use of an anonymous donor does not require secrecy about the use of gamete donation. Others may know that a couple has received a gamete, and yet they may not be aware of the identity of the particular donor. Further, secrecy about gamete donation does not require that an anonymous donor be employed. A couple can keep the fact that they have engaged in gamete donation hidden from others and yet know the identity of the gamete donor. For most couples, however, the use of an anonymous donor is part of a larger plan of secrecy. For this reason, anonymity will be taken to be associated with secrecy about gamete donation in the following discussion.

Several interrelated arguments have been given for donor anonymity. One that appears frequently is that recipients of gametes will be stigmatized socially, as will the resulting children unless the identity of donors is kept hidden. Those who are "barren" have been accorded little sympathy historically,[17] and discriminatory attitudes toward them still pervade our society. Recipients of donated sperm and eggs can find themselves victims of heightened stigmatization because they bring third parties into the creation of a child, an act that has traditionally involved only two natural parents. To avoid stigmatization and ostracization, those pressing this argument contend, recipient couples must make their immediate family seem as "normal" as possible.[18] They can do so by keeping their participation in gamete donation secret and by using anonymous donors.

The social stigmatization argument is also applied to the children born of gamete donation.[19] Defenders of anonymity maintain that these children would be socially isolated by their peers were their mode of conception known.[20] Donor anonymity, they maintain, protects children born of these procedures from social opprobrium. Curiously, the possibility that donors might also experience social stigmatization and need protection from negative reactions were their contribution known is not addressed as yet another reason for donor anonymity by those presenting this argument.

Family privacy provides the focus of a second argument for keeping the identity of gamete donors hidden. Its proponents postulate a need to protect the family from interference or harassment by those donors. They fear that known donors might enter the lives of children born of their gametes and, out of self-interest, attempt to seduce these children away.[21] Donor well-being does figure in this second argument, for some suggest that anonymity also protects donors from interference in their lives by offspring. Children born of their gametes will not know how to locate them should they wish to press claims for support and inheritance on them.

This argument, while acknowledging donor welfare as a factor that can enter into consideration, pictures donors in contradictory ways. On the one hand, they are seen as having such a keen and selfish interest in relating to the children born of their gametes that recipients must take precautions against their intrusions. On the other, they are viewed as having such a strong interest in avoiding all future contact with their children that their identity must be hidden. The privacy argument presents donors in conflicting and irreconcilable ways as selfish manipulators. It does not consider that donors might have an altruistic stake in knowing the fate of children who result from their gametes.

The need to maintain a large pool of gamete donors provides the basis for the third argument for donor anonymity. A concern has been raised, especially by infertility specialists, that if donors were known, they would be reluctant to provide gametes (presumably because children born of their gametes would later interfere in their lives) and that as a consequence there would be insufficient numbers of donors to meet the needs of infertile couples.[22] Here the predominant picture of donors is of self-interested individuals who wish to have nothing to do with the children born of their gametes once donation has taken place. They must be guaranteed anonymity or they will not provide their gametes.

The complexities of relations among family members provide grounds for yet another argument for donor anonymity. It has been suggested that relationships within families are necessarily disturbed when members donate gametes to one another. Children born of egg donation will receive the maternal attentions of both their biological and nurturing mothers and, as a consequence, will experience confusion about the identity of their "real" mother.[23] Openness about the family donor might blur the boundaries around parenthood and cause unresolvable identity conflicts for these children.[24] Further, relations within the family might be damaged by the hovering presence of the donor.[25] If family members are to be used as donors at all, it is argued, their identity should be kept strictly confidential so that the recipient couple can construct its own parental relation with the child without their interference. The picture of donors as potential self-serving intruders reemerges in this argument. The possibility they might play a positive role in the development of the child and in family relationships is not taken into consideration.

ARGUMENTS OF THOSE WHO FAVOR THE USE OF IDENTIFIABLE GAMETE DONORS

Several arguments have been given for using known, rather than anonymous, donors. A primary one is that truthfulness is a significant value that ought to be honored and protected. On this view, it is morally wrong to keep the truth about their origins, including the identity of the donor whose gamete brought them into life, from children born of gamete donation. To do so is to place a lie at the center of the relationship between parent and child that can ultimately form the seed of the relationship's undoing.[26] Donor anonymity is part and parcel of an ethically unacceptable plan of secrecy that denies the importance of the truth.

This argument is often supplemented by one found in the adoption litera- ture that to deceive children about their conception is to violate their right to know about their biological and family origins. One's biological inheritance and genealogy are significant social constructions essential to one's identity.[27] Warnock is among those who uphold the right of children born of donated gametes to know of their origins. She maintains that

> The child is being used as a means to the parents' ends, namely to have, or seem to have a "normal" family; and I do not think that using one person as a means to another's ends can ever be right, unless the person has consented to be so used. . . . I cannot argue that children who are told their origins . . . are necessarily happier, or better off in any way that can be estimated. But I do believe that if they are not told, they are being wrongly treated.[28]

Proponents of this argument hold that children should be informed about the basic circumstances under which they were conceived and the people who contributed to their creation.[29] To know about the interests, skills, and family histories of donors enables children born of gamete donation to identify with their genetic heritage and to develop a sense of self. This argument does not address any potential benefit that might accrue to donors were they to be open about their contribution.

It is not just children, but the recipient family on whom donor anonymity can have deleterious effects, proponents of this argument maintain. The use of anonymous donors is often part of a larger plan of secrecy about the use of oocyte donation. Yet those in favor of openness point out that there is growing documentation of the negative effects of secrecy within the family.[30] The parental anxiety that results from evasiveness and the fear of disclosure can create a significant barrier between parent and child that is detrimental to them both. Children who have learned of their origins accidentally have been shocked and hurt by the deception to which they have been subjected.[31] On balance, proponents of openness argue, secrecy may cause more harm to the child and the relationship between parents and child than it prevents.

Moreover, they contend, the norm for family relationships and kinship groups at the foundation of our society is one of trust.[32] If a major exception to this norm is to be made for gamete donation, a strong justification must be given. Yet no such justification has been provided by those who favor donor anonymity. Further, their approach would deny access to significant information about their social and individual identity to a group of people who could not be consulted about whether this should be allowed.[33] This concern raises basic questions, not only about fairness and consent, but about what we owe to the children born of gamete donation.

The truthfulness argument in its several forms holds that from the perspective of the recipients and the child born of gamete donation it is wrong to maintain donor anonymity on both deontological and consequentialist grounds. The fact that anonymous donors are also complicit in the deception of the child and that they might have some obligation of truthfulness toward that child is not addressed in this argument.

Another argument against donor anonymity is based on the negative psychological effects on recipients that could be created by keeping the donor's identity hidden. Those who receive donated gametes may use donor anonymity as part of a systematic denial of their infertile condition.[34] Keeping the donor's identity secret can inhibit their ability to mourn the loss of genetic connection with the child and serve to delay their acknowledgment of the pain and suffering they have experienced. Some argue that the emotional energy that parents spend in denying or hiding infertility might be better used to address the problems of infertility and gamete donation openly.[35] That anonymous gamete donation might also have negative psychological effects on the donor is not viewed as an additional factor to be taken into consideration by those who advance this argument.

THE MEANING OF GAMETE DONATION AND THE ROLE OF DONORS

Neither set of arguments appears to prevail over the other. This is because they are incomplete and exhibit no consistent and coherent understanding of the function of donors, who are essential participants in gamete donation procedures. Donors appear in these arguments as faceless surds who are granted no individual or social identity. They are taken into account instrumentally, insofar as they affect the size of the donor pool and impinge on the welfare of recipients and children. When they are viewed as persons in their own right, they are seen as self-interested manipulators with little regard for their effect on the children born of their gametes or the recipient parents. Donors are viewed as "types" in these arguments, rather than as ethically significant figures with personal identities and moral characters.

The relative invisibility of donors in the debate about donor anonymity reflects the view of gamete donation presupposed by many who favor donor anonymity. This view predominates by default, since the conception of the meaning of gamete donation presumed by those who are against anonymity often goes unrecognized and unacknowledged, even by those who hold it.

Many proponents of donor anonymity presuppose that gamete donation involves a transaction between strangers resulting in the delivery of a body product. The relation between the parties is governed by a contract that is designed to regulate the provision of this product while minimizing personal relationships among them.[36] Human gametes are to be removed from their possessors and distributed to recipients in an impersonal, even, mechanical way. Donors bear no responsibility for the disposition of their sperm or eggs, but supply bodily material that others are entitled to use in ways of their own choosing. On this view of gamete donation, anonymity provides the foundation of a permanent wall of separation between donors and recipients.

This view of the meaning of gamete donation is undergirded by a dynamic of fear.[37] Those who advance it fear social opprobrium and shame, unwanted intrusions into the lives of recipients and their children, and confusion on the part of the children about family relations and self-identity. Their fear is not groundless. The values and cultural orientations permeating the gamete donor system in this country have worked to create tremendous ambivalence toward it. While the use of new reproductive technologies is often applauded as beneficial to those who are childless, the participation of third parties in these technologies raises concerns about weakening the importance of the biological tie to the family and to society. This concern overpowers and negates perceptions of the benefits of gamete donation. The way in which to avoid the social stigmatization that results, those who favor donor anonymity contend, is to keep the act of donation secret and to ignore the donor's existence once donation has taken place. Ironically, the very secrecy that surrounds gamete donation contributes to the lack of social acceptance of the procedure. What is kept hidden must be shameful and wrong.

A fundamentally different conception of gamete donation and the role of donors is implicitly held by many who favor the use of gametes from known donors. On this second conception, gamete donation involves the bestowal of a gift from the body by one individual to another. Certain gifts are given in response to basic human needs of others. This is true of donations of tissue, blood, and organs; these are life-giving gifts that enable human persons to function as such. The provision of a gamete is also a life-giving gift that responds to the human needs of others. Yet it is life-giving in a distinctive sense, for it does not keep others alive, but facilitates their ability to create life.

Because gamete donation is a beneficent act performed by donors to enhance the good of recipients in this unique way, it establishes a special moral relation between them. This relation is more enduring in its impact on the participants than that between tissue, blood, or organ donors and recipients due to the nature of the gift involved. The child born of the gift does not become absorbed into the very being of the recipient, but remains a distinct individual with needs and interests of his or her own. Because of this, the act of gamete donation entails certain long-range obligations on the part of both recipients and donors. This alternate view captures more adequately and fully the nuances of meaning involved in gamete donation.

OBLIGATIONS OF GAMETE
DONORS AND RECIPIENTS

The moral relation between recipients and donors on this second view can be understood in closer detail within the moral framework governing gift giving.[38] The gift of a gamete creates a web of obligations that extends between recipients and donors and from them both to the resulting children. These obligations continue beyond the discrete point in time at which the gamete is given. A major obligation incurred by those who receive gifts is to express gratitude.[39] The gift of a gamete represents an especially significant and symbolic offering, in that it involves the provision of a life-*giving* gift of the body, the very means whereby the recipient can bring a child into existence. Consequently, it creates a special debt of gratitude in recipients. Although some gamete recipients may attempt to repay this debt by financially compensating donors for their time, risk, and inconvenience, this does not completely cancel their debt. This is especially true of oocyte donors because they must undergo a degree of bodily invasion and risk that sperm donors need not. The special nature of this gift—assistance in bringing a child into being—obliges recipients to express their gratitude by viewing donors as more than anonymous surds. It obliges recipients to view them as actual, characterizable, morally considerable persons who are deserving of respect and appreciation. Donors are individuals whose needs, interests, and rights ought to be taken into account in the process of gamete donation.

Givers also incur a moral obligation when they provide a gift—the obligation to give a complete gift, and not just part of one. The gift that gamete donors give includes their genetic material. To give a complete gift, donors must provide recipients, and ultimately the resulting children, with relevant information that may be carried in this genetic material. The sperm donor with a family history of heart disease has an obligation to provide this information to recipients, particularly if they have a male child. The oocyte donor whose mother and aunt had breast cancer should provide this information to recipients who have a female child. The donor who fails to give accurate information about his or her medical history bears direct moral responsibility for any relevant illnesses and disabilities that the resulting child suffers. Moreover, donors have an obligation to update the medical histories they provide to donors and recipients periodically to make them aware of any medical disorder that surfaces subsequent to donation.

AN ALTERNATE VIEW OF
GAMETE DONORS' OBLIGATIONS

Some argue that the duties of gamete donors go far beyond merely providing medical information. Callahan maintains that sperm donors are more than contributors of sperm that enable others to have children. As the biological fathers of the children who result from their donation, they have permanent and nondispensable duties toward them. Callahan claims:

> A sperm donor whose sperm is successfully used to fertilize an ovum, which ovum proceeds through the usual phases of gestation, is a *father*. Nothing more, nothing less. He is as much a father biologically as the known sperm inseminator in a standard heterosexual relationship and sexual intercourse.[40]

Because of the causal connection between their act of donation and the birth of these children, according to Callahan, gamete donors have full-fledged parental obligations toward the children born of their donation. One is responsible for what one causes. Donors cannot simply drop their sperm—or eggs—and leave.

It is incorrect, however, to assert that sperm donors cause the birth of their biological children. Although sexual intercourse and sperm donation may both result in the birth of a child who is biologically related to the source of the sperm, the causal pathway and persons bringing about the pregnancy in each case are different. The man who impregnates a woman by means of sexual intercourse is the cause of that pregnancy in that he directly injects his sperm into the woman's uterus. The act of the man is sufficient, and no intervening acts by others are necessary. The act of the sperm donor, however, is different. He does not directly introduce his sperm into the recipient's uterus. Instead, he provides it to others who must carry out many additional tasks before the sperm reaches the uterus—if it does. A set of intervening acts must take place before the donor's sperm can be used to assist in bringing about a pregnancy. The same is true of the oocyte donor. Her act of donation provides one necessary condition for the pregnancy, but does not constitute its sufficient condition. On Callahan's own axiom, since the donor does not cause the resulting child, he or she is not morally obligated to assume the full-fledged duties of parenthood.

Even if it were the case that gamete donors did cause the pregnancies that resulted from use of their gametes, this would not indicate that they were morally responsible for the care of the resulting children. We are not morally responsible for everything that we voluntarily cause. The person who causes an electric shock to his host when he turns on an electrical appliance in his host's home does not bear moral responsibility for that shock. The host does, as he is the person liable for keeping his home in good repair. It is true that, in distinction to the guest, who is not aware of the defect in the appliance, the gamete donor knows that his or her gamete will be used in an attempt to conceive a child. However, the donor's knowledge does not in itself make him or her morally responsible for the care of that child. We know that we cause sadness to those over whom we win an election, and yet we are not morally responsible for assuaging their feelings. We know that we may cause others to go without milk for a time when we purchase the last remaining container on the shelf, but we are not morally responsible for providing them with milk. Knowledge that one will cause an occurrence does not, in itself, render one morally responsible for all that results from it.

THE MORAL SIGNIFICANCE
OF BIOLOGICAL CONNECTEDNESS

Yet Callahan's underlying point that the biological relation between gamete donor and child has social and moral significance echoes a theme underlying the major arguments both for and against gamete donor anonymity. The primary argument for anonymity, that it is necessary to counter the social stigma that participants in gamete donation face because they sunder the biological connection between parent and child, recognizes the significance of the biological relation. The major argument for openness about the identity of gamete donors, that children born of gamete donation have a right to know the truth about their biological origins, also acknowledges the importance of the biological relation.

Why is the biological relation so important to parenthood? The family is composed of persons linked by a set of enduring relationships of which the most significant are affected by the birth process. We view ourselves as persons with a relation to previous generations of our family, with a connection to contemporary biologically linked relatives, and with expectations of relating to and contributing to future generations of our kin. The birth of a child has implications for a wider family group than the parents. Appropriate behavior of family members is defined by certain roles, such as mother and father, that are largely based on biological links, on connections through birth. While we may point to adoption as an indication that biological ties are not essential to parenthood, we must also note that adoptive parents acquire parental status only after the biological parents have given up their rights to the child. The biological role is recognized as important to parenthood even in adoption.

While the biological connection is of great significance to parenthood, however, it is not essential. We see this not only in the case of adoptive parents, but with stepparents, foster parents, and guardians. In such situations, when both the biological and the rearing relation between parent and child cannot be retained because of the contingencies of life, we give the rearing relation priority out of concern for the predominant interests of the child. While it is ordinarily in the interests of the child to be raised by biologically related parents, the cluster of other major interests of the child, such as those in basic nourishment and freedom from physical abuse, can predominate over this interest and outweigh it when they come into conflict. Although we accept the severance of the relation between the biological and the rearing parents in such instances, we do so reluctantly and out of necessity.

When gamete donation is used, however, we do not face a given situation in which children already exist and there is question about whether to retain their relation with their biological parents. Instead, we deliberately set out to bring children into the world who will not be raised by parents who both have some biological connection to them. While this can also be justified as a matter of necessity arising out of the contingencies of life for those who are infertile, the biological relation between children and gamete donors remains important in such circumstances.

Children born of gamete donation enter a situation in which they will lack something of significance in forming and sustaining their very selves. Our conception of who we are as individuals takes into account the hereditary links antecedent to and consequent on our birth. We define ourselves, in part, in terms of certain core characteristics that we share with our biological relatives. Nelson maintains that " . . . there really is an important kind of vulnerability to which children are exposed here, residing not in some brutely biological call of blood, but rather in the structures of meaning through which we try to make sense of our lives."[41] Part of what gives meaning and cohesiveness to our lives and helps us to feel recognized as individuals is our biological connectedness to others in our families.

THE MORAL SIGNIFICANCE OF BIOLOGICAL CONNECTEDNESS FOR DONORS

Gamete donation raises the possibility that not only the children born of it will face a loss of meaning and cohesiveness in their lives, but that donors will as well. Donors lose a connection with biological children who would have had a place within their structure of kinship relations and who still may have some significance for their own sense of selfhood. Gamete donors are beginning to recognize this. Recent emphasis on gaining their informed consent for donation has given many donors an opportunity to reflect upon the meaning of their participation in the procedure. As a result, some express interest in the children resulting from their gametes and concern about their obligations toward them. They reveal that they are not as eager to avoid contact with these children as has been assumed by proponents of donor anonymity. They appear to have a conception of themselves as givers of a gift with long-range consequences for which they are partially responsible.

In one study, for instance, younger sperm donors and those who had donated for adventuresome reasons often indicated that they had not adequately understood that they might have biologically fathered children whom they would never see or know.[42] Eighty-two percent of sperm donors in another study observed that they thought about their offspring and worried about their welfare.[43] In yet another study, 90% of sperm donors were willing to provide detailed information about their medical, social, educational, and personal histories in nonidentifying form to recipient families.[44] Almost three-fourths of these donors left a personal message to be given to any child born of their gametes.

Oocyte donors also express an interest in the recipients of their eggs and concern about the children born of their gametes. In one study, oocyte donors wanted to know whether a pregnancy had occurred as a result of their donation and wished to have some contact with the recipient couple after their donation.[45] In another study, 85% of volunteer egg donors indicated they would have liked to have known the outcome of the donation and over half were willing to have any child born of their oocyte contact them at maturity.[46] Over 80% of these donors had no objection to telling the recipients their names. In a study of 234 couples undergoing IVF, half said they would donate oocytes even if their names were made available to recipients.[47]

These responses indicate that a central reality of gamete donation is that donors feel it involves the provision of a gift in which they have a personal and altruistic stake. The biological connection between donors and the children born of their gametes creates ties between them that cannot be entirely erased by the presumption in favor of donor anonymity.

THE MORAL SIGNIFICANCE OF THE REARING RELATION

Yet families are meant to be places of privacy and intimacy from which third parties are excluded. They are set apart as places in which members foster close personal relationships whose nourishment requires that others keep a distance. The privacy argument for donor anonymity rightly emphasizes the need to insulate the family from intrusion by those outside it. Our legal tradition recognizes the importance of the family circle and its need to make decisions about personal matters according to its values and preferences with minimal intrusion by the state. How, then, should the recipient family and donor relate? How can recipients and donors meet their obligations to one another and to the children who result from gamete donation without violating family privacy?

Gamete recipients assume complete responsibility for the children born of gametes that have been donated to them. As part of this responsibility, they must ensure that the family in which they raise their children retains its domestic integrity. Although it is important to the development and identity of children to know about their biological origins, it is also necessary for their growth and sense of self that they form an integral part of their rearing family. Goldstein, Freud, and Solnit have argued that it is necessary to children's self-identity and emotional balance that they be brought up by a stable family grouping on a long-term basis—even if this is not their biological family.[48] Continuity of relationships, surroundings, and environmental influences are important to the physical, emotional, intellectual, social, and moral growth of children. Should their biological parents reappear after a long period of separation during which they have been raised by others, these psychologists claim, it would generally be detrimental to the well-being of these children to be given to their biological parents. We need not embrace the view of Goldstein et al. in its entirety to acknowledge that the family setting in which children are raised plays an important role in their development and view of who they are. When we are forced to choose which is more significant for the personal and social identity of children, however—the biological relation or the rearing relation—we must choose the rearing relation because of the overriding significance of the nurturing relationship to the well-being and development of the child.

Consequently, when we must decide between respecting the interest of children in having a stable family grouping as they grow to maturity and their interest in knowing about their biological origins, we must give greater weight to the former. If a choice must be made, it is more important for developing children to have continuity in the set of people who rear them than to have accurate information about their origins. This means that given the need to maintain family privacy, the choice whether and when to reveal the identity of gamete donors to these children should rest with the rearing parents. This decision is a profound moral one that should be made within a given family, rather than as a matter of public policy.[49]

Some gamete recipients may judge that their family is strong enough to be able to acknowledge the identity of the gamete donor while their child is still young. Indeed, some may wish to make the donor part of their extended family, as a sort of uncle or godmother. Others may wish to keep information about the donor hidden from their developing children, not just for their own ends, as Warnock suggests above, but for the sake of those children. They may be convinced that the social arrangement that can best ensure the optimal nurturing of children is the two-parent nuclear family, not a three-parent or extended family. Consequently, they may view the donor as a unique individual with rights and needs, and yet believe that they must put the interests of their young children, as they perceive these, above those of the donor. In such cases, this entails keeping the identity of the donor anonymous.

The question of what parents owe their children will have special poignancy for gamete donors who wish to know the children born of their gamete but cannot. Even though they have some degree of parental responsibility for the outcome of their gift, a living child, they may recognize that fulfilling this responsibility means allowing that child to develop without knowing who they are. Donors have an obligation to give a complete gift, and not just part of one. In circumstances where recipient parents judge it best for the child not to know the donor, giving a complete gift may involve remaining anonymous.

"MATCHING" RECIPIENTS AND DONORS

The situation changes, however, when the child reaches the age of maturity. The family will have played its essential role in the child's personal and social development, and the basic reason for keeping the donor in the background — to protect the integrity of the family — will have evaporated. Moreover, by this point in time most recipient families will be strong enough to address problems that might be created if the child wants to know the identity of the gamete donor. Recipients who have acknowledged to themselves that the donor is a real, characterizable person who stands in a special relation to their child because of his or her biological connection, will be prepared to accept the possibility that the donor may wish to know the child and that the child may wish to know the donor.

The relation between donors and recipients, consequently, should be structured so that at the time of donation, both donors and recipients choose whether they want to receive identifying or nonidentifying information about each other. Donors and recipients would be "matched," in part, on the basis of the degree of information about the donor and the recipient to be revealed to each other. Recipients have an interest in being given at least nonidentifying medical, personal, and social information about donors for the sake of the child born of gamete donation. Those who believe that their family would thrive were the donor's identity known would be paired with a donor willing to give identifying information. Donors also have an interest in having at least nonidentifying basic personal and social information about those who receive their gift and raise the child born of their gamete. Their interest derives from their biological relation with the child, which, as discussed above, can be important to their sense of selfhood and to the meaning and cohesiveness of their lives. The well-being of the child will be ineradicably affected by the family in which he or she is nurtured, and donors may therefore wish to know something about that family. This arrangement allows donors to fulfill their obligation to gamete recipients and the resulting children to provide relevant information that may be carried in their gamete about their medical history, and it allows gamete recipients to honor their debt of gratitude to donors. Finally, donors, at the time of donation, should be given the opportunity to choose whether they wish to reveal their identity to the child born of their gamete when that child reaches the age of 18. Some who choose to remain anonymous while the child is young may wish to be known by the mature child.

A nationwide registry should be developed with relevant information about gamete donors in which those who are willing to be identified at the time of donation are entered by name and those who wish to remain anonymous are given a code name or number. Statutory provisions should be enacted concomitant with the initiation of the registry stating that children born of gamete donation and the gestating women are prohibited from bringing paternity or maternity claims against gamete donors. Information about donors in this registry should be periodically updated and made available to the rearing parents during the children's developing years. When children born of gamete donation reach age 18, they should be given the opportunity to learn whatever is known about the donor that is listed in the registry if they have not already been told.

CONCLUSION

We are moving toward greater openness about the identity of gamete donors, as developments in sperm donation illustrate. Oocyte donation appears to be moving along a parallel path, albeit somewhat belatedly. It seems likely that the wall of separation between gamete donors and recipients will be torn down in the future and that they will engage in an exchange of important information that will allow children born of oocyte or sperm donation to develop a full identity while maintaining adequate boundaries. It would be preferable ethically if nonanonymous gamete donation were accepted, as the present cloak of secrecy inhibits free discussion and falsifies relationships.[50] Moreover, it distorts the very meaning of gamete donation as a unique gift with an enduring impact that creates a distinctive web of obligations on the part of donors and recipients. Until there is greater acceptance of openness about gamete donation, donors will have to recognize that giving a complete gift of a gamete in some circumstances may oblige them to remain anonymous, to be known, if ever, when their biological child reaches the age of majority.

NOTES

1. U.S. Congress, Office of Technology Assessment, *Infertility: Medical and Social Choices*, OTA-BA-358 (Washington, DC: U.S. Government Printing Office, 1988), p. 36.

2. David J. Handelsman, Steward M. Dunn, Ann J. Conway, Lyn M. Boylan, and Robert P. S. Jansen, "Psychological and Attitudinal Profiles in Donors for Artificial Insemination," *Fertility and Sterility* 43 (1983): 95–101; Mark V. Sauer, Ingrid A. Rodi, Michelle Scrooc, Maria Bustillo, and John E. Buster, "Survey of Attitudes Regarding the Use of Siblings for Gamete Donation," *Fertility and Sterility* 49 (1988): 721–22; Ken R. Daniels, "Artificial Insemination Using Donor Semen and the Issue of Secrecy: The Views of Donors and Recipient Couples," *Social Science and Medicine* 27 (1988): 377–83; Mark V. Sauer, M. J. Gorrill, K. B. Zeffer, and Maria Bustillo, "Attitudinal Survey of Sperm Donors to an Artificial Insemination Clinic," *Journal of Reproductive Medicine* 34 (1989): 362–64; Ken R. Daniels and Karyn Taylor, "Secrecy and Openness in Donor Insemination," *Politics and the Life Sciences*, 1993 (12): 155–70; Robert D. Nachtigall, "Secrecy: An Unresolved Issue in the Practice of Donor Insemination," *American Journal of Obstetrics and Gynecology* 168 (1993): 1846–51.

3. P. Lutjen, A. Trounson, J. Leeton, C. Wood, P. Renou, "The Establishment and Maintenance of Pregnancy Using In Vitro Fertilization and Embryo Donation in a Patient with Primary Ovarian Failure," *Nature* 307 (1984): 174.

4. Sauer, "Survey of Attitudes," pp. 721–22; Mary Warnock, *A Question of Life: The Warnock Report on Human Fertilisation and Embryology* (New York: Basil Blackwell, 1985), p. 37.

5. Ethics Committee of the American Fertility Society, "Ethical Considerations of

the New Reproductive Technologies," *Fertility and Sterility*, 53, Supplement 2 (1990): 5S; Warnock, *A Question of Life*, p. 37.

6. Andrea M. Braverman and the Ovum Donor Task Force of the Psychological Special Interests Group of the American Fertility Society, "Survey Results on the Current Practice of Ovum Donation," *Fertility and Sterility* 59 (1993): 1216–20; American Fertility Society, "Guidelines," 1S-9S.

7. Patricia P. Mahlstedt and Dorothy A. Greenfeld, "Assisted Reproductive Technology with Donor Gametes: The Need for Patient Preparation," *Fertility and Sterility* 52 (1989): 908–14.

8. Daniels, "Secrecy and Openness," p. 156; R. Snowden, G. D. Mitchell, E. M. Snowden, *Artificial Reproduction: A Social Investigation* (London: George Allen and Unwin, 1983), pp. 125–43; Robyn Rowland, "The Social and Psychological Consequences of Secrecy in Artificial Insemination by Donor (AID) Programmes," *Social Science and Medicine*, 21 (1985): 391–96.

9. Patricia P. Mahlstedt and Kris A. Probasco, "Sperm Donors: Their Attitudes toward Providing Medical and Psychological Information for Recipient Couples and Donor Offspring," *Fertility and Sterility* 56 (1991): 747–53.

10. Rona Achilles, "Donor Insemination: The Future of a Public Secret," in *The Future of Human Reproduction*, ed. Christine Overall (Toronto: Women's Press, 1989), pp. 105–19; Kurt W. Back and Robert Snowden, "The Anonymity of the Gamete Donor," *Journal of Psychosomatic Obstetrics and Gynaecology* 9 (1988): 191–98.

11. Jonathan Glover, *Ethics of New Reproductive Technologies: The Glover Report to the European Commission* (De Kalb: Northern Illinois University Press, 1989), p. 36; Erica Haimes, "Recreating the Family? Policy Considerations Relating to the 'New' Reproductive Technologies," in *The New Reproductive Technologies*, ed. M. McNeil, I. Varcoe, S. Yearley (New York: St. Martin's Press, 1990); Back and Snowden, p. 197.

12. Daniels, "Secrecy and Openness," p. 159; Rowland, "The Social and Psychological Consequences of Secrecy," p. 392.

13. W. H. Cary, "Results of Artificial Insemination with an Extra-Marital Specimen (Semi-Adoption)," *American Journal of Obstetrics and Gynecology* 56 (1948): 727–32.

14. Mahlstedt and Probasco, "Sperm Donors," pp. 752–53; B. Z. Sokoloff, "Alternative Methods of Reproduction: Effects on the Child," *Clinical Pediatrics* 26 (1987): 11–17.

15. Mark V. Sauer and Richard J. Paulson, "Human Oocyte and Preembryo Donation: An Evolving Method for the Treatment of Infertility," *American Journal of Obstetrics and Gynecology* 163 (1990): 1421–24.

16. Society for Assisted Reproductive Technology, "Assisted Reproductive Technology," p. 959.

17. G. Christie, "The Psychological and Social Management of the Infertile Couple," in R. Pepperrell et al., eds., *The Infertile Couple* (London: Churchill Livingston, 1980).

18. Nachtigall, "Secrecy," p. 1847; Achilles, "Donor Insemination," pp. 109–10.

19. Paul Lauritzen, *Pursuing Parenthood: Ethical Issues in Assisted Reproduction* (Bloomington: Indiana University Press, 1993), p. 85.

20. Snowden, Mitchell, Snowden, *Artificial Reproduction*, pp. 125–43.

21. Family Law Council, *Creating Children: A Uniform Approach to the Law and Practice of Reproductive Technology in Australia* (Canberra: Australian Government Publishing Service, 1985).

22. Daniels, "Secrecy and Openness," p. 157.

23. A. Raoul-Duval, H. Letur-Konirsch, R. Frydman, "Anonymous Oocyte Donation: A Psychological Study of Recipients, Donors and Children," *Human Reproduction* 7 (1992): 51–54.

24. Mahlstedt and Greenfeld, "Assisted Reproductive Technology with Donor Gametes," pp. 908–14.

25. Family Law Council, *Creating Children*, p. 7.

26. Mahlstedt and Greenfeld, "Assisted Reproductive Technology with Donor Gametes," pp. 908–14; Lauritzen, *Pursuing Parenthood*, pp. 86–88.

27. National Bioethics Consultative Committee, "Reproductive Technology: Final Report to Australian Health Ministers," August, 1989.

28. Mary Warnock, "The Good of the Child," *Bioethics* 1 (1987): 141–55.

29. Mahlstedt and Greenfeld, "Assisted Reproductive Technology with Donor Gametes," pp. 908–14.

30. Lauritzen, *Pursuing Parenthood*, p. 86.

31. Annette Baran and Reuben Pannor, *Lethal Secrets* (New York: Warner Books, 1989); Rowland, "The Social and Psychological Consequences of Secrecy," p. 395.

32. Daniels, "Secrecy and Openness in Donor Insemination," p. 159

33. Erica Haimes, "Gamete Donation and Anonymity," *Bulletin of Medical Ethics*, March 1991, pp. 25–27.

34. Nachtigall, "Secrecy," p. 1847; Baran and Pannor, *Lethal Secrets*, pp. 36–39.

35. R. D. Nachtigall, G. Becker, M. Wozny, "The Effects of Gender-Specific Diagnosis on Men's and Women's Response to Infertility," *Fertility and Sterility* 57 (1992): 113–21.

36. Thomas H. Murray, "On the Human Body as Property: The Meaning of Embodiment, Markets and the Meaning of Strangers," *Journal of Law Reform* 20 (1987): 1055–88.

37. Mahlstedt and Greenfeld, "Assisted Reproductive Technology with Donor Gametes," p. 911.

38. Marcel Mauss, *The Gift* (New York: W. W. Norton, 1967); Thomas H. Murray, "Gifts of the Body and the Needs of Strangers," *Hastings Center Report* 17 (1987): 30–38.

39. Paul F. Camenisch, "Gift and Gratitude in Ethics," *Journal of Religious Ethics* 9 (1981): 8–19.

40. Daniel Callahan, "Bioethics and Fatherhood," *Utah Law Review*, 1992 (1992): 735–746.

41. James Nelson, "Genetic Narratives: Biology, Stories, and the Definition of the Family," *Health Matrix* 2 (1992): 82.

42. Achilles, "Donor Insemination," pp. 112–13.

43. Ken R. Daniels, "Semen Donors: Their Motivations and Attitudes to Their Offspring," *Journal of Reproductive and Infant Psychology* 7 (1989): 121–27.

44. Mahlstedt and Probasco, p. 752.

45. L. R. Schover, R. L. Collins, M. M. Quigley, J. Blankenstein, and G. Kanoti, "Psychological Follow-Up of Women Evaluated as Oocyte Donors," *Human Reproduction* 6 (1991): 1497–91.

46. M. Power, R. Baber, H. Abdalla, A. Kirkland, T. Leonard, J. W. W. Studd, "A Comparison of the Attitudes of Volunteer Donors and Infertile Patient Donors on an Ovum Donation Programme," *Human Reproduction* 5 (1990): 352–55.

47. T. Oskarsson, E. S. Dimitry, M. S. Mills, J. Hunt, and R. M. Winston, "Attitudes toward Gamete Donation among Couples Undergoing *in vitro* Fertilization," *British Journal of Obstetrics and Gynecology* 98 (1991): 352–57.

48. Joseph Goldstein, Anna Freud, Albert J. Solnit, *Beyond the Best Interests of the Child* (New York: Free Press, 1973).

49. Ruth Macklin, "Artificial Means of Reproduction and Our Understanding of the Family," *Hastings Center Report*, 21 (1991): 10.

50. Allan Templeton, "Gamete Donation and Anonymity," *British Journal of Obstetrics and Gynaecology* 98 (1991): 343–45.

EIGHT

WHAT IS WRONG WITH COMMODIFICATION?

Ruth Macklin, Ph.D.

What, if anything, is wrong with paying money to egg donors? Some people see nothing wrong, from an ethical point of view; it has even been argued that it would be wrong *not* to pay women who choose to provide oocytes for infertile women. Others are hesitant to endorse such payments, yet stop short of ethical condemnation. Still others are more critical, arguing that paying women for eggs, like paying women to be surrogates, amounts to commodification of the human body and therefore demeans women and degrades that which is distinctively human.

Underlying these different positions are arguments that appeal to different considerations: comparisons with paying men to be sperm donors; worries about a slippery slope that begins with paying for eggs, slides to paying for embryos, and lands at the bottom with paying for babies; the question of fairness in compensating women who provide this service; and worries about damage to the fabric of society when bodily products or services are commercialized. Arguments on both sides of the issue are persuasive, making it difficult to arrive at a clear resolution of the problem. Also underlying the different positions are moral sentiments, against which it is hard to mount a rational argument.

My own conclusion is that commodification of human beings for any purpose is unsavory and ought to be avoided whenever possible. Yet "unsavoriness" is not a category of moral disvalue strong enough to warrant prohibition. If commodification does not involve a violation of a moral principle or the rights of any person or group, then it would be unwarranted to ban such commercial transactions. The account that follows explores the arguments surrounding the practice of paying egg donors, and ends by opting for the "least worst" resolution.

The well-established tradition of paying sperm donors (making them ven-dors, properly speaking, rather than donors) leads some to argue that women who donate their ova should similarly be compensated. Another long-stand-ing practice in the United States is that of commercial blood collection, which has been questioned in recent years more on grounds of the quality of the blood supply when paid donors are used than on the quite different premise that buying human body products is somehow wrong.

A great deal of criticism has been leveled at the practice of commercial surrogacy, wherein women are paid significant sums to bear a child for an infertile woman or couple. A number of states have enacted legislation pro-hibiting commercial surrogacy and assigning criminal penalties to brokers.[1] Although payment to surrogates has been charged with being a form of "baby selling" and therefore against public policy, defenders—and even some crit-ics—of commercial surrogacy deny that baby selling is a proper charac-terization. Paid surrogacy has been justified on the grounds that the money is for the surrogates' "time and inconvenience," not for the baby she eventually delivers and hands over. Payment for "time and inconvenience" is the same justification used for compensating normal, healthy volunteers to serve as subjects of biomedical or behavioral research. It is also the phrase that has been adopted to describe what ovum donors are being paid for.

The practice of surrogacy poses an array of ethical problems that go well beyond the issue of payment. For that reason, assisted reproduction using eggs from a third party is much more analogous to the use of donor sperm than it is to surrogacy. It is sufficient to note here that as a matter of public policy, it would not be inconsistent to argue that commercial surrogacy ought to be prohibited but that commerce in gametes ought to be permitted.

WHAT ARE DONORS PAID FOR, AND DOES IT MATTER?

A presumption appears throughout the literature that although it would be wrong to pay donors for their eggs, it is ethically permissible, if not required, to compensate them for the time they spend, the risks they undergo, and the inconvenience they experience. However, nowhere is an explanation offered for why payment for eggs is ethically suspect but monetary compensation for these other things is not.

An ethical advisory committee report issued by the American Fertility Society (AFS) in 1990 stated that "there should be no compensation to the donor for the egg."[2] The sentence that followed asserted that "This does not exclude reimbursement for expenses, time, risk and associated inconve-nience." The revised 1993 guidelines from AFS state that "Donors should be compensated for direct and indirect expenses associated with their participa-tion, inconvenience, time, risk and discomfort."[3] The implication of the wording is that it is at least suspect, if not ethically wrong, to pay women for their eggs. But it is not made clear just what is ethically problematic.

How can we tell if a woman is being paid for her eggs (and is thus a vendor) or for her inconvenience, time, risk, and discomfort? An interview with a woman who was an egg donor at an Austrian IVF clinic is revealing. The interviewers asked: "How much did you get paid per operation and how does the financial transaction take place?" The woman replied: "After the procedure I get os 10,000 (U.S. $800) no matter how many eggs they take out. If there are no matured eggs or they miss the ovulation I get no money except expenses like tramfare. But this has not happened to me so far. The doctors pay for the product 'egg.' "[4] In contrast, if a woman were paid the same amount of money whether or not any eggs are harvested, it would be reasonable to conclude that she is being paid for her time, inconvenience, and so on.

A report of the combined ethics committee of the Canadian Fertility and Andrology Society and the Society of Obstetricians and Gynaecologists of Canada includes the following recommendation: "The Societies endorse the payment of gamete donors to reimburse them in a reasonable fashion for the costs and inconvenience of donation and any screening procedures which are essential to the safe operation of donor gamete programs."[5] The combined ethics committee considered two other options. The first option was to permit no payment. The committee rejected this on grounds that it would likely result in shortages of donated gametes.

The second option was to permit unrestricted payment. This option was rejected on the grounds that an excessive financial incentive might tempt some individuals to lie about their medical or genetic history or previous gamete donations they had made.[6] The committee's refusal to allow unrestricted payment was not based on the ethical consideration of protecting *donors* from exploitation that might result from coercive offers of money. Instead, the ethical justification rested on the "harm principle," that is, protection of gamete *recipients* who might be harmed as a result of transmission of infection or genetic disease.

The combined committee's reasoning makes clear why they rejected the two extreme options—permitting no payment to donors or permitting unrestricted payment. Yet the recommendation the committee did adopt is silent on the matter of paying for the eggs. The recommendation is phrased in terms of reimbursement to donors: "to reimburse them in a reasonable fashion for the costs and inconvenience of donation." This wording carefully avoids any implication that donors are being paid for the eggs.

Apparently uncomfortable with the commercial aspect, Sherman Elias and George Annas contend that "the Warnock and Waller Commissions may well be on the right track in discouraging commerce in gametes and in limiting payment to out-of-pocket and medical expenses."[7] Yet this recommendation is incomplete since it leaves open the question of how to characterize the egg donor's "time, inconvenience, and discomfort." Payment for medical expenses obviously does not cover these items. Payment for the woman's transportation, tolls, parking, and so on obviously does count as "out-of-pocket expenses." If the donor punches a time clock and loses hourly wages as a result of her participation in egg donation that, too, would count as "out-of-pocket expenses." So we are left with the category of "time (other than lost wages), risk, discomfort, and inconvenience."

Even John Robertson, a staunch defender of payment to egg donors, avoids language implying that it is perfectly permissible to pay directly for the eggs: "Many persons would find payment for the egg donor's time and effort morally unobjectionable and appropriate, if not also obligatory."[8] In this passage and elsewhere, Robertson states that it would be unfair not to pay donors, but he is silent on the question of whether payment for the eggs would somehow be wrong.

The implication in all of these accounts seems to be that payment to people for their services is ethically permissible but paying them for bodily products is not. Payment to women for time and effort sounds like paying people for their work, surely an ethically acceptable if not obligatory social practice. Paying for risk and discomfort is like compensating normal, healthy volunteers of biomedical or behavioral research, also a widely accepted practice. Paying for human eggs begins to sound suspiciously like payment to live kidney donors, a transaction that gives rise to strong repugnance in many people.

It is, however, hard to find a basis for claiming that payment for the risks, discomfort, and inconvenience a donor undergoes is ethically sound but payment for the product extracted as a result of the process is ethically wrong. The only reason for subjecting women to these risks, discomforts, and inconvenience is to obtain the eggs. Perhaps it is the idea that paying for ova makes them into a commodity and that is somehow wrong. But it could equally well be maintained that payment for bodily services is also a form of "commodification." If there is something suspect about commodifying human reproductive products, it is similarly suspect to commodify human reproductive services.

GENDER PARITY:
PAYMENT FOR SPERM AND EGGS

One argument in favor of paying ovum donors contends that a woman's eggs should be treated just like a man's sperm. Since there is a long tradition of paying men for sperm donations, why not pay women to be egg donors? Both male and female gametes that are donated are not needed by their owners. Sperm are continuously produced in men, and although women are born with their entire supply of eggs, that supply contains many more than a woman will ever need in her reproductive lifetime. It has been stated that paying sperm donors but not egg donors would unfairly discriminate against women, who undergo greater risk in order to donate eggs.[9]

Others suggest that perhaps it is time to rethink the sale of sperm. For example, the Glover Report to the European Commission[10] offers several arguments against the established practice of paying semen donors. The report notes that "as with blood donation, payment may lead unsuitable people to apply, lying about their medical history (perhaps one of AIDS) in order to be paid."[11] The reply to this objection in regard to semen donation has already occurred in the United States in the regulations governing licensed sperm banks. All semen donors are tested for HIV at the time of the donation, the sample is stored, and the donors retested after six months to ensure that they have not seroconverted in the interim. Since it is not (yet) possible to store frozen ova, egg donors can be tested only initially, leaving open the possibility that "unsuitable" people may choose to donate for the money.

There are other differences between sperm and egg donation, however, not in the nature of the products (both are human gametes) but in the nature of the process that yields the products. Sperm donors may undergo some inconvenience, but it could hardly be maintained that they are submitting themselves to considerable discomforts or undertaking substantial risks. The question whether sperm donors are paid for their sperm or compensated for their time and inconvenience seems never to have been addressed. The presumption seems to be that they are paid for the "product," but worries about commodification have not traditionally been expressed.

In contrast to sperm donors, women who become egg donors undergo a minor surgical procedure. Also, they take hormones prior to extraction of their eggs in order to make the eggs suitable for fertilization and subsequent implantation in the recipient. This difference between sperm and ovum donors in the level of risk, discomfort, and inconvenience has prompted some people to claim that women should not only be paid for their eggs, as men are for sperm, but that the increased risk and discomfort to these women justifies paying them a lot more. In a conversation in which the sum of $2,000 paid to egg donors was cited, a leading researcher in techniques of assisted reproduction remarked that these women ought to be paid even more than that, considering all that they undergo.[12]

In one key respect, sperm and eggs are similar to one another and different from other bodily products. Gametes are human bodily materials from which other humans can be created. Whether this fact confers some distinct moral status on human gametes is unclear. It is surely true that people may care more about what happens to their donated gametes than to their donated blood. Yet the claim that their status as gametes makes it unethical to sell sperm or ova but permissible to donate them is puzzling without further argument.

EXPLOITATION OF WOMEN

The charge of "exploitation of women" has been leveled against paid surrogacy and payments for ovum donation. Since exploitation of human beings is, at least on one conception, a serious ethical wrong in violation of the Kantian imperative "never to treat persons merely as a means,"[13] it is important to determine whether paying egg donors can properly be charged with being a form of exploitation. This concern relates more to the amount of payment than to the simple fact of payment. The more money donors receive, the more it may become a coercive offer, one that is exploitive. If women were paid a nickel for their eggs, that could hardly be considered exploitation on the grounds that they are being paid *too much*, though it might be exploitive in paying *too little*. After all, when laborers are underpaid by their employers the latter are accused of exploiting the workers. This curious twist has occurred in the debates over paid surrogacy. It has been argued that the standard $10,000 fee paid to a surrogate is too *low*, that it is exploitive precisely because it is not a fair wage for services rendered. As an hourly wage, it comes to about $1.49 per hour. Whether egg donors are properly to be construed as "laborers" is one of the questions raised by the commodification argument.

Money is offered to men and women in order to induce them to be gamete donors. It can be assumed that without payment, the source of gametes from anonymous donors would dry up. The acceptability of this practice rests on the view that an inducement is ethically acceptable but an "undue" inducement is not. Whenever greater sums of money are involved, an undue inducement becomes elevated into a coercive offer. It can then be questioned whether the action is fully voluntary. Since voluntariness is a necessary condition for the ethical acceptability of a biomedical intervention such as egg retrieval, the more the voluntariness of the donor's decision can be questioned, the more ethically worrisome is the practice.

Here the contrast between the amount paid to sperm and egg donors is instructive. Intuitively, no one is likely to contend that $25 or $50 (the usual range) or even $100 paid to sperm donors is a coercive offer or undue inducement. That is partly because of the relatively low amount of money; and also because the donor is not being induced to engage in a form of behavior he might not do anyway. In contrast, $2,000 is a significant sum for students or for poor or lower-class women; and they are surely being induced to undergo something they would not otherwise be doing. This argument does not conclude that payment to donors is unethical, but simply that the amount to be paid is the important factor.

How can we determine when payment to egg donors is exploitive? John Harris identifies three issues: "The first involves the question of whether it is morally objectionable to use others as a means to our own ends, the second asks whether paying them for being such a means constitutes exploitation, and the third is of course whether in all the circumstances, exploitation is such a bad thing."[14] Harris argues persuasively that it is not wrong to use others as a means to one's own ends when those others have autonomously accepted that project as their own and have not been coerced in some way into becoming instruments.[15] Presumably, this reflects the Kantian notion that people must not be treated as a means *merely*. One may treat others as a means to one's own ends just so long as others' ends are also served in the process.

Harris proposes the following definition of exploitation: "Exploitation occurs when those exploited have not autonomously adopted their part in our projects as one of their own projects but have been coerced in some way into becoming instruments of ours."[16] It does not follow from this that whenever financial interests are involved, the situation is then exploitive. The key ingredient in this conception of exploitation seems to be that of coercive pressure, or absence of genuine autonomy, rather than the fact of remuneration.

An antipaternalist line of argument leaves the decision whether to bear pain or undergo inconvenience in exchange for money up to the individual who is most affected, rather than seeking to regulate the practice by prohibiting or setting upper limits on payments. John Hoff[17] contends that people constantly make judgments balancing pain/inconvenience and money. The coal miner undertakes filth and danger for money; the nightshift employee receives a bonus. If the donor chooses to undertake the procedure despite the pain, is that coercion or the satisfaction of a need in a manner acceptable to the donor? Indeed, Hoff maintains, it could be argued there is more "coercion" where the donor gives eggs to a relative out of "guilt" rather than for money. The former donation does not benefit the donor, other than alleviation of guilt; the latter does.

All this is true enough. But it leads us to consider just which actions and transactions can reasonably be regulated and which cannot. No one would really want to regulate intrafamilial goings on, whereas providing professional guidelines or state health department regulations for acceptable limits that infertility programs may pay to egg donors would not interfere in any way with family privacy.

The exploitation line of argument takes a more specific form in relation to wealthier individuals or couples paying money to poorer women for use of their bodies. Here the argument does not focus on women generally, but rather on women of lower socioeconomic status. Taking an antipaternalist stance, John Hoff says it seems somewhat "matronizing" to deny poor people the opportunity to earn money by giving up "excess" body tissue (provided they are informed of the risk). Every service in our economy is sold: academics sell their minds; athletes sell the use of their bodies. The best art in the world is the subject of commodification. If a pretty actress can sell her body for television, why should a fecund woman be denied the ability to sell her eggs? Why is one more demeaning than the other? If anything, why is not the sale of eggs, which has a more socially useful purpose, a more appropriate transaction. Surely, Hoff asserts, we are beyond the point where the sale of a service by itself taints the service.

As a factual matter, it has been questioned whether paid egg donors do or are likely to come from the poorer socioeconomic class. John Robertson observes that "the recipient's desire to receive good genes will place a premium on women who are healthy and appear to be of good stock. Donors— even repeat donors—are as likely to be middle as well as lower class women."[18] In addition, Robertson questions whether it follows that because donors are poorer than recipients, the arrangement therefore amounts to exploitation: "neither the risks nor the payments are so great that an unacceptable exploitation of poorer persons would occur."[19]

All things considered, it is implausible to conclude that paying egg donors is exploitive. The facts surrounding the socioeconomic status of ovum donors show that they do not come from the poorest class of society. And there is nothing to suggest that these women are coerced, or do not autonomously choose to become donors. This is one way, among many others, of making money. Even if receiving compensation is the primary motive for choosing to become a donor, that does not imply that the women are being exploited.

ETHICAL PRINCIPLES AND PAYING DONORS

An ethical analysis of any action or social practice is incomplete if it fails to address the question whether an ethical principle is violated. So, how about the practice of paying egg donors? The answer is not immediately evident because, as in almost all situations in which actions or practices are evaluated by appealing to ethical principles, the principles themselves must first be subjected to analysis and interpretation. The two leading principles of bioethics that are relevant in this context are respect for persons and justice.

Whether paying egg donors violates the principle of respect for persons depends on whether the principle is interpreted narrowly or broadly. According to the narrow interpretation, if the subject of a biomedical intervention grants voluntary, informed consent to the procedure, the person is respected and the principle is not violated. Since prospective egg donors are fully informed (we may assume, or at least hope) of the purpose, procedures to be performed, the time involved, the risks, and the benefits, paying the donors does not violate the principle. Along the same lines, paying donors is not a violation of individuals' right to liberty or privacy if we assume that there are no coercive practices involved in commercial egg donation. Here again, there is no failure to respect persons. The principle of respect for persons would be violated if paying egg donors constitutes a form of exploitation. However, as John Harris argues convincingly, it is not plausible to say that women who autonomously agree to donate their eggs for a sum of money are being exploited in virtue of the payment.

Nevertheless, a broader interpretation of respect for persons might yield a different conclusion. This interpretation looks to the value that underlies and justifies the principle: the notion that human beings as such are uniquely valuable. This broader principle requires special respect not only for the informed choices of individuals, but for that which is human.[20] It appears, then, that whether respect for persons is violated depends on whether the principle is given a narrow or a broad interpretation.

The same might be said for the principle of justice. In one respect, paying egg donors does not violate a principle of justice, since there appears to be no inequitable treatment of one group as opposed to another. Poorer women are paid for their eggs just like middle-class or wealthier women. If poorer and better-off women are paid the same amount for being donors, that seems fair since they are undergoing the same procedure and are thus subjected to the same risks, discomforts, and inconveniences. If payment is to be made as actual compensation for lost wages, working women who earn more would presumably get more money for the time they put in as donors than would women who earn less. That arrangement could be considered unjust because it violates the principle of "equal pay for equal work." To become clear about what is just in this realm seems to require a decision about precisely what women are being paid for: "the product egg"; risks, discomfort, and inconvenience; or what their time is worth on the labor market.

A different consideration of justice points to the fact that the pattern of commercial programs is one of better-off women as recipients and less-well-off women as donors, a pattern that results from the high cost of IVF and embryo implantation. That cost is beyond the reach of poorer women unless public funding for IVF becomes a matter of policy. According to this consideration, justice is violated because a wealthier class of women are the donors and a poorer class are the recipients. Here again, however, defenders of an interpretation of justice that allows the market to determine all transactions will view this class difference between donors and recipients as just another instance of the workings of the marketplace.

Appeals to ethical principles are thus quite complex, and argument employing them can cut both ways. Robertson observes that "objections to paying egg donors stem from a religious or moral view of human dignity that is not universally shared. . . . Indeed, refusing to pay donors for their efforts seems unfair and exploitative."[21] So, contrary to the view that it is exploitive for wealthier women to pay poorer women for their reproductive products or services, Robertson argues that it is exploitive *not* to do so. This is what is required in order "to treat donors fairly."[22]

COMMODIFICATION

If there is something wrong with paying money for bodily products or services, what is the nature of that wrong? One way of characterizing the wrong is *commodification* of the procreative process. The theory that there are some forms of exchange among human beings that should be prevented from being carried out for money has been put forth by a number of writers. For example, Michael Walzer has argued that some market exchanges should be blocked.[23] The fact that our society is capitalistic and is dominated by commercial transactions of all sorts does not compel the conclusion that therefore, anything whatsoever may be put up for sale. An illustration offered as uncontroversial is "the norm that citizens should be legally free to vote or not as they wish, but not to sell their votes or to vote a certain way for a price."[24] This general line of argument can be applied to the specific situation involving the sale of bodily parts and reproductive services.[25]

To quote an expression used by Leon Kass in discussing embryos produced by *in vitro* fertilization, the human body, its parts, and its reproductive products are not "mere meat."[26] Therefore, they should not be subject to the same market forces that govern the sale of pork bellies. Human organs are not like calves' livers or thymus glands, at least in the judgment of the U.S. Congress when it enacted a law prohibiting commercial procurement and distribution of organs for transplantation.[27]

Commercial traffic in frozen embryos would constitute another instance of unacceptable commodification, although it would surely be a mistake to characterize that as "baby-selling." Nevertheless, the line between selling babies and selling embryos is not sharp and distinct. Elias and Annas argue that "the problem with commerce in human embryos is that the sale of human embryos can become confused with the sale of human children. Accordingly, it seems reasonable to outlaw the sale of human embryos."[28] Laws have been enacted in Florida, Louisiana, and Massachusetts banning the sale of embryos. John Robertson contends that the terms of these laws would not cover the sale of unfertilized eggs.[29] Although Elias and Annas say that sale of sperm and ova does not present the same problem as the sale of human embryos, their remark quoted earlier suggests that they disapprove of commercial traffic in gametes.

Similarly, the Glover Report evinces a strong preference for a noncommercial ethos both for semen donation and for egg donation, but stops short of proposing a legal ban, "which would anyway probably be unenforceable."[30] The report urges strong public campaigns for altruistic donation, "bringing the plight of the infertile to the front of public attention."[31]

We are still left with the question whether paying egg donors constitutes an ethically suspect or unacceptable commercial traffic in human products. It is surely different from commercial traffic in organs, primarily because of the greater risks organ donors face from surgery and anesthesia as well as (in the case of kidney donors) their heightened risk of living with one rather than two kidneys. It is more like payment for blood, another bodily product, although blood donation requires less time and fewer risks and discomforts than egg retrieval.

Yet even the sale of blood, like other human bodily materials, is a form of commodification. The Glover Report offers arguments that weigh equally against payment to blood donors and to gamete donors. One is that payment is likely to incline donors to think less about the implications of what they are doing. A second is that payment "deprives donors of the chance of doing something purely for others."[32] Citing the remark of some blood donors that "paying for blood would debase the value of the act," the Glover Report observes that payment and nonpayment seem to lead to two different conceptions of donation.

The reasons the Glover Report gives for favoring a noncommercial approach to semen donation rest on values quite different from those of a market economy. The idea that gamete donors should think about the implications of what they are doing, and that altruism is a good thing, are sound premises in an argument that questions payment but are not likely to move those who see nothing amiss in making everything subject to market forces.

A point made by John Harris is illustrative in this connection: "In the case of gamete donation, if it is acceptable to make voluntary donations of such things, then the addition of a financial interest does not necessarily add anything to the *morality* of the practice."[33]

Although it seems correct to say that commodification does not violate any ethical principle, it can nevertheless be viewed as an unsavory feature of our society, a society in which almost everything is subject to market forces. Commodification is unsavory for the same sort of reason that public executions and public humiliation of criminals are unsavory. This is not an aesthetic judgment. It is a judgment about what kind of society we value.

THE FABRIC OF SOCIETY

Even if it can be convincingly argued that neither respect for persons nor justice is violated, it can still be maintained that the practice of paying for reproductive services is somehow demeaning or degrading to us as a society, that it ruptures the very fabric of society. Although the fabric of society is a hard concept to define, and although it is difficult to determine empirically just when the fabric is being torn and when it remains intact, it is a useful concept for thinking about what is undesirable about certain sorts of human interactions and societal practices. A practice in which women are paid to ingest hormones and to have their eggs extracted may not contravene an ethical principle or violate anyone's rights. Still, it reflects the extent to which our society is willing to accept the idea that if people are prepared to receive money to have their bodies invaded, it is just like any other commercial transaction.

Margaret Jane Radin provides an analysis in terms of our conception of personhood and human flourishing: "In our understanding of personhood we are committed to an ideal of individual uniqueness that does not cohere with the idea that each person's attributes are fungible, that they have a monetary equivalent, and that they can be traded off against those of other people."[34] Radin argues that if market rhetoric were adopted by everyone in many contexts, it would transform "the texture of the modern world."[35] That texture is another way of referring to the elusive concept of the fabric of society. Market rhetoric leads us to view "reproductive capacity as just a scarce good for which there is high demand." This way of talking and thinking fosters "an inferior conception of human flourishing." As an example of the "intuitive grasp of the injury to personhood involved in commodification of human beings," Radin cites baby selling and slavery. Her lengthy analysis of "market-inalienability" (not to be bought and sold on the market) and the wrongs involved in commodification of human beings cannot be replicated here, but it is sufficient to note that not everyone is likely to buy into her analysis.

Suppose one does not accept Radin's analysis and sees nothing wrong, in principle, with commodification. Is it acceptable to conclude, then, that the best public policy is simply to abandon any attempt to regulate the amount of money paid to egg donors? In that case, market forces would truly govern the practice, and clinics that perform the services would become truly competitive in this regard (if they are not already). Inevitably, this would raise the cost of the procedure to egg recipients, since the money to pay the donors will have to come from somewhere and it is unlikely to come out of the clinic's profit margin. Furthermore, we must recall the objection to unrestricted payment noted by the Canadian Combined Ethics Committee. The "harm principle" calls for protection of gamete recipients from transmission of infection or genetic disease by donors who are induced by excessive payments to lie about their medical or genetic history.

Those who argue for unrestricted payments to donors and letting the market govern egg donation have to face the question of consistency. Can an argument for prohibiting a commercial market in organs be consistent with an unregulated approach to commercial egg donation? Why not allow payment to kidney donors for their "risks, time, and inconvenience" and deny that payment is for the organ itself? If paying living persons for donation of one of their paired organs, or even for bone marrow, is ethically unacceptable but paying egg donors is ethically acceptable, wherein lies the difference?

One reply is that the difference lies in the degree of risk to the donor. The problem becomes one of drawing the line, with the need to specify where that line is and why it is appropriate to draw it there. If the reply is that blood and sperm are renewable resources, then we must contend with the fact that so, too, is bone marrow. Kidneys can certainly not be regenerated by the human body, but then neither can a woman's eggs. However, ova are plentiful and exist in much greater supply than any one woman could ever use. The same cannot be said of a kidney, since a donor's remaining kidney might be damaged in an accident. Is that the grounds for a public policy that prohibits selling human kidneys but can permit selling human eggs?

There is little doubt that most people feel a repugnance at the idea of allowing commercial traffic in human organs. Repugnance is a moral emotion, and if moral emotions are ever a guide to reasoned ethical judgment,[36] this is a good case in point. It may well be the case that people who are opposed to paying egg donors experience a similar, albeit weaker, moral emotion. We are left with the puzzlement of whether the strength of a moral emotion provides a justifiable ground for drawing ethical lines governing matters of public policy.

CONSEQUENTIALISM: PROHIBITING VERSUS PERMITTING PAYMENT

With so many other concepts brought into play—exploitation, commodification, respect for persons, altruism, and justice—it is easy to overlook a fundamental approach to ethics and public policy. That approach calls for an assessment of the consequences of alternative courses of action, in this case prohibiting versus permitting payment to egg donors.

The leading consequentialist argument is that if women are not paid to donate eggs, who would do it? The source of eggs for donation would disappear, and fewer infertile women could then be assisted in this way. How great a loss this would be depends on one's assessment of the social and personal importance of enabling couples to have children who are biologically related to at least one parent, or of a woman's undergoing the experience of pregnancy and childbirth.

Recall that the Canadian Combined Ethics Committee rejected the option of permitting no payment to gamete donors on grounds that altruism would not encourage sufficient donors "to meet the need unless these individuals *at least* received fair compensation for their costs in terms of time and inconvenience." John Robertson uses the same justification, contending that "the ethical objections to payment must be balanced against the need to pay women to assure an egg supply for needy recipients. . . . "[37] Indeed, Robertson goes further in surmising that moral objections to payment would not constitute "the compelling need necessary to justify interference with the reproductive freedom of infertile couples."[38] "Moralistic" or symbolic reasons for prohibiting payment could not count as sufficient justification for interfering with a fundamental right, that is, the infertile couple's right to form families noncoitally.[39]

One likely consequence of legally prohibiting payments to egg donors is to drive the practice underground.[40] Private arrangements or transactions "off the books" might flourish, thereby making the practice more difficult to monitor or regulate. A system that could lead to a black market in human ova would create more ethical problems than one like the current practice of permitting payment to donors for their "time, risk, inconvenience, and discomfort."

It is hard to predict whether the consequences of prohibiting payment would be to encourage an underground economy in sale of gametes, to deny procreative rights to infertile couples, or to perpetuate the existing imbalance between poorer women as donors and wealthier women as recipients. One consequence of allowing payment is to increase the available options to poorer women, enabling them to earn money by a method that is no more degrading than alternative means they might choose.

Regulation, rather than prohibition, would likely lead to the best overall consequences. Regulatory measures should include at least three key elements. First, adequate screening safeguards need to be established to ensure that paying egg donors does not compromise the quality of the product, as has occurred in the case of paid blood donors. Second, an upper limit should be set on the amount of payment to guard against the possibility of exploitation. And third, women who agree to be donors must be paid for their time, risk, inconvenience, and discomfort regardless of whether eggs are successfully retrieved and regardless of the number of eggs obtained.

If, in the end, the consequences of prohibiting payment to egg donors would cause more damage to the fabric of society than allowing such payments, then as unsavory as commodification may be it remains the lesser of two evils. As an ethical conclusion, this is unsatisfying. It does not endorse payment to oocyte donors as a good thing. Nor does it dismiss the ethical concerns about degrading women, commodifying the human body, or perpetuating the unjust distribution whereby poorer women provide the eggs and wealthier women receive them. Opting for the "least worst" solution is the only sound way to resolve ethical debates about policy when reasonable people disagree. Regulation of the practice of paid egg donation is a reasonable middle ground between free-market commercialization and outright prohibition of payment.

CONCLUSION

The debate over the ethics of paying egg donors comes down to a disagreement over commodification. Some, like Radin, hold that treating reproductive capacity as just another market force leads to "an inferior conception of human flourishing" and is damaging to the texture of the modern world. Others, like Robertson, view these reasons for prohibiting payment as "moralistic" or "symbolic," and therefore find it appropriate to pay women "to assure an egg supply for needy recipients." The most serious ethical objections to paying egg donors are those that rest on the prospect of exploitation. Yet the facts relating to the relative wealth of egg donors and recipients do not support the contention that payment to donors is a form of exploitation of poor women by the rich.

Considerations of justice may still apply, however. Even though individual women may not be exploited in receiving payment for their oocytes, the class of women who are donors is, in general, less well-off financially than the class of women who receive the eggs. But, it is argued, this disparity is no different from that which obtains in a wide variety of other situations in a market-driven society. So we are left with the question of whether the values of market-driven societies should permeate every aspect of those societies, the debate over commodification. It is hard to find fault with the point made by Harris, noted above: " . . . if it is acceptable to make voluntary donations of [gametes], then the addition of a financial interest does not necessarily add anything to the morality of the practice."

My conclusion is that although commodification is not immoral, it is nonetheless "unsavory." This category of disvalue does not involve a violation of ethical principle; yet it rests on the conviction that not every human exchange ought to be subject to market forces. Although unsavoriness is not a full-blooded moral category, it serves to remind us that there are degrees of ethical value and that reasonable people disagree about the ethical accept-ability of practices that fall in the middle of a continuum ranging from evil incarnate, at one end, to supreme moral virtue, at the other.

NOTES

1. Examples include Florida, Kentucky, Michigan, New Hampshire, Utah, and Washington. Cited in the New Jersey Commission on Legal and Ethical Problems in the Delivery of Health Care, *After Baby M: The Legal, Ethical and Social Dimensions of Surrogacy*, 1992.

2. Quoted in Machelle M. Seibel and Ann Kiessling, "Compensating Egg Donors: Equal Pay for Equal Time?" (letter), *New England Journal of Medicine*, 328 (1993): 737.

3. Ibid.

4. Johanna Riegler and Aurelia Weikert, "Product Egg: Egg Selling in an Austrian IVF Clinic," *Reproductive and Genetic Engineering* 1 (1988): 222.

5. A Report of the Combined Ethics Committee of the Canadian Fertility and Andrology Society and the Society of Obstetricians and Gynaecologists of Canada, "Ethical Considerations of the New Reproductive Technologies" (September 1990), p. 41.

6. Ibid.

7. Sherman Elias and George J. Annas, *Reproductive Genetics and the Law* (Chicago: Year Book Medical Publishers, 1987), p. 240.

8. John A. Robertson, "Technology and Motherhood: Legal and Ethical Issues in Human Egg Donation," *Case Western Reserve Law Review* 39 (1988–89): 31.

9. Ibid.

10. Jonathan Glover and others, *The Glover Report to the European Commission* (De Kalb: Northern Illinois University Press, 1989).

11. Ibid., p. 83.

12. Jacques Cohen in personal conversation.

13. See John Harris, *Wonderwoman and Superman* (Oxford: Oxford University Press, 1992), p. 121, and Harris's citations of Feinberg and Warnock Report.

14. Harris, p. 123.

15. Ibid., p. 124.

16. Ibid., p. 124.

17. These comments were made during discussion of an earlier draft of this paper by John Hoff, a member of NABER.

18. Robertson, p. 31.

19. Ibid.

20. I owe the phrasing of this broader interpretation of the principle of respect for persons to Cynthia Cohen.

21. Robertson, p. 31.

22. Ibid., p. 31.

23. Michael Walzer, *Spheres of Justice* (New York: Basic Books, 1983).

24. Richard J. Arneson, "Commodification and Commercial Surrogacy," *Philosophy & Public Affairs* 21 (1992): 133.

25. See generally, Margaret Jane Radin, "Market-Inalienability," *Harvard Law Review* 100 (1987): 1849–1937.

26. See Leon R. Kass, " 'Making Babies' Revisited," *The Public Interest* 54 (1979): 32–60.

27. National Organ Transplant Act of 1984, 42 U.S.C. Para. 274(e) (1982).

28. Elias and Annas, p. 240.

29. Robertson, p. 29.

30. Glover Report, p. 85.

31. Ibid.

32. Ibid., p. 84.

33. Harris, p. 128.

34. Radin, "Market-Inalienability," p. 177. Pages cited here are from an excerpt of Radin's original article, published in Kenneth D. Alpern (ed.), *The Ethics of Reproductive Technology* (New York: Oxford University Press, 1992).

35. Ibid., p. 177.

36. See Sidney Callahan, *In Good Conscience: Reason and Emotion in Moral Decision Making* (New York: Harper Collins, 1991).

37. Robertson, p. 31.

38. Ibid., p. 32.

39. Ibid., p. 30.

40. This possibility was suggested to me by John Hoff.

NINE

GENETIC SCREENING IN OOCYTE DONATION

Ethical and Legal Aspects

Carson Strong, Ph.D.

Rapid advances are being made both in genetic testing and the technology of assisted reproduction. Where these two areas overlap, difficult and potentially far-reaching issues demand our attention. A case in point is genetic screening of oocyte donors. If such screening is to be carried out, what tests should be performed? Should potential donors be tested for cystic fibrosis carrier status if not all who might transmit a defective gene can be detected? Should they be tested for susceptibility genes for such common diseases as colon cancer, breast cancer, and coronary artery disease? Who should make these decisions? Should prospective parents be allowed to seek oocyte donors with superior genetic endowment, as a way to enhance the characteristics of their offspring?

It will be helpful to consider current practices concerning genetic testing in gamete donation before I address these issues. After discussing the ethical presuppositions and legal framework of such practices, I shall consider ethical and legal issues likely to arise in the not-too-distant future.

CURRENT PRACTICE AND GUIDELINES

During the past several decades, discussions of genetic screening in gamete donation have focused on sperm donation; only recently have they extended to oocyte donation. "Genetic screening" refers to taking a genetic history and carrying out appropriate genetic tests. A 1979 survey of practitioners offering artificial insemination revealed that genetic screening of semen donors was inadequate.[1] A number of commentators maintained there was a pressing need to remedy this situation and raised the question of what form such screening should take.[2] In 1981, Timmons and colleagues proposed guidelines for genetic screening of sperm donors in which they emphasized the need to obtain a genetic history from both the sperm donor and recipient.[3] At about the same time, Fraser and Forse[4] also proposed a set of guidelines; other authors[5] soon followed with guidelines of their own.

A set of guidelines was put forward by the American Fertility Society[6] (AFS) in 1993 that applies to both sperm and oocyte donation. Since these are currently in use, they merit special attention. The AFS guidelines recommend excluding donors with any of the following conditions: a major Mendelian disorder; a major multifactorial or polygenic malformation; a familial disease with a major genetic component; a chromosomal rearrangement; carrier of an autosomal recessive gene known to be prevalent in the donor's ethnic background and for which carrier status can be detected; or advanced age (females 35 or older, males 40 or older). In addition, the AFS guidelines propose that donors be rejected if they have a first-degree relative (parents or offspring) with any of the following: a major multifactorial or polygenic disorder; a major autosomal dominant or x-linked disorder with late age of onset or reduced penetrance; an autosomal recessive disorder, if the disorder has a high frequency in the population and the donor's gametes will be used on many occasions; or a chromosomal abnormality, unless the donor has a normal karyotype.

The AFS guidelines state that the same genetic screening carried out on sperm donors should be offered to the female recipients of donated sperm. However, in addressing oocyte donation, the guidelines fail to state that genetic screening should be offered to the male partner who provides the sperm. This seems to be an oversight; if the objective is to avoid genetic disease in the offspring, then the male partner also should be offered screening.

Although there is considerable agreement among the various sets of guidelines that have been put forward, there also are notable differences. For example, Fraser and Forse[7] recommend that first-degree relatives of donors be free of major psychoses, epileptic disorders, juvenile diabetes mellitus, and early coronary disease, but the 1993 AFS guidelines[8] do not include this recommendation. Timmons and colleagues[9] recommend that if two or more stillbirths, fetal deaths, or unexplained neonatal deaths occur in a first-degree relative of the donor, then further investigation should be carried out to rule out a genetic etiology; however, neither Fraser and Forse nor the AFS guidelines[10] include this recommendation. Selva and coworkers[11] recommend routine karyotyping of donors, but Fraser and Forse claim that routine karyotyping is not justifiable.

It is worth noting several features of this occasionally conflicting body of literature. First, the various authors and committees do not distinguish their guidelines from previously published guidelines, nor do they defend their version over others. For example, the Ethics Committee of the AFS does not explain why its 1993 guidelines drop the recommendation in its previous guidelines that donors should be rejected who have first-degree relatives with major psychoses, epileptic disorders, juvenile diabetes mellitus, or early coronary disease. Similarly, Verp and colleagues[12] do not explain why they chose not to include Fraser and Forse's recommendation that a donor be rejected if there is a first-degree relative with a chromosomal abnormality, unless the donor is known to have a normal karyotype. Thus, there has been little critical assessment of opposing views in this literature.

Moreover, little attention has been given in these guidelines to identifying the ethical principles upon which genetic screening in gamete donation should be based. Such ethical principles would be useful not only in assessing the differences in the various proposed guidelines, but in addressing issues that will be faced in the future. Their omission creates a significant void that must be filled if certain practices related to genetic screening are to be justified ethically.

ETHICAL FRAMEWORK

Therefore, let us consider what ethical principles guidelines for genetic screening in gamete donation should follow. What are the ethical reasons for performing genetic screening of gamete donors in the first place? Several reasons can be given. First, doing so helps promote the autonomy of the recipient and her male partner in making reproductive decisions. In order to make an informed decision to proceed with gamete donation, the recipient and her partner need to know about any significant genetic risks that may be involved.

Second, genetic screening can prevent harm to the couple that might be caused by having a child with serious genetic diseases. A number of studies have documented that care of a handicapped child can involve serious problems for families, including emotional and economic difficulties, an increased incidence of divorce, behavioral problems in the child's siblings, and major sacrifices concerning education, careers, and travel.[13] Prevention of harm can be addressed at two levels. Patients generally lack knowledge about genetics and do not themselves know what tests should be performed. Thus, they need information and recommendations by those who counsel them. In deciding what these recommendations should be, we might ask what degree of protection from risks of transmitting genetic disease a reasonable person in the patient's position would want. At the second level, we should recognize that some patients are more risk averse than others and might be interested in testing beyond a minimal standard. Thus, at this level there might be room for individual patient judgment concerning what tests to perform in the attempt to prevent harm to them.

A third reason to offer genetic screening is to prevent harm to a child who would be born with serious genetic disease. However, if we understand harming persons as making them worse off than they otherwise would have been,[14] then preventing harm to the child would seem possible only in those rare cases in which the anomalies are so severe that it can reasonably be argued that nonexistence is objectively preferable to the life the infant would have.

Although these values provide the ethical justification for genetic screening in gamete donation, several other important ethical values are involved in such screening. The participation of a third-party donor introduces several concerns. First, the well-being of the donor might be adversely affected by genetic screening. The physical risks to the donor are not especially great, since genetic screening can be accomplished by drawing blood. In fact, the risks of oocyte retrieval typically would be greater than the physical risks of genetic screening for the donor. However, the donor's well-being could be adversely affected by inappropriate use of the information obtained. There is a risk that employers or insurance companies might discriminate against the donor on the basis of such information.[15] Test results might also have implications for the donor's own health. If, for example, genetic conditions involved in multifactorial diseases were found, changes in lifestyle might become advisable for the donor. Because genetic information has the potential to affect the donor's life in significant ways, informed consent for genetic screening is necessary. Thus, donor autonomy also is a relevant ethical consideration.

Another relevant value is the autonomy of the physician carrying out genetic screening. Physicians must make judgments about how to perform their professional duties, including the duty to do no harm. Such judgments often are evaluative in nature. An example would be a judgment about how much risk the physician is willing to allow the patient to take in achieving a certain end. Such judgments might differ from those of patients. Physicians should be allowed to refuse patient requests that would violate their conscientious judgments about such matters. Thus, a physician might have views concerning what genetic tests should be performed or whether a donor should be rejected that reflect the physician's judgment about what level of risk is acceptable. Conscientious objection should not be so broad, however, as to include refusal to inform patients about significant risks of transmitting genetic diseases.

Having identified these values, we are better able to understand the differences in the various proposed guidelines. One approach to formulating guidelines is to put forward minimal standards. Such guidelines are based on judgments about what tests patients reasonably should be offered, given patients' general lack of knowledge about genetics. The 1993 AFS guidelines,[16] for example, can be interpreted as an attempt to put forward such minimal standards. However, some physicians might find it appropriate, based on their own conscientious judgment, to go beyond minimal standards. An example might be the preference expressed by Selva and colleagues[17] for doing routine karyotyping of donors. A similar example might be the recommendation by Timmons and colleagues[18] that if two or more stillbirths, fetal deaths, or unexplained neonatal deaths occur in a first-degree relative, then further investigation should be carried out to rule out a genetic etiology. It should be considered acceptable for physicians to go beyond minimalist approaches, provided the couple and donor give consent based on adequate information, including information about whatever costs might be involved.

Minimal standards should identify genetic diseases that are relatively severe and/or relatively likely to occur, compared to other genetic diseases. Making such determinations is a matter of judgment, as differences between the various proposed guidelines reflect. In addition, some couples might request a particular test, even though they realize that the disease in question is not among the most severe or most frequently occurring. This is an example of the sort of decision that might appropriately be left to the couple, to be based on their personal values.

LEGAL FRAMEWORK

Legal liability for negligence in genetic screening and counseling is based on principles of tort law. To establish that a tort has occurred, it is necessary to prove that a *breach of duty* resulted in an *injury* and that the breach of duty was the *proximate cause* of the injury. Compensation can be obtained only if the harm is one for which the law provides a remedy.[19] Lawsuits claiming negligence in genetic screening and counseling typically arise following the birth of a child with genetic disease.

Two types of suits can be distinguished. *Wrongful birth* suits are brought by parents, who claim that the birth of the child would have been prevented had it not been for the negligence of the health care providers. The parents typically claim that they have been denied the opportunity to make an informed decision concerning conception or termination of pregnancy.[20] Examples of such negligence include failure of the physician to recognize genetic risks, failure to inform the parents of the availability of genetic or prenatal tests, and improper performance of tests. In wrongful birth suits, parents usually seek damages for the costs of raising the handicapped child. They might also seek damages for their own pain and suffering.[21]

Wrongful life suits are brought by the handicapped infant and assert that the infant would not have been born had it not been for the negligence of the health care providers.[22] In deciding whether there has been a breach of duty in wrongful birth and wrongful life lawsuits, courts assess the plaintiff's behavior against the standard of care of the profession. In general, physicians "must have and use the knowledge, skill and care ordinarily possessed and employed by members of the profession in good standing. . . . "[23] Several qualifications should be made concerning this standard. First, the knowledge and skill required varies with the physician's training. Specialists practicing within their specialty are held to a higher standard than general practitioners would be concerning that area. Moreover, there is a trend to hold specialists to a national standard of care, although general practitioners sometimes are held only to the standards of the local community.[24] The courts permit some flexibility and recognize differing views concerning national standards, as long as each view is espoused by a "respectable minority." Standards concerning disclosure of information to patients usually are derived from case law concerning informed consent. A widely held standard requires the physician to disclose the information that a reasonable person in the patient's position would want to know.[25]

The question of the liability of the oocyte donor and the recipient's male partner also deserves attention. To my knowledge, no lawsuits or statutes have addressed the question of gamete donor liability. Robertson states that oocyte donors could be legally liable for withholding information about their genetic histories that poses risks for the recipient or offspring.[26] If failure to reveal leads to avoidable congenital anomalies, the donor could be sued for wrongful birth or wrongful life. Similarly, a wrongful life action could be brought by a child against the male parent for congenital disease resulting from withholding genetic information. Children can sue their parents in tort for personal injuries resulting from negligent or intentional acts during the prenatal period.[27] There is no reason to think that parental negligence prior to conception could not also give rise to legal action, given that physicians have been found legally liable for preconception negligence.[28] Presumably, the child's anomalies would have to be severe in order to argue successfully that nonexistence is objectively preferable to life with the anomalies.

ROUTINE TESTING OF ALL OOCYTE DONORS

As the number of available genetic tests increases with advances in genetics, what changes should be made in guidelines for screening in gamete donation? One might ask for each new test whether it should routinely be carried out on all donors as part of a minimal standard for testing. In deciding this, several factors should be considered: the prevalence of the defective gene in the population; the likelihood that the child would acquire the disease, given that one or both genetic parents carry the defective gene; the severity of the disease; and the accuracy and reliability of the genetic test in question. The prevalence of the defective gene is relevant for several reasons. First, the greater the prevalence, the greater the risk to parents and offspring. Second, the higher the prevalence, the higher the positive predictive value of the test. In a population with very low prevalence, the test would have a low positive predictive value, meaning that there would be a relatively high ratio of false positives to true positives.

Two areas in which special screening issues will arise in the near future are testing for the cystic fibrosis gene and testing for susceptibilities to common diseases such as colon cancer, breast cancer, and coronary artery disease. Let us consider these two areas.

Cystic fibrosis (CF) is the most common lethal autosomal recessive disease among whites in the United States. In this population, the disease occurs in approximately one in 2,500 live births, and approximately one in 25 persons carries the defective gene.[29] In 1989 the nucleotide sequence in the most prevalent defective allele, known as ΔF508, was identified.[30] This allele accounts for approximately 75% of all defective CF genes among whites in the United States.[31] Since then, over 200 additional defective alleles with lower prevalence have been identified.[32] The discovery of the ΔF508 allele raised the issue of when population screening for CF should begin. An important consideration was the fact that screening for ΔF508 would detect only about half of all couples at risk of transmitting CF to offspring. Properly counseling patients about the significance of CF test results therefore would require some discussion of the complexities of CF testing, which would create problems for patient understanding. It became obvious that population screening would require substantial resources, including personnel for the provision of counseling.

The National Institutes of Health[33] (NIH) and the American Society of Human Genetics[34] (ASHG) issued statements expressing the view that it was premature to begin population screening. Several arguments in support of this position were put forward.[35] First, the available test would not be capable of detecting a large percentage of couples at risk. Second, the disease frequency and mutations vary according to ethnic and racial background, so that laboratory and counseling modifications would be required in different populations. Third, there are limitations on the ability to educate patients concerning the use of an imperfect test. Fourth, couples in which one partner has a positive test and the other has a negative test would have an increased risk (approximately 1 in 400) of bearing a child with cystic fibrosis. Presumably, the concern is that this would be an ambiguous situation involving a risk high enough to create anxiety, but not high enough to lead to prenatal diagnosis or other intervention. According to the NIH statement, population screening should not be undertaken until tests are capable of detecting at least 90 to 95% of carriers.

Since the NIH statement was issued, advances have been made in detecting some of the less frequently occurring alleles. Now it is possible to detect 85 to 90% of carriers of mutations.[36] A question that arises is whether it is now appropriate routinely to offer CF testing in oocyte donation, as part of the minimal standard of genetic screening. The earlier arguments against population screening do not seem to hold persuasively against screening in oocyte donation at this time. Approximately 72 to 81% of cases in which both genetic parents are heterozygotes can be detected. In addition, the number of oocyte donors would be relatively small, compared to the number of couples who would be tested in population screening, and therefore the demand for resources to provide testing and counseling would not be as great. Problems associated with differing prevalence and mutations among different ethnic groups should not preclude testing that focuses on whites in the United States at this time.

The problems in explaining test results to patients would be less formidable, given the smaller group of patients and the improved detection rate. Moreover, if the donor's test were positive and the male partner's test negative, there would be ways of responding that help reduce risks and avoid anxiety. The donor could be rejected in favor of a donor whose test is negative. If the donor's test is negative and the male partner's positive, this would provide meaningful information that the couple could use in deciding whether to go forward with oocyte donation. This situation would arise in less than 3% of cases, which seems too low to justify withholding CF screening in oocyte donation generally.

Because there are costs involved, the test should be offered as optional at this time, thereby allowing couples to decide whether they wish to incur these costs. Although the future holds the promise of genetic therapy, at present CF is not curable. In the absence of a cure, the severity of the disease is great enough to justify offering the test in oocyte donation at this time. Of course, this argument does not imply that population or routine prenatal screening is justifiable at this time.

TESTING DONORS FOR SUSCEPTIBILITY TO COMMON DISEASES

Another issue likely to arise in the not-too-distant future is whether donors should be tested for susceptibilities to common diseases. These familial diseases typically are not autosomal recessive, but are transmitted by autosomal dominant, x-linked, or polygenic inheritance. A genetic history often will identify donors at risk of transmitting such diseases. According to current guidelines, such donors would be rejected. In the future, as tests for susceptibility genes become available and costs decrease, testing donors at risk may become preferable to outright rejection, especially if the supply of oocytes is scarce. Eventually, it might become reasonable to screen prospective donors routinely for certain familial diseases, even where there is a negative family history, for several reasons. First, a few donors might not be well informed concerning the health status of family members. Second, some familial diseases might have reduced penetrance or variable expressivity, and the donor might report a negative history, even though the defective gene is carried in the donor's family.

For some susceptibility genes, the severity of the disease and likelihood that the child would acquire the disease might be relatively low. This raises the question concerning what degree of severity and likelihood would be required to justify including a test in the minimal standard, assuming a low-cost reliable test. One might answer by using as a benchmark those diseases that have a high enough severity and likelihood of occurrence that we *currently* routinely test for them, at least in defined populations. An example is sickle-cell anemia, which has a carrier frequency of one in 10 to 12 among American blacks. Similarly, Tay-Sachs disease has a carrier frequency of one in 30 among Ashkenazi Jews. Both are autosomal recessive, so there is a 25% chance of transmitting the disease if both parents are carriers. A strong argument could be made for including in a minimal standard common famil-ial diseases with a severity and likelihood of occurrence comparable to, or higher than, the above-mentioned diseases. An example might be hereditary nonpolyposis colorectal cancer, for which it is estimated that one in 200 Americans carry the defective gene.[37] An individual who carries the gene is estimated to have a 70 to 90% chance of getting colon cancer.[38] Thus, it is a serious disease with a likelihood of occurrence comparable to sickle-cell anemia. Currently the cost of testing for the gene for hereditary nonpolyposis colorectal cancer is approximately $1,000.[39] At present it would be more reasonable simply to reject donors at risk than to incur the expense of testing, but as costs come down this might change.

Other familial diseases have an extremely low prevalence. Even if tests for them are available, they need not be routinely carried out or even discussed with the patient. Between these rare diseases and those for which routine screening clearly should be performed there is a continuum in terms of severity and likelihood of occurrence. There will be a gray area involving familial diseases with severity and likelihood of occurrence somewhat lower than those for which routine screening clearly is warranted. Here it would be appropriate to let the recipient and her male partner decide whether they want testing. A minimal standard might include informing them of the availability of such tests. As the number of tests in this gray area increases, informed consent might become more difficult, because of the increasing number of tests that must be discussed. However, if sufficient time were devoted to the informing process, informed decisions should be possible.

A minimal standard, therefore, would involve several categories of tests. For some tests—those involving diseases with relatively high severity or likelihood of occurrence—the physician would *recommend* that the tests be carried out. For other tests, the physician would discuss the availability of the test, but encourage the recipient and male partner to make their own decision. The question of what tests should be included in these two categories is best decided by an interdisciplinary group. The Ethics Committee of the AFS has assumed a leadership role in this area[40] and provides an example of an appropriate body to address these questions as new tests arise. Such a body can periodically update guidelines for minimal standards.

LEGAL LIABILITY AS NEW TESTS EMERGE

Let us consider what legal liabilities there *should* be in the near future for failure to offer available tests for CF or susceptibility genes in oocyte donation. We will begin with CF and consider whether each of the elements of tort in wrongful birth could reasonably be held to exist when failure to offer the test in oocyte donation is followed by birth of a child with CF. Causation is an element that could be established in such a situation. It could be argued that had the tests been offered, the couple would have wanted them performed. Moreover, the couple might claim that if both potential genetic parents had been found to be carriers, then the donor would have been rejected. It also could be argued that harm occurred. As yet, there is no cure for CF, and in the absence of a cure or highly effective treatment CF involves serious impairments to health leading to early death. These impairments can give rise to significant burdens on parents who provide care to affected children. I argued above that patients should be told about CF tests, as part of a minimal standard for oocyte donation at this time. That argument supports the view that there is a breach of duty when testing is not discussed. Finally, it can be argued that the law should provide a remedy for this tort. In previous court decisions the law has provided a remedy in cases involving Tay-Sachs disease,[41] autosomal recessive polycystic kidney disease,[42] and neurofibromatosis,[43] among other genetic diseases. If a remedy should be provided for these diseases, then it would be difficult to justify an exception for CF, in the absence of a cure. Thus, it seems that legal liability could follow from failure to inform about CF tests in oocyte donation leading to the birth of a child with CF.

What about susceptibility genes? Again let us consider whether each of the elements of tort for wrongful birth would exist when failure to offer the test is followed by onset of the disease in the offspring. Causation could be established by arguing that had the test been offered, the couple would have requested that it be performed, and that if a defective gene had been detected, the child would not have been conceived. It might be possible to establish a breach of duty based on whatever minimal standards are followed at the time of the putative tort. A failure by the physician to inform patients of the availability of tests included in a minimal standard could be taken to constitute a breach of duty. Establishing that harm occurred would depend in part on the age of onset of the disease in question. Adult onset is common for many familial diseases. In such cases, parents bringing wrongful birth lawsuits might have difficulty establishing that they have been economically harmed. Although it might be argued that they have been emotionally harmed, courts often consider such harm to be offset by the benefits of having a child.[44] This might be especially so in cases of assisted reproduction. These considerations suggest that it would be difficult to establish legal liability for wrongful birth, at least in cases of late-onset diseases.

If the disease has relatively early onset and the parents suffer economic burdens, then harm might be established. In such situations it would be reasonable to impose legal liability on physicians who had deviated from minimal standards.

Wrongful life suits brought by the offspring would not be reasonable, however, regardless of whether the disease has early or late onset. Although many familial diseases are serious, generally they are not so devastating as to make nonexistence objectively preferable to a life in which the disease occurs. Thus, the element of harm could not reasonably be established.

SELECTION OF OOCYTE DONORS TO ENHANCE THE QUALITY OF OFFSPRING

Another issue likely to arise involves whether gamete donors should be selected in order to enhance the characteristics of offspring. Recipients might request donors on the basis of intelligence, height, or beauty. This practice raises two major questions: Is such selection ethically justifiable? Should it be legally permitted? Because artificial insemination by donor (AID) has been a relatively widespread practice in the United States for several decades, it will be helpful to begin by considering the extent to which selection for superior characteristics has been a part of the practice of sperm donation.

In 1988 the Office of Technology Assessment published the results of a survey that involved a national sample of sperm banks and physicians who provide AID.[45] Several survey questions dealt with matching the characteristics of the sperm donor to those of the social father. According to an estimate based on a weighted sample of 367 physicians, 72% of physicians who provided AID were willing to "select donor characteristics to recipient specifications." Among those, 90% would match for height, 82% for body type, 66% for educational attainment, 57% for I.Q., and 45% for special abilities, such as athletic skill. All 15 sperm banks surveyed allowed recipients or their physicians to specify donor traits. Among the 15 sperm banks, 14 would match for height, 14 for body type, 11 for educational attainment, 11 for special abilities, and 7 for I.Q. One sperm bank, The Repository for Germinal Choice, specializes in semen samples from donors who are highly educated and accomplished.[46] Thus, a substantial percentage of physicians who provide AID and sperm banks are willing to engage in selection that could be described as enhancement. However, this selection purportedly is carried out to match characteristics of donor and social father. Given the widespread tendency in AID to maintain secrecy concerning the offspring's genetic origins,[47] it is reasonable to assume that social fathers often desire matching because it serves the goal of secrecy. It is unclear to what extent recipients' specification of donor characteristics is motivated by the hope of enhancement as opposed to secrecy. Of course, in selecting mates people often consider what the offspring would be like. Sometimes mates are chosen, in part, because it seems likely that they will transmit desirable characteristics. Clearly, such selection constitutes a method of enhancing the quality of offspring. It seems fair to conclude, therefore, that even when selection of sperm donors is motivated by secrecy, it sometimes indirectly serves enhancement because it matches a male partner who was himself selected in part because of enhancement considerations.

It is worth noting that, according to the survey, 20% of physicians who provide AID were unwilling to select donor characteristics based on the recipient's specifications.[48] Also, among the 72% who were willing to do so, a number were unwilling to fulfill certain types of specifications. Specifically, 29% were unwilling to select for educational attainment, 37% were unwilling to select for I.Q., and 50% were unwilling to select for special abilities. Also, most of the respondents from the 15 sperm banks surveyed were opposed to the type of semen banking performed by The Repository for Germinal Choice.[49] Thus, although some selection for enhancement seems to occur, there is a lack of consensus among professionals involved in AID that enhancement is acceptable.

Oocyte donation is relatively new, and there is little data concerning selection of donors. Published reports suggest that selection of donors based on education[50] or other characteristics requested by recipients[51] occurs to some degree. However, the relatively small number of oocyte donors,[52] compared to sperm donors, may limit the extent to which selection for enhancement takes place at present. In the future, technical advances such as primordial follicle donation[53] might increase the supply of oocytes. This would increase the feasibility of selection for enhancement.

Is selection of oocyte and sperm donors to enhance the quality of offspring ethically justifiable? Several arguments can be given in support of such selection. First, as mentioned above, such selection commonly is a consideration in choosing mates. This seems to be ethically justifiable. If we value personal autonomy, including reproductive liberty, then we should value the freedom of individuals to select mates based on their personal preferences, including preferences that take into account the possible characteristics of offspring. If it is ethically permissible to take such considerations into account in selecting mates, then it would seem ethically permissible to take them into account in selecting gamete donors. Both types of situations involve reproductive liberty in choosing a genetic parent for one's offspring, and this is an important aspect of procreative freedom.

Second, from the point of view of the offspring's interests, selection of oocyte and sperm donors with superior characteristics seems to be defensible, as it is likely to give the offspring qualities that would be advantageous. Third, having a child with superior characteristics is likely to promote the happiness of the parents, especially when parents seek such qualities in their offspring.

On the other hand, several arguments can be given against selection of gamete donors for superior characteristics. First, those who are economically advantaged are more likely to use this method of enhancement because they are better able to afford the costs of assisted reproduction. Thus, such enhancement would be skewed among different socioeconomic and ethnic groups. Because enhancement can increase a child's opportunities for improved socioeconomic status, unequal access to it would exacerbate current social and economic inequities. Second, allowing parents to choose enhancement through selection of gamete donors might set a precedent that will lead to social harms in the future associated with positive eugenics. Abuses might occur similar to those of previous eugenic programs. Possibly, efforts might be made to redesign human nature, resulting in more harm than benefit.

Responses can be made to these arguments against selection of donors. Admittedly, positive eugenics could lead to harmful social consequences, but we should not assume that this would necessarily be the case. There is too much uncertainty to be confident about predictions concerning this matter. Even if we decide that it is important to set a precedent against positive eugenics, there are ways of setting precedents other than banning selection of gamete donors. For example, a policy that discourages prenatal testing and abortion for enhancement purposes could constitute such a precedent.[54] Similarly, a policy that discourages testing preembryos for enhancement would serve as a precedent. Assuming, for the sake of argument, that we should take a stand against positive eugenics, several considerations suggest that selection of gamete donors is not the best place to take one's stand. First, selection of gamete donors for enhancement purposes is similar to the justifiable and deeply entrenched practice of selecting mates partly on the basis of enhancement considerations. As stated above, it is difficult to argue that the latter is justifiable but the former is not. Second, matching gamete donors to social parents seems justifiable, independently of the pros and cons of maintaining secrecy about the child's genetic origins. Even parents who would not be secretive about the child's origins might reasonably want the child to resemble the social parents in certain ways. Race and ethnic background are obvious examples. Tall parents might reasonably prefer tall children, and highly intelligent parents might reasonably prefer intelligent children. Moreover, it is difficult to permit matching without enhancement being implicated. From a practical point of view, the two cannot entirely be separated.

Although the concern about inequity is important, there may be a better way to address this problem. Making assisted reproduction, including oocyte donation, available to all couples with a medical need as part of a basic health care plan would avoid the skewed access that exacerbates inequities. Assuming that assisted reproduction is an important enough service, it seems reasonable—perhaps even obligatory—to expand access to it. The above arguments support the view that selection of oocyte donors for enhancement purposes is ethically acceptable and should legally be permitted.

CONCLUSION

The many issues raised by oocyte donation include those pertaining to genetic screening of donors. This essay has dealt with at least three areas that deserve further discussion. First, although a number of guidelines for genetic screening in gamete donation have been put forward, they have made divergent recommendations, and little attention has been given to articulating the ethical purposes of such screening. I suggest that a satisfactory set of guidelines should serve two purposes: to identify minimal standards for recommendations for testing; and to identify tests that go beyond minimal recommendations that should be presented to the infertile couple as options to be performed if the couple and donor wish. Second, with advances in the technology of genetic testing, there will be an ongoing need to reexamine the question of what tests should correspond to each of these two purposes. Third, offspring enhancement is one of the most profound issues arising from the overlap between genetic and assisted reproduction. Although enhancement raises serious concerns that suggest we should discourage it, I have argued that selection of gamete donors is not an appropriate place to draw a line against it.

NOTES

1. Martin Curie-Cohen, Lesleigh Luttrell, and Sander Shapiro, "Current Practice of Artificial Insemination by Donor in the United States," *New England Journal of Medicine* 300 (1979): 585–90.

2. William G. Johnson, Robin C. Schwartz, and Abe M. Chutorian, "Artificial Insemination by Donors: The Need for Genetic Screening," *New England Journal of Medicine* 304 (1981): 755–57.

3. M. Chrystie Timmons, Kathleen W. Rao, Carol S. Sloan, et al., "Genetic Screening of Donors for Artificial Insemination," *Fertility and Sterility* 35 (1981): 451–56.

4. F. Clarke Fraser and R. Allan Forse, "On Genetic Screening of Donors for Artificial Insemination," *American Journal of Medical Genetics* 10 (1981): 399–405.

5. See, for example, Joe Leigh Simpson, "Genetic Screening for Donors in Artificial Insemination," *Fertility and Sterility* 35 (1981): 395–96; Marion S. Verp, Melvin R. Cohen, and Joe Leigh Simpson, "Necessity of Formal Genetic Screening in Artificial Insemination by Donor," *Obstetrics and Gynecology* 62 (1983): 474–79; J. Selva, C. Leonard, M. Albert, et al., "Genetic Screening for Artificial Insemination by Donor (AID)," *Clinical Genetics* 29 (1986): 389–96; Ethics Committee of the American Fertility Society, "Ethical Considerations of the New Reproductive Technologies," *Fertility and Sterility* 46 Suppl. 1 (1986): 36S–44S, 83S–84S; Ethics Committee of the American Fertility Society, "Ethical Considerations of the New Reproductive Technologies," *Fertility and Sterility* 53 Suppl. 2 (1990): 43S–50S, 88S–89S.

6. American Fertility Society, "Guidelines for Gamete Donation: 1993," *Fertility and Sterility* 59 Suppl. 1 (1993): 1S–9S.

7. Fraser and Forse, "On Genetic Screening of Donors," p. 403.

8. American Fertility Society, "Guidelines for Gamete Donation: 1993."

9. Timmons, Rao, Sloan, et al., "Genetic Screening of Donors," p. 452.

10. Ethics Committee of the American Fertility Society, "Ethical Considerations" (1986); Ethics Committee of the American Fertility Society, "Ethical Considerations" (1990); American Fertility Society, "Guidelines for Gamete Donation: 1993."

11. Selva, Leonard, Albert, et al., "Genetic Screening," p. 394.

12. Verp, Cohen, and Simpson, "Necessity of Formal Genetic Screening."

13. Carson Strong, "The Neonatologist's Duty to Patient and Parents," *Hastings Center Report* 14 (1984): 10–16.

14. Joel Feinberg, "Wrongful Life and the Counterfactual Element in Harming," *Social Philosophy and Policy* 4 (1987): 145–78.

15. Paul R. Billings, Mel A. Kohn, Margaret de Cuevas, et al., "Discrimination as a Consequence of Genetic Testing," *American Journal of Human Genetics* 50 (1992): 476–82.

16. American Fertility Society, "Guidelines for Gamete Donation: 1993."

17. Selva, Leonard, Albert, et al., "Genetic Screening," p. 394.

18. Timmons, Rao, Sloan, et al., "Genetic Screening of Donors," p. 452.

19. Ellen E. Wright and Margery W. Shaw, "Legal Liability in Genetic Screening, Genetic Counseling, and Prenatal Diagnosis," *Clinical Obstetrics and Gynecology* 24 (1981): 1133–49.

20. Kathryn J. Jankowski, "Wrongful Birth and Wrongful Life Actions Arising from Negligent Genetic Counseling: The Need for Legislation Supporting Reproductive Choice," *Fordham Urban Law Journal* 17 (1989): 27–62.

21. Leslie P. Francis, "Recent Developments in Genetic Diagnosis: Some Ethical and Legal Implications," *Utah Law Review* 1986 (1986): 483–93.

22. Jankowski, "Wrongful Birth and Wrongful Life," p. 30.

23. Jankowski, p. 38.

24. Wright and Shaw, "Legal Liability," p. 1136.

25. Wright and Shaw, p. 1137; Jankowski, p. 39.

26. John A. Robertson, "Technology and Motherhood: Legal and Ethical Issues in Human Egg Donation," *Case Western Reserve Law Review* 39 (1988–89): 1–38.

27. Bonnie Steinbock, *Life Before Birth* (New York: Oxford University Press, 1992), pp. 95–100.

28. *Park v. Chessin* 88 Misc. 2d 222, 387 N.Y. S. 2d 204 (Sup. Ct. 1976), 60 App. Div. 2d 80, 400 N.Y. S. 2d 110 (1977), Modified sub nom. *Becker v. Schwartz*, 46 N.Y. 2d 401, 386 N. E. 2d 807, 413 N.Y. S. 2d 895 (1978).

29. President's Commission for the Study of Ethical Problems in Medicine and Biomedical and Behavioral Research, *Screening and Counseling for Genetic Conditions* (Washington, DC: U.S. Government Printing Office, 1983), p. 13.

30. John R. Riordan, Johanna M. Rommens, Bat-sheva Kerem, et al., "Identification of the Cystic Fibrosis Gene: Cloning and Characterization of Complementary DNA," *Science* 245 (1989): 1066–73.

31. Benjamin S. Wilfond and Norman Fost, "The Cystic Fibrosis Gene: Medical and Social Implications for Heterozygote Detection," *Journal of the American Medical Association* 263 (1990): 2777–83.

32. Aubrey Milunsky, "Commercialization of Clinical Genetic Laboratory Services: In Whose Best Interest?" *Obstetrics and Gynecology* 81 (1993): 627–29.

33. NIH Workshop on Population Screening for the Cystic Fibrosis Gene, "Special

Report: Statement from the National Institutes of Health Workshop on Population Screening for the Cystic Fibrosis Gene," *New England Journal of Medicine* 323 (1990): 70–71.

34. American Society of Human Genetics Board of Directors, "The American Society of Human Genetics Statement on Cystic Fibrosis Screening," *American Journal of Human Genetics* 46 (1990): 393.

35. NIH Workshop on Population Screening for the Cystic Fibrosis Gene, "Special Report," p. 70.

36. ASGH Ad Hoc Committee on Cystic Fibrosis Carrier Screening, "Statement of the American Society of Human Genetics on Cystic Fibrosis Carrier Screening," *American Journal of Human Genetics* 51 (1992): 1443–44.

37. Natalie Angier, "Scientists Isolate Novel Gene Linked to Colon Cancer," *New York Times*, Dec. 3, 1993, p. A1.

38. Ibid.

39. Ibid.

40. Ethics Committee of the American Fertility Society (1986); Ethics Committee of the American Fertility Society (1990).

41. *Gildiner v. Thomas Jefferson Univ. Hospital*, 451 F. Supp. 692 (E. D. Pa. 1978).

42. *Park v. Chessin*.

43. *Speck v. Finegold*, 408 A. 2d 496 (Pa. Super. 1979).

44. Jankowski, "Wrongful Birth and Wrongful Life," pp. 43–44.

45. U.S. Congress, Office of Technology Assessment, *Artificial Insemination: Practice in the United States: Summary of a 1987 Survey—Background Paper* (Washington, DC: U.S. Government Printing Office, 1988), pp. 40–41, 64, 65, 67, 72–73.

46. U.S. Congress, Office of Technology Assessment, *Artificial Insemination*, p. 67.

47. See, for example, Susan C. Klock and Donald Maier, "Psychological Factors Related to Donor Insemination," *Fertility and Sterility* 56 (1991): 489–95; Leslie R. Schover, Robert L. Collins, and Susan Richards, "Psychological Aspects of Donor Insemination: Evaluation and Follow-up of Recipient Couples," *Fertility and Sterility* 57 (1992): 583–90.

48. U.S. Congress, Office of Technology Assessment, p. 41.

49. U.S. Congress, Office of Technology Assessment, pp. 72–73.

50. Martin M. Quigley, Robert L. Collins, and Leslie R. Schover, "Establishment of an Oocyte Donor Program: Donor Selection and Screening," *Annals of the New York Academy of Sciences* 626 (1991): 445–51.

51. Andrea Mechanick Braverman, "Survey Results on the Current Practice of Ovum Donation," *Fertility and Sterility* 59 (1993): 1216–20.

52. See, for example, Quigley, Collins, and Schover, "Establishment of an Oocyte Donor Program," p. 450; Mark V. Sauer and Richard J. Paulson, "Human Oocyte and Preembryo Donation: An Evolving Method for the Treatment of Infertility," *American Journal of Obstetrics and Gynecology* 163 (1990): 1421–24.

53. Christine Kilgore, "Egg Donation Programs Facing Ethical Issues, Donor Shortage: Potential for Ovum Banks," *Ob. Gyn. News*, Feb. 1–14, 1990, p. 1.

54. I have argued elsewhere that, at present, we should discourage prenatal testing and abortion for enhancement purposes. See Carson Strong, "Tomorrow's Prenatal Genetic Testing: Should We Test for 'Minor' Diseases?" *Archives of Family Medicine* 2 (1993): 1187–93.

TEN

TOWARD A FEMINIST PERSPECTIVE ON GAMETE DONATION AND RECEPTION POLICIES

Rosemarie Tong, Ph.D.

Egg donation, a technique that enables a fertile woman to donate one of her eggs to an infertile woman, is one of the most recent additions to so-called infertility services. According to John A. Robertson, egg donation is not nearly as ethically problematic as either surrogate motherhood or embryo freezing.[1] He is probably correct. Whatever regrets an egg donor might have about parting with her genetic material, they will not be as severe as those a surrogate mother might have about relinquishing a child she has gestated for nine months.[2] Moreover, whatever "potential" for personhood eggs have, they do not have the potential for personhood that embryos or newborn infants have.[3] A gamete seems much more akin to an actual body part (blood, bone marrow, a kidney) than a potential person (embryo or newborn infant).

Still, egg donation is not altogether ethically unproblematic. In the first place, infertility specialists usually offer the option of egg donation to infertile couples who have tried just about everything else to get pregnant. Not wanting to let any stone go unturned, such couples often find it extremely difficult to say "no" to this one last chance. Very likely they will think, or be caused to think, that were they to forsake this final opportunity, they might never forgive themselves.[4] Second, since egg donors subject themselves to considerable inconvenience, discomfort, and even pain on behalf of others' well-being, questions immediately arise about whether this level of self-sacrifice should be encouraged. Although egg donation is not as perilous as kidney donation, for example, it is certainly more risky than either blood donation or its analogue, sperm donation. Third, it is unclear whether current egg donation policies serve the best interests of women in the way current sperm donation policies allegedly serve the best interests of men. Several commentators have already noted two gender disparities between the treatment of egg and sperm donors, both of which *might* have more adverse effects on women than on men: (1) Whereas sperm donors are almost always anonymous,[5] a considerable number of egg donors are known to their recipients;[6] and (2) whereas almost all sperm donors are paid for their services,[7] a considerable number of egg donors are either not paid at all[8] or undercompensated for their services.[9]

Predictably, it is the fact that sperm donors and egg donors are treated differently that has attracted feminists' attention. What the public might not realize, however, is that there is no *single* feminist position on current gamete donation and reception policies. Instead, a variety of feminists, including liberal, Marxist, radical, and cultural feminists, have offered divergent analyses of current gamete donation and reception policies. The primary task of this paper is, therefore, to determine whether differently minded feminists (to say nothing of feminists *and* nonfeminists) can develop a mutually agreeable gamete donation and reception policy. Toward this end, I will first discuss *why* it is that feminists disagree about fundamental human-relations issues, and *how* these disagreements affect their respective analyses of gamete (especially egg) donation and reception policies. Having done this, I will suggest that we feminists need to reconsider the empirical truth of some of our more stereotypic assumptions about male and female identity and behavior. Finally, focusing on issues of screening, counseling, and matching, I will sketch a feminist policy for gamete donation and reception that seeks to incorporate the values and concerns of as many different kinds of feminists as possible without dismissing as entirely irrelevant the values and concerns of nonfeminist thinkers.

SOME FEMINIST PERSPECTIVES ON THE SELF-OTHER RELATIONSHIP

Since gender relations are currently being reassessed in our society, this is a propitious time to reconsider our policies for gamete donation and reception. Feminist theorists provide some important insights into just how deeply our gender assumptions run. They believe that our views on the self-other relationship shape our understanding of men's and women's gender identities and behavior in general as well as the motivations of sperm and egg donors in particular.

As feminist legal theorist Robin West sees it, a "separation thesis" informs virtually all aspects of our legal, moral, and political life. According to this thesis, "a 'human being,' whatever else he is, is physically separate from all other human beings."[10] Human beings are autonomous, atomic, separate, and boundaried individuals who proceed with their own private lives. West describes what she regards as the two main strains of "masculine" or "male" thought: a "liberal-theory" strain and a "critical-theory" strain. While both of these strains enunciate the separation thesis, the thesis manifests itself differently in each.

Proponents of liberal theory emphasize that what they regard as the natural human state of separation brings with it the precious gift of freedom. Freedom, which allows individuals the right to pursue their own separate ends, is the official value of liberal theory.[11] However, the very separation that makes individuals free also makes them vulnerable. Given that human beings are separate, their goals tend not only to differ, but also to conflict. The subsequent competition frequently leads to suffering, injury, or even death: "Annihilation by the other, we might say, is the official *harm* of liberal theory, just as autonomy is its official value."[12]

Agreeing with proponents of liberal theory that separation is *man's* fate, proponents of critical theory bemoan, rather than celebrate, the loneliness of the human condition. Man's isolation haunts him. He craves community. He wants to transcend the separation that is "natural" to him. Alienation, not annihilation by the other, is the real harm to lament, just as community, not freedom to be one's self, is the real value to cherish.[13] Separation is man's tragic destiny—the original sin for which redemption is sought.

The separation thesis is not the exclusive possession of men, however. West argues that in their desire to secure for women the same opportunities, occupations, rights, and privileges men have had, liberal feminists have tended to embrace the separation thesis, especially the form that values autonomy and fears annihilation (the power of sisterhood apparently notwithstanding). Indeed, in their drive for sameness with men, some liberal feminists have downplayed their sameness with women. They have cautioned women against emphasizing their differences from men, viewing these biologically produced and/or culturally shaped differences as traps that limit women to maintaining the human species, while men strive to push it on to greater heights. For most liberal feminists, especially the most "male-identified" ones, *real* choice is always a possibility for women.

In contrast, cultural, Marxist, and radical feminists have rejected the "male" view of the self-other relationship that guides liberal feminist thought. In its stead they have endorsed "female" metaphysics, a view of human relationships that is oriented by a connection thesis. Indeed, it is the central insight of cultural, Marxist, and radical feminists, says West, "that women are 'essentially connected,' not 'essentially separate,' from the rest of human life, both maternally, through pregnancy, intercourse, and breastfeeding, and existentially, through the moral and practical life."[14] Yet, as West also observes, cultural, Marxist, and radical feminists, have reacted very differently to women's capacities for "connectedness."

Cultural feminists follow the lead of thinkers like Carol Gilligan[15] and Nel

Noddings,[16] whose so-called feminine approaches to ethics valorize the traits and behaviors traditionally associated with women (sharing, giving, empathy, sympathy, nurturance, and so on). Feminists stress women's capacities of caring; they believe that women, much more than men, value personal relationships, striving to create and maintain them. The connection thesis, filtered through the lens of cultural feminism, produces a completely different picture of morality than does the separation thesis, filtered through the lens of liberal feminism: "Intimacy and the ethic of care constitute the entailed *values* of the existential state of connection with others, just as autonomy and freedom constitute the entailed values of the existential state of separation from others for men."[17] Thus, separation is cultural feminism's ultimate harm, and connection its fundamental good.

Marxist and radical feminists typically paint another, darker side of the connection thesis. They agree with cultural feminists that connection is women's fundamental reality, but they do not believe this capacity for relationships is a cause for celebration. On the contrary, they believe that women's connections set women up for exploitation and misery: "Invasion and intrusion, rather than intimacy, nurturance and care, is the unofficial story of women's subjective experience of connection."[18]

Marxist feminists emphasize that all too often women are involuntarily connected to men because they are not economically self-sufficient. They argue that for a variety of reasons, capitalists and patriarchs have united to keep women out of the workplace where they could earn their own money. Women do men's housework, take care of their children, and provide them with a variety of emotional and sexual services in exchange for financial support. As long as a woman loves her husband and he her, and/or as long as she regards him as a good father and provider, a woman might term her marriage relationship a "good" one. Should her husband begin to abuse her or her children verbally and physically, however, she might change her assessment, regarding herself as trapped in a bad marriage from which she cannot easily escape simply because she has no marketable skills.

In contrast to Marxist feminists, radical feminists stress that even worse than men's economic control over women is men's sexual control over women. Women might dream pleasant thoughts about "making love" and "having babies," but when the sugar-coating is licked off the *realities* of heterosexual intercourse and pregnancy, all too often these "connecting" experiences taste of women's violation. According to radical feminists, this kind of sexual harm, as opposed to economic harm, is unique to women. Whereas men fear annihilation, isolation, or disintegration of their artificially constructed communities, women fear *occupation*: "Both intercourse and pregnancy are literal, physical, material invasions and occupations of the body. The fetus, like the penis, literally occupies my body."[19] Thus, radical feminists suggest that women actually value and crave "individuation"—the freedom to pursue their own ends and gain "solitude, self-regard, self-esteem, linear thinking, legal rights, and principled thoughts."[20] But this is a personal goal women dare not express. In a society that rewards self-sacrificial women and frowns upon independent ones, self-realization can be a dangerous goal for women. Since society so often puts "uppity women" in their place, it seems safer for women to acquiesce to society's norms: to be docile, obliging, and compliant no matter what the costs to them.

SOME FEMINIST POSITIONS ON GAMETE DONATION AND RECEPTION POLICY: A STUDY IN DIFFERENCE

Clearly, an analysis of the differences between "male" and "female" perspectives on the self-other relationship helps us understand why feminists do not have *one* position on gamete donation and reception in general or on egg donation and reception in particular. Because they rely on the "male" separation thesis, and because they view men and women as essentially the same, liberal feminists want to use existing sperm donation policy as the paradigm for egg donation policy. They reason that if it is in sperm donors' best interests to remain anonymous and to be paid for their genetic material, then it is probably in egg donors' best interests to remain anonymous and to be paid for their genetic material. Liberal feminists think it is a mistake to assume that unlike sperm donors, egg donors have a strong interest in maintaining control over the ultimate destiny of their genetic material, in creating and maintaining bonds with the people who use their eggs or the children who are produced from them. They also think it is a mistake to assume that unlike men, women do not wish to be paid for their genetic material; that they want to make a true gift (rather than sale) of their eggs to infertile couples. However, liberal feminists do not think it is a mistake to require more stringent informed-consent policies for egg donation than for sperm donation, since egg retrieval is far more risky, inconvenient, and painful than sperm retrieval. There is, after all, considerable difference between submitting to a laparoscopy and engaging in masturbation. Indeed, so great is this difference and several others—including the fact that women's supply of eggs is *very* small compared to men's supply of sperm—that liberal feminists insist that women be paid far more for their eggs than men are paid for their sperm.

Interestingly, liberal feminists do not think that egg *recipient* policies should be modeled on what they regard as problematic *sperm recipient* policies. Currently, a sizable percentage of physicians provide artificial insemination by donor (AID) only to heterosexual women in stable, preferably married relationships.[21] Liberal feminists claim that physicians exceed the limit of their authority when they refuse to provide single heterosexual women or lesbian women with AID on the grounds that it is morally wrong for a woman to become a single parent deliberately or to rear her child in an "abnormal" (translation = "lesbian") family. In liberal feminists' estimation, any such refusal constitutes an unjustified restriction on women's procreative liberty, since there is no conclusive evidence that unless children are reared by heterosexual couples, they will suffer great harm.[22] Married or not, heterosexual or not, all women should have access to the sperm, or, as the case may be, the eggs they need to procreate. Moreover, it is also liberal feminists' view that a woman's age, in and of itself, should not be used as an automatic reason to prevent her from either selling (giving) her eggs or buying (receiving) another woman's eggs. Provided that a woman is legally competent and a medically appropriate candidate for gamete donation or, as the case may be, gamete reception, it is her business whether she decides to sell her eggs to help pay her way through college or, whether at the postmenopausal age of 55, she decides to purchase an egg in order to get pregnant.

Marxist feminists react negatively to liberal feminists' reasoning. They argue that even if a policy of *anonymous* egg donation might serve women's interests, it is far more dubious that a policy of *commercial* egg donation is likely to do the same. Unless women who have the best interest of other women at heart gain control over the egg donation industry, chances are that profiteers will use to their advantage one of the basic lessons capitalists, as well as patriarchs, teach women; namely, that when all else fails, a woman can always sell her body: her sexual services, her reproductive services. In an ever shrinking and increasingly lower-paying job market, an unskilled woman, or a woman who needs money fast, might be tempted to sell her oocytes for a $750-to-$3,000 fee even if the process constitutes a threat to her health,[23] as it must in the case of those whom the "industry" terms "super donors" (women who sell their eggs fairly routinely). Marxist feminists stress the fact that egg recipients are, for the most part, far more wealthy than egg donors—an economic disparity that can easily destroy women's "connections" to each other. Regrettably, when money enters a relationship, the feminist vision of a powerful sisterhood is sometimes replaced by a decidedly nonfeminist picture of a rich woman going to market to purchase just the right eggs she needs to "cook" herself a baby—a baby, whom a poor woman dares not have, lest she not be able to support it. Thus Marxist feminists conclude that if society thinks it is wrong to permit a market in certain organs because people might take risks they would not take were they financially secure, then it should think twice about permitting a market in eggs (though not necessarily sperm) for the same reason. To say that women *choose* to sell their eggs is, in Marxist feminists' estimation, simply to say that when a woman is forced to choose between poverty and exploitation, she sometimes chooses exploitation as the lesser of two evils.

Not surprisingly, liberal feminists have questioned the logic behind Marxist feminists' opposition to commercial egg donation. They ask why it is exploitative to *pay* a woman for eggs, but not to take them as a gift. In asking this question, they draw parallels between a woman's decision to sell her eggs and a woman's decision to sell her reproductive services. With respect to the latter decision, liberal feminist Lori Andrews has reasoned that if gestational motherhood, for example, is not inherently exploitative but becomes so only when women are economically coerced into it, then the "focus should not be on banning payment but on making sure the surrogates get paid more."[24] In practice, says Andrews, most of the women who serve as gestational mothers do so not because they are in desperate need of food, clothing, or shelter, but because they want what she terms "luxuries": a private-school education for their children, a redecorated house, or a second car.[25] Liberal feminists extend Andrews's comments about gestational mothers to egg donors. Most of the women who sell their eggs are not desperately poor. On the contrary, many of them describe themselves as "middle-class" women who want to do something good for people *and* earn a little money on the side while doing it.

Marxist feminists dismiss Andrews's and other liberal feminists' understanding of economic exploitation as simplistic. They observe that the *more* money society offers relatively poor women for their reproductive services or products, the *more* difficult it will be for them to say "no" to an arrangement that might be opposed to their best interests.[26] Some temptations are simply too difficult to refuse.

Agreeing with Marxist feminists that not only commercial gestational motherhood but also commercial egg donation are morally dubious practices, radical feminists broaden the Marxist feminist analysis of exploitation to include cases of non-economic exploitation. Radical feminists claim that just because a woman has no *economic* reasons for serving as a gestational mother or egg donor does not mean that her decision to offer one or both of these services is an entirely free one. Because we live in a society that repeatedly teaches women that it is women's role to be the givers par excellence, radical feminists claim that many women feel guilty if they are not as self-sacrificial as possible—if they are not giving other people everything they can give them, including their sexual and reproductive services. Appeals are made to generous, loving, altruistic women to give "the gift of life" to sorrowing, lovely, childless couples; and the more direct and immediate these appeals are, as in the case of egg donors known to their recipients, for example, the harder they are to resist.[27] Women typically find it very difficult to disappoint friends and relatives—to refuse to help them in their hour of need. Similarly, women typically find it very difficult to ignore what society tells them they must do in order to be "normal" and "fulfilled." In the past, *infertile* women were excused from mothering if, for example, they could not find a child to adopt—a child their husbands also wanted. Today, however, the "good tidings" of assisted reproduction are brought to infertile women—even postmenopausal infertile women. Now it is never too late to become a "normal" or "fulfilled" women—a mother—unless, of course, one lacks the funds to pay for the "best" that medicine can provide.

What also concerns radical feminists about all forms of egg donation is that, unlike sperm donation, it is a process under the control of both the medical establishment and profiteering infertility clinics. Through the Self-Insemination Movement and the establishment of feminist sperm banks, women have been able to secure some control over AID,[28] since it is rather easy to inseminate oneself. But egg donation and transfer is a practice that demands considerable medical expertise. Given that women do not control the practice of egg donation and transfer, radical feminists favor tight restrictions on it—indeed, even a ban on it.

Predictably, liberal feminists are not any more impressed by the radical-feminist than the Marxist-feminist case against egg donation. In the first place, liberal feminists argue that women can control this nation's infertility clinics. Women who are infertility patients can simply refuse to take their business to clinics that treat women in anything other than respectful ways. Like the man's wallet, the woman's pocketbook is a mighty weapon in a capitalist society. Moreover, women who are considering a career in medicine can choose to specialize in fields such as reproductive health and infertility treatment. They can develop styles of medical practice that serve the interests of women and men equally.

Secondly, and even more to the point, liberal feminists fault radical feminists for acting "maternalistically"—that is, for assuming that they know what is *really* best for the women who currently choose to be gamete donors or recipients. Liberal feminists concede that in a society such as ours which has over-emphasized women's capacities for self-sacrifice and women's "need" to mother, it is reasonable to worry that some egg donors and recipients might be making less than fully voluntary decisions about their roles in procreation. Yet, liberal feminists reject the view that all egg donors and recipients are mindless robots whom society has programmed to act in potentially self-destructive ways. As they see it, provided that a woman has given her informed consent to serve as an egg donor or to be an egg recipient, her decision must be recognized as voluntary. Liberal feminists agree with philosopher Joel Feinberg that a decision is voluntary to the degree that a person has considered:

> (1) the degree of probability that harm to oneself will result from a given course of action, (2) the seriousness of the harm being risked, i.e., "the value of importance of that which is exposed to the risk," (3) the degree of probability that the goal inclining one to shoulder the risk will in fact result from the course of action, (4) the value or importance of achieving that goal, that is, just how worthwhile it is to one (this is the intimately personal factor, requiring a decision about one's own preferences, that makes it so difficult for outsiders to judge the reasonableness of a risk), and (5) the necessity of the risk, that is, the availability or absence of alternative, less risky, means to the desired goal.[29]

Rather than encourage medical professionals or, worse, legal authorities to "save" women from their supposedly misguided maternal instincts, liberal feminists think that all feminists should instead simply encourage women to ask themselves *why* they want to be mothers, no matter how dearly they have to pay for this privilege.

In contrast to both liberal and radical feminists, cultural feminists see in egg donation, as well as sperm donation, possibilities for increased human connection—the kind of collaborative reproduction that, in the 1960s, was supposed to defeat the view that children are "genetic possessions." Stressing women's differences from men and emphasizing the *positive* side of the connection thesis, cultural feminists favor *open*, as opposed to anonymous, egg donation policies, and *noncommercial*, as opposed to commercial ones. They believe that collaborative reproduction is possible, and that sperm donors and egg donors have a legitimate stake in the outcome of the pregnancies they make possible. If gamete donors are interested, they should at least be kept posted on their genetic child's development, and at some point in time, perhaps when the child has reached the age of majority, at least be introduced to him or her. Ideally, however, gamete donors should play an even more active, indeed parental, role in their genetic child's life—assuming, of course, that doing so would not harm the child.[30]

To the degree that cultural feminists recommend that gamete donation be open, they recommend that it be noncommercial. They argue that if some men and women are inclined to *freely* give their bodily fluids, tissues, and organs to the people who need them, there is no reason to think that this group of generous people would insist on payment for their *gametes*. In the estimation of cultural feminists, generous impulses are to be affirmed and fostered among human beings, since self-giving is a particularly good way to create and maintain strong relationships.

Radical and liberal feminists fear that cultural feminists might be romanticizing *women's* capacities for creating and sustaining human relationships in particular. Not all women value intense personal relationships, including the mother-child relationship. Moreover, even women who regard themselves as "maternal" types and who seek to mother collaboratively with other women, might discover the limits of their generosity after their mutual child is born. Two strangers, two friends, two sisters, or even a mother and daughter might agree to an arrangement intended to permit both of them to play a relatively equal role in rearing their mutual child only to discover that they cannot live up to terms of their arrangement. Sharing a child is easier in theory than in practice.

In addition, liberal feminists claim that in the same way that relatively few men are willing to give their sperm to strangers for no compensation, relatively few women are willing to give their eggs to strangers for no compensation. Short of convincing the members of this highly individualistic society that their organs, tissues, and bodily fluids are "natural resources" to be shared by one and all, a good number of women as well as men will insist that their gametes are not community property but personal property. These women will be inclined to reason that it is discriminatory to pay men for their sperm but not to pay women for their eggs. After all, like most men, most women cannot afford to provide their services for free.

A UNITARY FEMINIST POSITION ON GAMETE DONATION AND RECEPTION: WORKING TOWARD A CONSENSUS

As we reflect on liberal, Marxist, radical, and cultural feminist positions on gamete donation and reception in general and on egg donation and reception in particular, it becomes apparent that feminists as well as nonfeminists sometimes assume things about male and female identity and behavior that are less a reflection of empirical fact than an expression of ideology. One assumption is that sperm donors want to remain anonymous—that they have no interest in what happens to their sperm after they leave the lab, and that they wish to avoid any knowledge of or contact with their genetic children, lest their genetic children make financial or, perhaps worse, personal claims on them. Although it is true that sperm donors do not wish to be the objects of paternity suits, a variety of psychologists and counselors have noted that a sizable percentage of sperm donors would at least like to know whether they have "fathered" any children. Indeed, several recent studies indicate that an increasing number of sperm donors are willing to share *identifying* as well as *nonidentifying* information about themselves with their recipients and children.[31]

Another assumption is that sperm donors are not about to make true *donations* of their gametes—that they are strictly "in it for the money." As it so happens, however, there is growing evidence that many men have a less crass view of the meaning of sperm donation. Indeed, some commentators believe that even if the profile of the typical sperm donor had to change from carefree, unmarried college student to responsible married man in the United States, as it did in France when some sperm banks in France stopped paying their donors and adopted policies of nonanonymity, enough U.S. men would be willing to donate sperm to meet the current demand.[32]

A third assumption is that egg donors want to know their recipients and vice versa. In point of fact there is no clear evidence that this is so. When egg donation techniques were first developed, most recipients knew their donors, since infertility centers typically required each potential egg recipient to find her own potential egg donor, usually a friend or relative. As more and more IVF specialists became concerned that some women in need of eggs were not above "guilt-tripping" their friends and relatives to provide them, they began a search for anonymous egg donors. Few of these anonymous egg donors have shown a strong interest in knowing the identities of their recipients, or vice versa.[33]

A fourth assumption is that even anonymous egg donors are willing to make true donations of their gametes. As it so happens, this is not the case. Although few anonymous egg donors are in desperate need of money, most of them are not willing to donate their eggs gratis.[34]

If what I have just noted above is true—if both men *and* women have interests in separation *and* connection, taking *and* giving—toward what kind of gamete donation and reception policy should all feminists work? What policy is most likely to expand the range of women's genuine procreative choices, minimize capitalism's and patriarchy's control over women's reproductive powers, and increase women's ability to create and maintain only those generic, gestational, and rearing connections that are compatible with women's freedom and well-being? In general, should this policy be open or anonymous, commercial or noncommercial? In particular, how should the recruitment, screening, counseling, and matching of gamete donors and recipients be handled?

TOWARD SOME GENERAL FEMINIST RECOMMENDATIONS ABOUT GAMETE DONATION AND RECEPTION POLICY

In general, a feminist gamete donation and reception policy should permit but not require openness, with the possible exception of the kind of disclosure rules that increasingly characterize adoption law and are intended to serve the best interests of adopted children. The ideal of truly collaborative reproduction—of more than two persons procreating and rearing a child—is one that most feminists affirm in theory, even as they debate about whether this vision can ever be realized in practice. Therefore, the law should make it *possible* for women (and men) to constitute families consisting of an egg donor, an egg recipient, and the egg recipient's husband (partner), or a sperm donor, a sperm recipient, and the sperm recipient's husband (partner). Currently, women (and men) must think long and hard before constituting such alternative families not only because of the possible personal problems that might be generated but also because there are few clear legal rules about the parental rights and responsibilities of each of the adults in such families, to say nothing of the child's rights.

Similarly, a feminist gamete donation and reception policy should permit, but not require, payment. Only if (1) increasing evidence firmly establishes that society is best served by an entirely noncommercial system of bodily fluid, tissue, and organ donation, and (2) legal developments conclusively affirm that the right to procreate does not include total access to all means of procreation,[35] should payment for gametes be forbidden. For now, gamete donors should be encouraged to donate their sperm and eggs gratis. Should the supply of gametes fail to meet the demand because of donors' lack of generosity, however, a reasonable payment system should be developed. Donors should be given enough compensation to offset the inconveniences, discomforts, and, in the case of egg donation, risks they experience. Under no circumstances, however, should payment be so high as to induce a gamete donor to act against his or her best interests.

TOWARD SOME PARTICULAR FEMINIST RECOMMENDATIONS ABOUT GAMETE DONATION AND RECEPTION

A. GAMETE RECEPTION POLICY

1. *Medical screening of gamete recipients.* The primary reason to *medically* screen women who want to use donor sperm or eggs should simply be to assess their physical health so that they, in consultation with medical professionals, can determine whether they are good candidates for alternative reproduction. When patients seem desperate to get pregnant, even conscientious physicians will be susceptible to their entreaties "to try anything, just in case it works," while less responsible physicians will be tempted to take advantage of their vulnerability. Thus, it is especially important that policymakers recommend against infertility services likely to expose women, especially women between the ages of 40 and 55, to serious medical and obstetrical risks.[36]

2. *Psychological screening of gamete recipients.* The primary reason to *psychologically* screen gamete recipients and, very importantly, their partners should simply be to determine whether they are both capable of (1) giving their informed consent to using an alternative mode of reproduction, and (2) handling the emotional stress that typically accompanies certain infertility treatments. Infertility centers should not use psychological screening for the purposes of ascertaining whether a gamete recipient and her partner are "good" parent material. Even *if* it is appropriate for professionals to screen for "good" parent material in the adoption situation, there are major differences between adoption and alternative reproduction that argue for not doing so in the latter situation. Feminist lawyer Lori B. Andrews has commented:

> In adoption, there is no biological bonding determining who should be allowed to parent a child. In contrast, with alternative reproduction, there is a biological tie between one or both of the prospective parents and the child. Traditionally, society has considered that biological tie to be a sufficient indication of parental merit to let a person reproduce and rear a child without prior restraint.[37]

3. *Counseling gamete recipients.* The primary reason for counseling gamete recipients, and very importantly, their partners, should simply be to support them in their decision *to use* or *not to use* an offered alternative mode of reproduction. Not nearly enough supportive counseling is offered gamete recipients, despite the fact that individuals and couples frequently report a desire for such services. Among the issues that many gamete recipients would

welcome help resolving are: emerging problems in their marital relationship, sexual dissatisfaction, crisis reactions, anxiety surrounding efforts to achieve a pregnancy, and alternative solutions to involuntary childlessness.[38] Clearly, responsible infertility centers will want to steer a midcourse between the Scylla of underemphasizing the likelihood of something "going wrong," on the one hand, and the Charybdis of overemphasizing this likelihood, on the other. Although infertility centers should refrain from counseling gamete recipients and their partners that donor conception is utterly unproblematic—that it "will be the same as having your own," "that once conception occurs, you will forget how it happened," and "that no one needs to know"[39]—they should also refrain from counseling gamete recipients that donor conception is so arduous and fraught with difficulty that only the strongest of the strong should consider it.

B. GAMETE DONOR POLICY

1. *Medical screening of gamete donors.* One of the two equally important purposes of gamete donation should simply be to make certain that gamete donors are healthy enough to withstand the physical rigors of gamete donation. Such certitude is relatively easy to achieve with respect to sperm donors, but not with respect to egg donors. Special emphasis should be put on ascertaining and then not worsening the health status of the "super donors" mentioned above. Common sense would suggest that if a woman is repeatedly primed with hormones and vaginally aspirated, her overall health might be negatively affected.

In addition to *medically* screening gamete donors for their own benefit, it is just as crucial to screen gamete donors for the benefit of those who will be using their genetic material (to say nothing of the child who will come into existence as the result of it being used). Clearly, physicians, sperm banks, and infertility centers have an obligation to provide gamete recipients with "safe" gametes, but how disease free and "genetically correct" must gametes be to merit the label "safe"? In order to safeguard the line between the negative selection of major genetic disorders or diseases and the positive selection of "better" human attributes, it would seem that sperm and egg donors should be screened only for those diseases, defects, and disorders that the public generally regards as serious enough to constitute a reason not to procreate or to terminate a pregnancy. Thus, physicians, sperm banks, and infertility centers should probably regard the current American Fertility Society guidelines for "minimal" genetic screening for gamete donors[40] as "maximal" for all practice purposes. Similarly, it would seem that whatever items constitute the *minimal* items for the appropriate genetic matching of recipients and donors, they should also ordinarily be regarded as the *maximal* items. It is one matter to enable an infertile couple to conceive a child that resembles the one they might have conceived "naturally" and quite another to enable them to conceive a child appreciably "better" than that one.

2. *Psychological screening of gamete donors.* In the same way that the medical screening of gamete donors is twofold, so too is the psychological screening of gamete donors. It is important for physicians, sperm banks, and infertility centers to protect gamete recipients from gamete donors whose mental state might lead them to break their promise not to enter their genetic child's life. However, it is equally important to protect gamete donors both from gamete recipients who might be emotionally harassing them to be "generous," and from the psychic phantoms that might be pressuring them to act against their own best interests. Nevertheless, physicians, sperm banks, and infertility centers should proceed on the assumption that most gamete donors are normal, well-intentioned people who should not have to submit to an insultingly high number of embarrassing personal questions. In most instances, a standard personality test coupled with a professional interview should be enough to reassure medical practitioners that the gamete donor is a stable person. Importantly, physicians, sperm banks, and infertility centers should require sperm as well as egg donors to submit to whatever method of psychological screening is decided upon. Men are not necessarily more psychologically strong than women or better able to keep their promises.

3. *Counseling of gamete donors.* As important as it is to screen gamete donors both for the sake of others and for themselves, it is even more important to counsel gamete donors. Minimally, the purpose of such counseling should be to secure truly informed consent. Maximally, it should be to help gamete donors explore the nature and consequences of their action for themselves, the gamete recipients, and any child born as the result of their collaborative project.

Counseling should begin with a candid and thorough discussion of the physical, psychological, and social risks and benefits of gamete donation. Responsible counseling will, of course, vary depending on whether one is addressing a sperm or egg donor. There is, after all, no need to discuss the virtually nonexistent physical risks of sperm donation with a man, while there is great need to discuss candidly the quite serious physical risks of egg donation with a woman. Indeed, in its efforts to thoroughly explain the egg donation process, one infertility center does more than *verbally* communicate the emotional risks, inconveniences, and hardships of this process to potential egg donors. It also shows these women *videos* of vaginal aspiration (the procedure by which their oocytes will be removed), underscoring the fact that the procedure is painful enough ordinarily to require the administration of a general anesthetic.[41] Just how graphic an informed-consent presentation ought to be is, of course, debatable. Nevertheless, feminists might wish to encourage clinicians to err on the side of being more rather than less explicit, especially when a woman takes major risks in return for relatively modest benefits.

Beyond counseling egg donors in particular about the medical risks of gamete donation, physicians, sperm banks, and infertility centers should counsel both sperm donors and egg donors about the psychological risks and emotional stresses and strains of gamete donation. Responsible medical practitioners should strive to strike a balance between overemphasizing the feelings of "loss" a donor might experience, for fear of inducing them, and under-emphasizing these possible feelings, for fear of trivializing them.[42]

CONCLUSION

Finally, any proposed feminist policy for the regulation of gamete donation and reception should take care neither to unfairly burden infertile people, as compared to fertile people, nor to unfairly assist infertile people, as opposed to fertile people. When a *fertile* couple choose to procreate, they are not required to be medically screened either for their own good or for the good of the child who will be the recipient of their genes (however disordered or defective) and/or the possible recipient of some of their diseases (HIV).[43] Nor are they required to be psychologically screened for their own good or for the good of the child who will be subject to their care, however adequate or inadequate. In contrast, when an *infertile* couple decide to procreate with the assistance of third parties, they are screened for a wide range of medical and psychological conditions, and, if found fundamentally "unfit," sometimes denied access to the reproductive materials and services they need to procreate.

In defense of this disparity, physicians argue that because it is *their* science that enables infertile people to procreate collaboratively with fertile people, they have a responsibility to ensure that these people do not willfully harm others (for example, by hiding their diseases and defects) or themselves (by entering into situations that they cannot handle psychologically and/or physically). In addition, physicians argue that, for the same reason, they are partially responsible for the well-being of a child who would not have existed were it not for the interventions of medicine. (This is a point that is better made, however, with respect to egg donation than sperm donation, since it is, as we noted above, possible for a *woman* to secure sperm through nonmedical channels and to inseminate herself.)[44]

Clearly, the case for physicians having some control over the use of reproductive technologies is a reasonable one, especially because the people who seek infertility services expect to be protected from excessive physical and psychological risks and to be shielded from emotionally and financially draining legal battles. Still, from a feminist perspective, it is doubtful that it is the role of *physicians* to develop criteria for *adequate* parenting, given that ours is a pluralistic society that espouses diverse standards of good parenting.[45] Rather than exceeding the limits of their expertise, or misusing their expertise in an authoritarian manner, physicians should instead seek to set the threshold for participating in alternative modes of reproduction at the same level as that for participating in the traditional mode of reproduction. To do otherwise might well constitute an unnecessary as well as excessive limit on *infertile* individuals' procreative liberties, since the people who conceive their children through alternative means of reproduction generally want those children very much and fully intend to provide them with a nurturant environment.[46] Significantly, physicians should also take care not to provide infertile people with genetic material measurably better than their own, unless, of course, the genetic material of these people is widely viewed as seriously diseased or defective. To enhance, as opposed to correct for, the genetic endowment of infertile people might constitute an unfair genetic benefit for infertile people, an opportunity that might induce fertile people to reject traditional modes of procreation in favor of assisted reproduction.

Although it is challenging to forge a feminist policy for gamete donation and reception that does not reinforce gender stereotypes that impede women (and also men) from procreating freely and responsibly, it is necessary to do so. Feminists have an obligation to come to a consensus—or to something that resembles a consensus—about what kind of policies are most likely to increase women's genuine reproductive choices; that is, to permit women to connect with each other, with men, and with children in ways that serve their *own* best interests rather than those of "capitalism" or "patriarchy." As important as it is for feminists to emphasize diverse issues of choice, control, and connection, it is even more important for feminists to work together to forge policies that serve all sorts of women. To be sure, such policies are not likely to address all the different concerns of liberal, Marxist, radical, and cultural feminists equally well, but they are likely to address most of these concerns to approximately the same degree. Clearly "most" is not "all"; but, for this feminist, "most" would still be a lot: a practical goal toward which I, at least, intend to work.

NOTES

1. John A. Robertson, "Ethical and Legal Issues in Human Egg Donation," *Fertility and Sterility* 52 (1989): 354.

2. Ronald Munson, *Intervention and Reflection: Basic Issues in Medical Ethics*, 4th ed. (Belmont, CA: Wadsworth Publishing Co., 1992), p. 463.

3. Peter Singer and Deane Wells, *Making Babies: The New Science and Ethics of Conception* (New York: Charles Scribner's Sons, 1985), p. 74.

4. Judy Berlefein, "Searching for Fertility," *Los Angeles Times*, October 6, 1991, p. 20.

5. George Annas, "Artificial Insemination: Beyond the Best Interests of the Donor," *Hastings Center Report* 4 (1979): 14–15.

6. Andrea Mechanick Braverman, "Survey Results on the Current Practice of Ovum Donation," *Fertility and Sterility* 59 (1993): 1219.

7. Machelle M. Seibel and Ann Kiessling, "Compensating Egg Donors: Equal Pay for Equal Time?" *New England Journal of Medicine* 328 (1993): 737.

8. Braverman, pp. 1218–19.

9. Seibel and Kiessling, p. 737.

10. Robin West, "Jurisprudence and Gender," *University of Chicago Law Review* 55 (1988): 1.

11. Ibid., p. 6.

12. Ibid., p. 7.

13. Ibid., p. 12.

14. Ibid., p. 3.

15. Carol Gilligan, *In a Different Voice* (Cambridge: Harvard University Press, 1982).

16. Nel Noddings, *Caring: A Feminine Approach to Ethics and Moral Education* (Berkeley, CA: University of California Press, 1984).

17. West, p. 18.

18. Ibid., p. 29.

19. Ibid., pp. 34–35.

20. Ibid., p. 35.

21. U.S. Congress, Office of Technology Assessment. *Artificial Insemination: Practice in the United States: Summary of a 1987 Survey—Background Paper*, OTA-BP-BA-48 (Washington, DC: U.S. Government Printing Office, August 1988), p. 29.

22. Maureen McGuire and Nancy J. Alexander, "Artificial Insemination of Single Women," *Fertility and Sterility* 43 (1985): 184.

23. See, e.g., Gena Corea, *The Mother Machine* (New York: Harper and Row, 1984); Barbara Katz Rothman, "How Science Is Redefining Parenthood," *Ms.* 154, July 1982, p. 34; R. Arditti, R. G. Klein, and S. Minden, eds., *Test-Tube Women: What Future for Motherhood?* (London: Pandora Press, 1984); Norma Wikler, "Society's Response to the New Reproductive Technologies: The Feminist Perspectives," 59 *Southern California Law Review* (1986): 1043; Women's Bureau, Grael in the Rainbow, "Documentation of the Feminist Hearing on Genetic Engineering and Reproductive Technologies," Brussels, March 6–7, 1986; Helen B. Holmes, Betty B. Hoskins, and Michael Gross, eds., *The Custom-Made Child: Women-Centered Perspectives* (Clifton, NJ: Humana Press, 1981).

24. Lori B. Andrews, "Alternative Modes of Reproduction," in *Reproductive Laws for the 1900s*, Sherrill Cohen and Nadine Taub, eds. (Clifton, NJ: Humana Press, 1989), p. 371.

25. Ibid.

26. Mary Gibson, "The Moral and Legal Status of 'Surrogate' Motherhood," presented at the Eastern Division Meeting of the American Philosophical Association, 1988 (unpublished).

27. Patricia A. Avery, "Surrogate Mother: Center of a New Storm," *U.S. News and World Report*, June 6, 1983, p. 76.

28. Renatte Guelli Klein, "Doing It Ourselves: Self Insemination," in R. Arditti, R. G. Klein, and S. Minden, eds., *Test-Tube Women: What Future for Motherhood?* (London: Pandora Press, 1984), pp. 382–90.

29. Joel Feinberg, *Social Philosophy* (Englewood Cliffs, NJ: Prentice-Hall, 1973), p. 47.

30. Marge Piercy develops some of these ideas in her feminist science-fiction classic, *Women on the Edge of Time* (New York: Fawcett Crest Books, 1976).

31. Robyn Rowland, "The Social and Psychological Consequences of Secrecy in Artificial Insemination by Donor (AID) Programmes," *Social Science and Medicine* 21 (1985): 394.

32. Simone B. Novaes, "Semen Banking and Artificial Insemination by Donor in France: Social and Medical Discourse," *International Journal of Technology Assessment in Health Care* 2 (1986): 92.

33. L. R. Schover, R. L. Collins, M. M. Quigley, J. Blankstein, and G. Kanoti, "Psychological Follow-up of Women Evaluated as Oocyte Donors," *Human Reproduction* 6 (1991): 1491.

34. Ibid., p. 1490.

35. Christine Overall, *Human Reproduction: Principles, Practices, and Policies* (Toronto: Oxford University Press, 1993.)

36. American Fertility Society, *Guidelines for Gamete Donation, 1993, Fertility and Sterility*, Supplement 1, 59 (1993): S75.

37. Andrews, p. 375.

38. Patricia P. Mahlstedt and Dorothy A. Greenfeld, "Assisted Reproductive Technology with Donor Gametes: The Need for Patient Preparation," *Fertility and Sterility* 52 (1989): 909.

39. Ibid.

40. AFS *Guidelines for Gamete Donation*, Appendix B, 9S.

41. Schover et al., "Psychological Follow-up of Women Evaluated as Oocyte Donors," p. 1491.

42. Mahlstedt and Greenfeld, pp. 908–14.

43. Anne Finger, "Claiming *All* of Our Bodies: Reproductive Rights and Disability," in R. Arditti et al., eds., *Test Tube Women: What Future for Motherhood?*, 281–97.

44. Andrews, p. 379.

45. Ibid., p. 374.

46. Ibid.

ELEVEN

PRIVATE AND PUBLIC POLICY ALTERNATIVES IN OOCYTE DONATION

Andrea L. Bonnicksen, Ph.D.

Oocyte donation adds new options to the growing array of reproductive technologies. It gives women without ovarian function the chance to bear children genetically related to their partners; it predicts improved pregnancy rates for older women trying *in vitro* fertilization (IVF); it gives couples at high genetic risk new conception options; and, if intrafamilial donation is used, it lets conception stay within the family.[1] First successfully tried in 1984, by 1993 oocyte donation was offered at 135 IVF programs in the United States. In that year, physicians initiated 2,766 IVF cycles using donor oocytes and reported 716 deliveries.[2]

Oocyte donation is a safe procedure that has led to births in families that might not otherwise have had children outside of adoption.[3] It has not been accompanied by contentious lawsuits such as those associated with embryo freezing or surrogate motherhood,[4] although recent pregnancies of postmenopausal women through the aid of oocyte donation have raised ethical questions.[5] Serving a relatively small clientele, oocyte donation tends to be open and nonsecretive because in a significant minority of cases donors and recipients know one another.[6] If oocyte freezing becomes available, this option may reduce the need to freeze embryos and therefore diminish the quandaries that arise when tens of thousands of embryos are stored.

Despite the relatively uneventful practice of oocyte donation thus far, ethical questions remain and new techniques suggest future dilemmas. The "need" for donors has been assumed, rather than persuasively argued, and egg donation is promoted with little systematic review of its merits or risks as an answer for women over 40 who wish to have children. Postmenopausal pregnancies and the potential use of fetuses or cadavers as sources[7] suggest that a framework is needed to integrate variations in egg donation as they arise. As an unfolding option in assisted conception, egg donation raises questions about whether lines should be drawn and, if so, when and by whom.

This chapter first identifies issues relating to informed consent, compensation, the definition of parenthood, and new techniques. It then considers alternative policy responses in the private and public sectors, highlighting a tension that arises in all forms of assisted conception. On the one hand, public policy deals with reproduction—a matter of personal privacy—in which government involvement is not necessarily constitutional or wise. On the other hand, self-monitoring by clinicians might not be sufficiently rigorous to protect those involved with oocyte donation. The chapter thus proposes that clinicians and professional associations accelerate their self-monitoring efforts and that policymakers craft laws clarifying parent-child relationships in oocyte donation. In the meantime, despite the general absence of comprehensive laws on assisted conception in the United States, cross-cultural reports can help shape expectations of ethical and appropriate practices in oocyte donation.

ISSUES RELATING TO OOCYTE DONATION

SECURING INFORMED CONSENT

Depending on how the donor is recruited, the effects of donation range from minimal to significant. Women who donate incidental to their own IVF attempts undergo no additional medical procedures, although one cannot discount the possibility that they will experience emotional hardship if they do not conceive but know that others may have conceived with their eggs. Women who donate incidental to other medical procedures, such as hysterectomies or tubal ligations, women recruited to donate anonymously, and friends or relatives who give to designated recipients, all undergo a variety of procedures. Among other things they take powerful hormones to increase the number of oocytes available for retrieval, give blood samples, have ultrasound tests, undergo local or general anesthesia for the oocyte retrieval itself, and engage in pre- and postdonation interviews. The risks of hormonal stimulation, especially for only one cycle, are thought to be minimal, but side effects are possible, such as ovarian cysts, which can rupture and require hospitalization.[8]

While practitioners may warn donors of physical risks and inconvenience, they know less about emotional effects. Anonymous sperm donors have felt unsettled about having sired children they do not know, and one oocyte donor was quoted as saying she would not try to find out if her oocytes resulted in children, but she would wonder if "there may be children related to me somewhere in the world."[9] Neither can one predict how known donors will feel watching their genetic children being raised by friends or relatives.

Recipients also face physical and emotional uncertainty. The recipient needs medication to prepare her endometrium to receive an embryo and must be brought to menstrual synchronicity with the donor. She may face risks associated with the cause of her infertility itself. If more than one embryo is transferred, she risks a multiple pregnancy. In one reported case, a woman died during the pregnancy of twins conceived from donor oocytes, leading the authors to propose careful monitoring of multiple pregnancies and special attention to the condition of pre-eclampsia, which "may be in some way related to unfamiliar genetic material."[10] Some practitioners encourage oocyte donation for women over 40 whose oocytes are not as receptive to a continuing pregnancy as those of a younger woman.[11] Pregnancies in women over 40 or 45 pose special risks, such as pregnancy-related hypertension, which may be aggravated by a multiple pregnancy.[12]

Because the impact of donation on donors, recipients, resulting children, and family members is uncertain, only partial warnings can be conveyed to participants before they decide whether to proceed. Some information needs to be given to all donors; for example, it cannot be assumed that a sister eager to donate to her sibling needs a less detailed description of the emotional and physical risks than an anonymous donor.[13] Useful items for informed consent are descriptions of the IVF process, the problem of attaining synchronicity, statements about legal rights, a warning of unknown emotional impacts, pregnancy and birthrates at the clinic, details on medical screening of donors, and a statement of who takes responsibility if the donor or infant has complications.

Clinics vary widely in oocyte donation procedures. A survey conducted by a subgroup of the American Society for Reproductive Medicine (ASRM—formerly the American Fertility Society) showed that clinics varied in whether they screened donors for such things as sexually transmitted diseases, genetic history, drug use, and psychological stability.[14] This variation also arises in sperm donation. Oregon is one of the few states regulating screening for sperm donors; it forbids donation by any person who "has any disease or defect known by him to be transmissible by genes; or knows or has reason to know he has a venereal disease."[15]

DECIDING COMPENSATION

Two compensation errors are possible: overcompensation, which suggests trafficking in body tissues, and undercompensation, which downplays the intrusiveness of donation. Policy across nations advises against commercialism in egg donation. The Council of Europe Document on Human Artificial

Procreation recommends that ova, sperm, or embryo donors should be reimbursed only for expenses and that "no profit shall be allowed" for donation by agencies that offer gametes.[16] Spain's law on assisted conception states that "donation shall never have a profit-making or commercial nature."[17] The Swiss Academy of Medical Sciences recommends that gamete donation "must be made free of charge."[18] Overcompensation also risks economic exploitation in which women feel pressured to donate because of the lure of the money. The ASRM Guidelines for Oocyte Donation note that "[f]inancial payments should not be so excessive as to constitute undue inducement."[19]

Some observers point to undercompensation as a problem. Oocyte donation involves a demanding protocol, and access to oocytes is limited by the fact that women normally release only one oocyte a month. Donors, who are hyperstimulated to produce multiple oocytes, face a rigorous protocol, one so rigorous that Canada's Royal Commission advised against any recruitment of anonymous donors who were not donating incidental to another medical procedure or to their own IVF attempts.[20]

Of 82 clinicians responding to a survey on oocyte donation (hereinafter cited as PSIG survey), 13 used only volunteers undergoing IVF as donors and did not compensate. Those responding to the survey who did compensate paid anonymous donors between $750 and $3,500, with an average of $1,548.[21] Seibel and Kiessling suppose that a man spends two hours and receives around $50 for donor insemination, which amounts to $25 per hour. They estimate that women recruited to donate oocytes spend approximately 56 hours at the task; at $25 per hour, they should expect to receive around $1,400.[22] Laws in some states prohibit compensation for organ donation, but sperm, ova, and blood might be considered to be regenerative tissues and therefore not organs.[23] Women who donate as part of their own IVF attempts may be compensated through reduced fees. Of those clinics surveyed that used as donors women undergoing IVF, six paid one-half the costs of a single IVF cycle and one paid the entire cost of an IVF cycle for donors.[24]

Not to pay recruited donors for time and effort would be "unfair and exploitative," according to Robertson, and also discriminatory in that men are paid to donate sperm.[25] The ASRM Guidelines conclude that compensation is needed for expenses, time, inconvenience and, "to some degree," for risk and discomfort. Practitioners agree that if payment is made it should be for services rather than for the product of healthy oocytes. In addition, the ASRM Guidelines recommend that payment should not be based on the number of oocytes retrieved.[26] If women donate relative to other medical procedures, such as a hysterectomy, payment must not be an inducement for the procedure.

Oocyte donation reveals a tension in economic liberty. On the one hand, a woman's liberty is furthered if she donates eggs for financial gain; on the other hand, her liberty is diminished if economic hardship places her in the position of "selling" part of her body. In addition, to put a value on the "products" of egg donation is arguably to depersonalize and commercialize conception in a way harmful to societal interests.

Among guidelines from agencies studying the matter are these: (1) Payment must not depend on the number of oocytes retrieved or fertilized, (2) parties should specify ahead of time who takes responsibility for the donor's medical care in the event of complications, (3) clinic policies should explicitly state when and how the donor is compensated, and (4) the donor should be given ample time to weigh the proposed compensation scheme.[27] Concluding that it is "unethical to allow people to risk their health to sell parts of their bodies," the Canadian Royal Commission on New Reproductive Technologies recommended against any recruitment of donors other than those undergoing IVF or incidental medical procedures and against any payment for egg donation.[28] The Human Embryo Research Panel set up by the U.S. National Institutes of Health reached a similar conclusion that advised against egg donation for research purposes by any woman not undergoing IVF or an incidental medical procedure.[29]

DEFINING RELATIONS AMONG PARTIES

Not infrequently, egg donors and recipients know each other; of the 1,802 IVF cycles initiated with donor eggs in 1992, 429 involved known donors and 1,373 involved anonymous donors.[30] Although trust underlies situations in which friends or relatives donate eggs, one can imagine scenarios in which conflicts arise. For example, if the recipient's marriage falters during the pregnancy, it is not unrealistic to suppose the donor will seek custody of the child. If a woman in an IVF program does not conceive, but another couple has conceived with one of her oocytes, a custody attempt is imaginable. Or if the baby is born with severe disorders, a dispute in which both parties disclaim parenthood might occur, as happened in one unhappy case involving surrogate motherhood.[31]

Assisted conception has made complex the legal status of relations between parents and children. The oft-predicted five parent scenario turned into reality recently when one donor's oocyte and one donor's sperm were combined externally to produce an embryo that was transferred to a surrogate who then gave the baby to prearranged adoptive parents. This gave the child a genetic mother, a genetic father, a gestational mother, and a legal mother and father.[32] The difference between gestational and genetic parenthood has provoked legal disputes in surrogate motherhood. In the case of *In Re Baby M*, the New Jersey Supreme Court held that state policy was violated when the gestational mother's status as "mother" was terminated ahead of time by contract without cause.[33] In the case of *Johnson v. Calvert*, however, the California Supreme Court ruled that a surrogate who gave birth to a baby conceived with the egg and sperm of a contracting couple (surrogate gestational motherhood) was not the child's legal mother. Rather, under California law, she who intends to procreate is the mother.[34]

Oocyte donation increases this complexity by allowing unusual ties between mothers, daughters, sisters, and other family members. Decades after sperm freezing made sperm donation relatively common, only half of the states specify by law that the consenting husband is presumed to be the natural father. The Uniform Parentage Act of 1973 frees a sperm donor from the duties and privileges of paternity and gives those duties and privileges to the male partner, who is presumed to be the natural father if he is married to the recipient and consents in writing to donor insemination and if a physician performs the procedure.[35]

The clarification of parent-child relationships with oocyte donation is more elusive than with sperm donation. In 1988, the National Conference of Commissioners on Uniform State Laws approved the Uniform Status of Children of Assisted Conception Act (USCACA) as a model for state legislatures to adopt in whole or modified form.[36] The framers' goal was to draft a "child oriented" act that would "effect the security and well being" of children born from assisted conception. Section 4a states that "a donor is not a parent of a child conceived through assisted conception." An explanatory note clarifies that "an egg donor would not [under 4a] be the child's mother." Five states have adopted laws stipulating that the donor will not be the child's mother: Oklahoma, Texas, Florida, North Dakota, and Virginia. The laws of the rest of the states are silent on the question of maternity under oocyte donation.

This silence, which leaves unclear the legal status of children born following oocyte donation, prompted a warning in the ASRM Guidelines that donors and recipients should "be made fully aware of the legal situation, including legal uncertainty, existing in their jurisdiction." The guidelines advise parties in oocyte donation to "execute documents" in which the donor gives up the rights and duties of parenthood and the recipient takes on those rights and duties and to "consult an attorney" to protect their "legal interests."[37]

Goode and Hahn found that few patients know about legal issues in oocyte donation.[38] As such, clinics may helpfully develop a checklist of legal matters to be discussed among participants and lawyers and may require participants to sign contracts before starting the donation process. Among the legal matters to be resolved are agreements about when the donor's claims to her oocytes end; the claims, if any, she has over embryos frozen as a result of the fertilization of her donated oocytes with the sperm of the contracting male; and arrangements about confidentiality, anonymity, and record keeping at the clinic.[39]

NEW TECHNIQUES, NEW DILEMMAS

At the same time practitioners are proposing egg donation as a way of extending a woman's reproductive years, the pool of donors expands only slowly. Egg donation is more complex than sperm or embryo donation because eggs cannot safely be frozen and stored for later use. If the demand exceeds the supply, the shortage can be alleviated by either putting brakes on the demand in the first place or deciding how to increase the supply.

Demand can be reduced by not presenting egg donation as a solution to infertility or age-related problems. Yet the opposite happens in clinics, where clinicians offer egg donation not just to recruit women with anovulation or other primary causes of infertility, but also to recruit new categories of women, including those at risk of genetic disorders and those whose eggs are less fertilizable due to their age. Another way to reduce demand is to focus on the women with primary infertility so as to improve their chances of conceiving with their own eggs. Some researchers have proposed retrieving immature eggs from women before ovulation and maturing them *in vitro* as a way of circumventing their ovulation problems. *In vitro* maturation would eliminate the need for hormonal hyperstimulation, thus making IVF easier for all women by allowing new groups of women to conceive with their own eggs and easing the burden on recruited egg donors.

Proposals for increasing the supply are more contentious. In one, researchers have proposed using the eggs of aborted fetuses as donor sources.[40] As proposed, the pregnant woman and her male partner would be approached about donation after the decision to terminate the pregnancy has been reached. Each would consent to donate the fetus's eggs after abortion. A number of eggs would then be extracted from the fetal ovary, matured *in vitro*, fertilized with the prospective father's sperm, and transferred as fertilized eggs to the prospective mother's uterus in an IVF procedure. A variation of this would involve transplanting ovaries from aborted fetuses to women without ovaries with the expectation that the ovaries would begin releasing eggs within a year and lead to *in vivo* conception.[41]

Fetal egg donation raises a plethora of ethical and legal dilemmas, not the least of which is that an infant might have a genetic mother who was never born, with unsettling impacts on the infant and on the "natural order of generations."[42] Britain's Human Fertilisation and Embryology Authority announced it would not approve projects using fetal eggs in IVF, and the members of the NIH Human Embryo Research Panel also concluded that fetal egg donation was ethically unacceptable.[43] Still, some clinicians have presented this as an answer to the supposed shortage of eggs.

It has also been suggested that women could donate eggs along with their organs when they sign organ donor forms. The NIH Human Embryo Research Panel regarded cadaver egg donation for research purposes as appropriate, with provisions for informed consent, but it did not approve of clinical transfer of fertilized eggs from women or girls who had died.[44]

A third possibility is to fertilize donor eggs with the male partner's sperm and then twin the resulting fertilized eggs, which would at least double the number of embryos available from any one donor egg. The prospect of human embryo twinning met with what has been called an "ethical hullabaloo" when attempted in an experimental setting with research embryos.[45] No public national commissions have approved twinning in the clinical setting. The National Advisory Board on Ethics in Reproduction (NABER), a private national bioethics commission, issued a report indicating that it could find nothing wrong per se with embryo splitting if the resulting embryos were not damaged or destroyed in the process.[46] Virtually all NABER members agreed that certain clinical applications of embryo splitting, such as improving the chances of initiating pregnancy in those undergoing IVF, were ethically acceptable, whereas others, such as providing an adult with an identical twin to raise as his or her own child, were not. The board could not reach consensus on whether research on duplicate embryos is ethically acceptable. Embryo splitting has been proposed primarily as a way of improving success rates in IVF, however, and it is likely to remain a debatable issue.[47]

Today's egg donation, in which adult women are recruited, hyperstimulated, and compensated for their services, may well, with hindsight, turn out to be a basic model surrounded by numerous variations. Each prospect adds to the layers of consent required, complicates the blend of parent-child relations, and increases the number of matters over which guidelines are appropriate. All of this may occur to pursue a technological goal that beckons to be pursued, rather than to further a concrete need after all alternative solutions have been exhausted. Categories of potential recipients and donors are expanding, which in an extreme scenario could lead to postmenopausal women giving birth to infants fertilized from the eggs of never-born mothers. This prospect would extend procreation from the very early to the later stages of the life span.

POLICY RESPONSES TO OOCYTE DONATION

Practices in oocyte donation vary across clinics, legislation is virtually nonexistent, and appellate courts have not entertained legal conflicts. As donation becomes more common and varied, additional disputes and a heightened recognition of effects on all parties can be expected. Policy revolves around the question of whether egg donation raises pragmatic issues of low urgency that are best left to incremental and voluntary rulemaking in the private sector or serious and urgent issues best dealt with promptly and preemptively by state or national legislatures.

PRIVATE-SECTOR RULEMAKING

Private-sector rulemaking places responsibility on practitioners and their professional associations to develop guidelines on donor compensation, donor screening, age limits, and other matters relating to the daily operation of an oocyte donation program. Four loci for such rulemaking are clinics, institutional committees, professional associations, and new organizations.

Clinic-based rulemaking leaves discretion with IVF practitioners. Rules are varied, flexible, and at times intuitive. For example, the decision at one clinic to offer donors $500 was a fee, according to the clinic's director, "pulled out of the air."[48] The range of practices revealed in the PSIG survey illustrates trial and error, clinic-based rulemaking, which also guided IVF and embryo freezing.[49]

A key advantage of clinic rulemaking is that clinicians see dilemmas first-hand and they can identify some problems earlier than outside observers or policymakers. Incentives for self-monitoring include desires to avoid lawsuits, preempt governmental policy, maintain integrity in a controversial field, and attract patients through proven track records. On the other hand, the narrow medical setting and a reluctance to weigh broader ethical issues confine the clinician's perspective. Clinicians sell a service and are not impartial arbiters of how that service should be marketed and carried out. Practices at private clinics may be influenced by the need to maintain a financially viable program.[50]

The perspectives of rulemaking broaden when cross-disciplinary review boards or ethics committees contribute to clinic policies. These committees can suggest changes in written consent forms and clinic procedures. Clinicians may not be inclined to consult with ethics committees, however. While 73% of the respondents to the PSIG survey had access to an institutional ethics committee, only 31% used that committee to plan their oocyte donation programs.[51] Moreover, ethics committee members may be unduly sympathetic to the hospital's goals, and private IVF clinics may not have ethics committees with which to consult.

Professional associations, such as ASRM and the American College of Obstetricians and Gynecologists (ACOG) also contribute to private-sector rulemaking. Guidelines drafted by these associations reflect coherent beliefs about how assisted conception is to be administered, they are distributed to clinicians, and they provide a reasonably detailed set of standards to be followed. It is questionable whether practitioners read them carefully, however, and, as documents reached by consensus and meant for general as well as professional readership, committee reports are not necessarily rigorous nor is their logic developed in great detail.

A third level of rulemaking involves organizations created specifically to oversee assisted conception. For example, in 1984 physicians set up a group later renamed the Society for Assisted Reproductive Technology (SART). Directors of IVF clinics apply for membership and are accepted if their programs meet minimum standards. Among other things, SART maintains a registry to gather data annually from member programs on such matters as the number of patients, IVF cycles started, embryo transfers, clinical pregnancies, and abnormal births.[52] Data gathering expands in scope as new techniques, such as oocyte donation, join the repertoire of assisted conception.

The National Advisory Board for Ethics in Reproduction (NABER) is another private group, this one a cross-disciplinary, nonpartisan organization formed by the ASRM and ACOG and now a separate legal entity funded by private foundations. Among other activities, NABER reviews ethical questions raised by reproductive technologies and prepares reports and guidelines for use by policymakers, practitioners, and the general public. The Nuffield Council on Bioethics, set up in Great Britain in 1991, also weighs bioethical issues of public interest.[53] National governments can empower such groups to develop ethical guidelines for research and practice, which gives governmental imprimatur to the organization while avoiding direct governmental involvement.

Private-sector rulemaking has pragmatic merit. One alternative to private-sector monitoring, restrictive legislation, is of doubtful constitutionality in the United States if it intrudes on reproduction and privacy. For example, laws in Sweden and Norway forbid oocyte donation altogether. Sweden's Law No. 711 (1988) forbids the transfer of an embryo to a woman if the oocyte is not her own or if the sperm is not that of her partner, and Norway's Law No. 68 (1987) states that "[t]he fertilized egg may be placed only in the woman in whom it originated."[54] The Swiss Academy of Medical Sciences has issued guidelines recommending that ova and sperm donation take place only if the recipients are married and if donor ova or sperm are used, but not both together.[55]

Such restrictions would probably not withstand constitutional scrutiny in the United States. Although the U.S. Supreme Court has not explicitly defined a constitutional right to procreate, Court decisions arguably confer implicit constitutional protection on citizens' interest in procreating.[56] Courts have concluded that procreative autonomy includes both the right to procreate and the right to avoid procreation,[57] which places on the government the burden of justifying substantive restrictions on oocyte donation. Moreover, many issues in oocyte donation warrant discussion, data gathering, introspection, and publicity, but arguably are not so compelling as to merit substantive restrictions at this time.

Procedural limits on the time, place, and manner of oocyte donation might, on the other hand, be justified as proper state powers to protect the citizens' health and welfare. For example, Spain's law on donor insemination states that no one sperm donor may sire more than six children, and the Swiss Medical Academy recommends that only ten children be born from gametes from any one ovum or sperm donor.[58] Still, states in the United States have been slow to enact laws monitoring donor insemination, which leads one to question the alacrity with which states will monitor oocyte donation. The realities of interest-group politics caution against expecting state legislation in the near future. Although some observers see egg donation as immoral and illicit and others criticize variations such as postmenopausal pregnancies and cross-sibling donation,[59] no organized, policy-oriented voice advocates restrictive legislation. On the contrary, the popular press depicts intrafamilial ovum donation sympathetically. Because legislators tend to react to rather than anticipate crises, the absence of a visible opposition, medical mishaps, and judicial disputes works against regulation. Without an "attentive public," regulation is not a high policy priority for lawmakers. This makes private-sector oversight a feasible alternative, if done carefully and with attention to the broader societal interests over assisted conception.

In the absence of state laws, clinicians and their associations have developed somewhat detailed recommendations. For example, clinics have put age limits on donors and recipients and have barred donation between children and parents.[60] The ASRM recommends that clinicians limit the number of children born from any one donor and requires donors to be of legal age.[61] Although not legally enforceable, such limits will be ignored by clinics only at some risk. For example, obtaining oocytes from 16-year-old donors would attract negative publicity, and using older women as donors would hinder pregnancy rates. When some IVF clinics distorted pregnancy and birthrates, IVF colleagues themselves called attention to the distortions, presumably to protect the integrity of the profession, avoid alienating clients, and prevent restrictive legislation.[62] On the other hand, a number of years ago, Curie-Cohen and colleagues revealed limited self-policing at donor insemination facilities.[63] Even after the authors published these findings, clinics only sporadically screened donors for genetic disorders and venereal diseases,[64] thus showing that negative publicity does not automatically translate to stringent self-monitoring by clinics.

If motivated to do so, clinics and professional associations can contribute to an emerging consensus about appropriate and inappropriate egg donation practices. This, in effect, becomes an egg donation policy, defined as a "general direction of thought and action, providing a basic framework for making decisions."[65] Private-sector policy is incremental, after-the-fact, and pragmatically geared to clinic protocols. Egg donation provokes concerns about aggressive recruitment of anonymous donors and overeager recruitment of older recipients, however, that might not best be addressed by practitioners themselves. Moreover, some proposed techniques provoke ethical concerns that extend beyond the parties in assisted conception to include broader public interests. In addition, donation raises legal quandaries that cannot be resolved in the private sphere no matter how great the motivation. For practices undergirded by ethical and legal uncertainty, public-sector rulemaking provides alternatives.

PUBLIC-SECTOR RULEMAKING

Several layers of public involvement, ranging from exploratory and voluntaristic to specific and legalistic, can be identified: setting up a national commission, establishing a national licensing authority, tapping existing regulations, waiting for court interpretations, and enacting state or federal legislation.

Commissions set up by national governments to review and make recommendations about assisted conception are common in Western industrial nations.[66] In 1984 the British Warnock Commission produced, after lengthy deliberation, a report that formed the basis for a government White Paper and eventually a parliamentary law.[67] In 1989 the Canadian government set up the Royal Commission on New Reproductive Technologies, the members of which conducted surveys, focus groups, and personal interviews, set up toll-free telephone numbers, and held highly publicized meetings. In all, they contacted 40,000 Canadians and then disseminated the findings of their two-volume, 1,000-page report through 1,000 media interviews and the distribution of one-quarter million information kits.[68] The French National Consultative Ethics Committee on Life and Medical Sciences was set up by presidential decree in 1983 to advise the government on bioethical matters. It has 41 members from varied disciplines, and it has published over 30 reports and statements on such practices as surrogate motherhood and embryo research.[69]

In Canada, the National Council on Bioethics, set up in 1989, also issues advisory guidelines on problematic areas of biomedicine.[70] Not infrequently, commission reports lead to the creation of national regulatory bodies that frame accreditation standards and license facilities engaging in assisted conception and/or embryo research. According to Andrews and Elster, seven of eleven countries in which commissions issued reports on assisted conception mention a cross-disciplinary body for overseeing reproductive technologies and embryo research.[71] The British Licensing Authority, enacted into law with the Human Fertilisation and Embryology Act of 1990, issues licenses to clinics for infertility treatment, storage of gametes, and research. It sets preconditions of and limits to research and practice.[72] Canada's Royal Commission on New Reproductive Technologies also recommended that a permanent regulatory and licensing body be set up to oversee all reproductive technologies.

A licensing authority allows flexibility because it sets up a system in which experts from multiple disciplines can integrate new technical developments without having to craft laws for each new technique. As Andrews and Elster note, "One way in which legislation can accommodate the dynamic nature of science and the questions new technologies raise would be to set general bounds and appoint a regulatory body to address specific issues as they arise."[73]

In the United States review boards have been ad hoc and short-lived. In 1979, members of the Ethics Advisory Board, appointed by the director of the Department of Health, Education and Welfare, concluded that *in vitro* fertilization was ethically acceptable and open to funding from the federal government with limits.[74] The board was disbanded and not reappointed, however, which imposed a de facto moratorium on funding for projects involving human embryos, inasmuch as federal policy required review by an ethics board for funding to take place. The disbanding had a secondary effect of eliminating a national forum through which issues relating to IVF could have been weighed. In 1984, witnesses testifying on IVF and embryo transfer in the U.S. Congress spoke with "remarkable unanimity" of the need to set up a national body to review, oversee, and educate citizens about reproductive technologies.[75] An effort by Congress to set up the Biomedical Ethics Board in 1985 failed when members of Congress could not agree on its composition, which also foreclosed the chance of a national forum for weighing issues raised by reproductive technologies.

In 1993, the Office of Technology Assessment recommended that a national agency be formed to review issues relating to biomedical technologies.[76] Then the NIH Revitalization Act of 1993 repealed the section of the Public Health Service Act that required a biomedical ethics board to review research proposals relating to embryos.[77] This lifted the de facto funding moratorium. The director of the NIH then appointed a panel to recommend guidelines that divided research into three categories: ethically acceptable, ethically unacceptable, and needing further review.

President Clinton disagreed with one of the panel's conclusions, namely, that embryos could, within limits, ethically be generated solely for research.[78] Researchers who have submitted proposals must wait for the NIH Director to act on the recommendations before learning what will and will not be funded by the government. While the government might refrain from funding projects involving the deliberate fertilization of eggs for research, such fertilization is not illegal. Withholding of funds denies legitimacy to the research, however, and it forecloses a forum for weighing the merits of research involving embryos. It has implications for egg donation, too, in that it slows research designed to test the safety of *in vitro* maturation of eggs or of egg freezing. For example, the need for egg donors might be lessened if multiple eggs are retrieved from each donor, frozen, and stored. An important step in making sure egg freezing is safe is to freeze eggs and then thaw and fertilize them to check such things as cleavage rates, morphology, and chromosomal composition. These fertilized research eggs would then be discarded, rather than transferred. Such studies are precluded if researchers believe they cannot fertilize eggs solely for research purposes because they do not have the funding for it or because they are wary of conducting studies without governmental imprimatur.

In the absence of a national review procedure for monitoring assisted conception, existing administrative regulations present a policy alternative. In 1992, Congress passed the Fertility Clinic Success and Certification Act, setting a structure for data gathering and the monitoring of IVF programs under the auspices of state medical agencies.[79] The Food and Drug Administration has taken steps to regulate tissue banks,[80] and it recommends that clinicians use only frozen sperm so donors can be tested for the human immunodeficiency virus.[81] Congress has considered bills to regulate the handling of tissues for transplantation, which could be interpreted to include gamete freezing banks.[82] The Federal Trade Commission has filed charges against IVF clinics for alleged misrepresentation of pregnancy rates.[83] These activities monitor clear and preventable injuries, such as those arising from inadequate laboratory conditions or unqualified personnel, and presumably do not intrude on constitutional rights.

Another policy model looks to the courts to craft and refine principles. Although judges reluctantly frame policy in matters that state legislatures normally oversee, their rulings provide authoritative guidance if state legislatures are silent or if the issue is novel. Appellate courts in assisted conception have proposed principles such as the relative burden test of *Davis v. Davis* and the intentionality principle of *Calvert v. Johnson*. Judicial decisions framed the principles in another area of medicine—end-of-life decision making—where cases, beginning with *Matter of Quinlan,* defined issues and proposed tests for making decisions and procedures for carrying them out.[84] Today, two decades after the Quinlan case, areas of consensus are identifiable,[85] and policy has spread from state legislatures and lower courts to the U.S. Congress and U.S. Supreme Court.[86] A similar model of incremental policy, in which state legislatures and lower courts experiment with alternatives, is not unlikely for defining parent-child relationships in assisted conception.

A final policy model enacts specific laws at either the state or federal level. The USCACA has prompted states to define relations between others and children in egg donation. The Royal Commission in Canada recommended that the provinces and territories amend existing family law to clarify relations in assisted reproduction.[87] At the federal level in the United States, no national law on assisted reproduction is in view, partly because of deep-seated political differences in matters involving reproduction. A number of European nations have passed laws ranging from strict (e.g., Norway) to more permissive (e.g., Great Britain).[88]

CONCLUSION

Issues in oocyte donation suggest that limits are appropriate, but debate revolves around what should be limited and by whom. For example, in response to news about pregnancies in postmenopausal women, French lawmakers introduced restrictive legislation to bar the practice.[89] In the United States, some commentators voiced concern for maternal health and for the needs of children born to older women, but others saw the reversal of a woman's age-related "precipitous fall in fecundity" through donor eggs[90] as a legitimate extension of reproductive liberty. To forbid oocyte donation to postmenopausal women in the United States would raise constitutional challenges regarding Fifth and Fourteenth Amendment liberty interests and also equal protection guarantees if the law barred the pregnancies of women past a certain age, but not fatherhood by men.

Substantive limits on reproductive technologies in the United States require a compelling need that does not seem to be met, at least in the context of the few women who elect to bear children past the age of 50. Procedural limits for age-related and other issues are more easily imposed, but the motivation and constituency to do so appear to be minimal. In the absence of regulations, therefore, clinics and professional associations bear the responsibility for developing rules and limits.

New techniques and new dilemmas in egg donation point to the need for accelerated incrementalism in which practitioners and their professional associations plan and implement cross-clinic rules about acceptable donors and recipients, the scope of medical and psychological screening, the content of consent forms, compensation schemes, and confidentiality practices. Private-sector organizations, such as the Nuffield Council in Britain or NABER in the United States, provide welcome direction, as do reports commissioned by governments in Canada and several European nations. Among other things, agencies independent of the medical sector can question assumptions that drive egg donation, such as the largely untested assumption that there is an urgent shortage of eggs. In the meantime, state legislatures may adopt laws, such as the USCACA, to clarify parentage for gamete donation, which has become an established part of assisted conception.

The relative absence of legislation in the United States cannot excuse any failure to develop systematic practices about oocyte donation in light of cross-national agreement that, among other things, great care must be taken to make sure donors freely consent to give eggs, women who donate incidental to hysterectomies or other surgeries must give independent consent for each procedure, women must not be placed at risk during donation, and eggs must not be bought or sold. While explicit rulemaking eventually might be advisable for assisted conception as a whole, minimum lawmaking today does not connote an absence of cross-cultural expectations about appropriate and inappropriate practices in oocyte donation.

NOTES

1. Mark V. Sauer, Richard J. Paulson, and Rogerio A. Lobo, "Reversing the Natural Decline in Human Fertility: An Extended Clinical Trial of Oocyte Donation to Women of Advanced Reproductive Age," *Journal of the American Medical Association* 268 (1992): 1275–79; Paul F. Serhal and Ian L. Craft, "Oocyte Donation in 61 Patients," *Lancet* I/8648 (1989): 1185–87.

2. Society for Assisted Reproductive Technology, American Society for Reproductive Medicine, "Assisted Reproductive Technology in the United States and Canada: 1993 Results Generated from the American Society for Reproductive Medicine/

Society for Assisted Reproductive Technology Registry," *Fertility and Sterility* 64 (1995): 13–21.

3. Martin M. Quigley, "The New Frontier of Reproductive Age," (Editorial) *Journal of the American Medical Association* 268 (1992): 1320–21.

4. *Davis v. Davis*, 1992 Tenn. Lexis 400; *York v. Jones*, 717 F.Supp. 421 (E. D. Va 1989); *In the Matter of Baby M*, 537 A.2d 1227 (1988); *Stiver v. Parker et al.*, 975 F.2d 261 (6th Cir. 1992).

5. Andrea Borini, Gabriella Baforo, Flavia Violini, Liana Bianchi et al., "Pregnancies in Postmenopausal Women Over 50 Years Old in an Oocyte Donation Program," *Fertility and Sterility* 63 (1994): 258–61.

6. American Fertility Society, "Guidelines for Oocyte Donation," *Fertility and Sterility* 59 (1993): 5S-7S.

7. Asher Shushan and Josef G. Schenker, "The Use of Oocytes Obtained from Aborted Fetuses in Egg Donation Programs," *Fertility and Sterility* 62 (1994): 449–51.

8. Martin M. Quigley, "Screening Providers of Gametes and Embryos," in *Emerging Issues in Biomedical Policy: An Annual Review*, ed. Robert H. Blank and Andrea L. Bonnicksen (New York: Columbia University Press, 1989): I, pp. 238–51.

9. Nadine Brozan, "Babies from Donated Eggs: Growing Use Stirs Questions," *New York Times*, January 18, 1988, pp. A1, A17.

10. Susan Bewley and Jeremy T. Wright, "Maternal Death Associated with Ovum Donation Twin Pregnancy," *Human Reproduction* 6 (1991): 898–99. For information on the risk of preeclampsia in women pregnant after egg donation, see C. T. Lee, P. Patrizio, M. Morgan, J. P. Balmaceda, and R. H. Asch, "Obstetric Outcome of Pregnancies from Donor Oocytes," Abstracts of the 43rd Annual Meeting of the Pacific Coast Fertility Society, April 26–30, 1995. Program Supplement, P. A32.

11. Sauer et al.

12. Ethics Committee of the American Fertility Society, "Ethical Considerations of the New Reproductive Technologies," *Fertility and Sterility*, Supplement 2, 53 (1990): 49S; Borini et al.

13. For a discussion of the special dilemmas facing the intrafamilial donor, see Jennifer Gunning and Veronica English, *Human In Vitro Fertilization: A Case Study in the Regulation of Medical Innovation* (Brookfield, VT: Dartmouth Publishing Company, 1993), pp. 75–76, 78.

14. Andrea Mechanick Braverman, 1993, "Survey Results on the Practice of Ovum Donation," *Fertility and Sterility* 59 (1993): 1216–20.

15. Amy L. Fracassini, "The Regulation of Sperm Banks and Fertility Doctors: A Cry for Prophylactic Measures," *Journal of Contemporary Health Law and Policy* 8 (1992): 275–307; Or. Rev. Stat. Sec. 677.370 (1989).

16. "Council of Europe Publishes Principles in the Field of Human Artificial Procreation," *International Digest of Health Legislation* 40 (1989): 907–12.

17. "Law No. 35/1988 of 22 November 1988 on Assisted Reproduction Procedures. Boletin Oficial del Estado, 24 November 1988, No. 282, pp. 33373–33378," reprinted in *International Digest of Health Legislation* 90 (1989): 82–93.

18. "Swiss Academy of Medical Sciences Issues Medico-Ethical Guidelines on Medically Assisted Procreation (1990 Version)," *International Digest of Health Legislation* 42 (1991): 346–50.

19. American Fertility Society, "Guidelines," p. 6S.

20. Royal Commission on New Reproductive Technologies, *Proceed with Care:*

Final Report of the Royal Commission on New Reproductive Technologies (Ottawa: Minister of Government Services, Canada, 1993), p. 592.

21. Braverman, p. 1218.

22. Machelle M. Seibel and Ann Kiessling, "Compensating Egg Donors: Equal Pay for Equal Time?" Letter to Editor, *New England Journal of Medicine* 328 (1993): 737.

23. John A. Robertson, "Ethical and Legal Issues in Human Egg Donation," *Fertility and Sterility* 52 (1989): 353–63.

24. Braverman, p. 1218.

25. Robertson, p. 360.

26. American Fertility Society, "Guidelines," p. 6S.

27. Guidelines published by the Interim Licensing Authority in Britain, for example, recommend that when donors are recruited among women undergoing medical procedures; any inducement of reduced or no charges should be offered only after the medical care is decided. Gunning and English, p. 203.

28. Royal Commission, p. 594.

29. National Institutes of Health, "Report of the Human Embryo Research Panel. Final Draft," September 27, 1994, p. 69.

30. Society for Assisted Reproductive Technology, American Fertility Society, "Assisted Reproductive Technology in the United States and Canada: 1992 Results Generated from the American Fertility Society/Society for Assisted Reproductive Technology Registry," *Fertility and Sterility* 62 (1994): 1121–28, at 1125.

31. *Stiver v. Parker et al.,* 975 F.2d 261 (6th Cir. 1992).

32. "California Baby Is Group Effort," *Chicago Tribune,* August 2, 1993, p. 3.

33. *In the Matter of Baby M,* 537 A.2d 1227 (1988).

34. *Johnson v. Calvert,* 1993 Cal. LEXIS 2474 (May 20, 1993).

35. Uniform Parentage Act, 9B U. L. A. 287 (1973).

36. Uniform Status of Children of Assisted Conception Act, 9B U. L. A. Suppl. 87 (1988).

37. American Fertility Society, "Guidelines," p. 7S.

38. Colleen J. Goode and Sandra J. Hahn, "Oocyte Donation and In Vitro Fertilization: The Nurse's Role with Ethical and Legal Issues," *Journal of Obstetric, Gynecologic and Neonatal Nursing* 22 (1993): 106–11.

39. For a discussion of secrecy in oocyte donation, see John A. Robertson, "Technology and Motherhood: Legal and Ethical Issues in Human Egg Donation," *Case Western Reserve Law Review* 39 (1988–1989): 1–38, 14–16.

40. Shushan and Schenker.

41. UK Human Fertilisation and Embryo [*sic*] Authority, "Donated Ovarian Tissue in Embryo Research and Assisted Conception: Public Consultation Document," *Human Reproduction* 9 (1994): 931–35.

42. National Institutes of Health, p. 72.

43. UK Human Fertilisation; National Institutes of Health.

44. National Institutes of Health, p. 72.

45. Howard W. Jones, Jr., Robert G. Edwards, George E. Seidel, Jr., "On Attempts at Cloning in the Human," *Fertility and Sterility* 61 (1994): 423–26; J. L. Hall, D. Engel, P. R. Gidoff, G. L. Mottla, R. J. Stillman, "Experimental Cloning of Human Polyploid Embryos Using an Artificial Zona Pellucida." Paper presented at the 1993 annual meeting of the American Fertility Society. Program Supplement.

46. National Advisory Board on Ethics in Reproduction, "Report on Human

Cloning through Embryo Splitting: An Amber Light," *Kennedy Institute of Ethics Journal* 4 (1994): 251–81, 266.

47. Andrea Bonnicksen, "Ethical and Policy Issues in Human Embryo Twinning," *Cambridge Quarterly of Healthcare Ethics* 4 (1995): 268–84.

48. Brozan, p. A17.

49. Andrea L. Bonnicksen, *In Vitro Fertilization: Building Policy from Laboratories to Legislatures* (New York: Columbia University Press, 1989), pp. 36–45.

50. Glenn Kramon, "Infertility Chain: The Good and Bad in Medicine," *New York Times*, June 19, 1992, p. C1.

51. Braverman, pp. 1217–19.

52. See, e.g., Society for Assisted Reproductive Technology.

53. U.S. Congress, Office of Technology Assessment, *Biomedical Ethics in U.S. Public Policy—Background Paper*. OTA-BP-BBS-105. Washington, DC: U.S. Government Printing Office, 1993, pp. 51–52.

54. Sweden. "Law No. 711 of 14 June 1988 on Fertilization Outside the Human Body," reprinted in *International Digest of Health Legislation* 40/1 (1989): 93; "Law No. 68 of 12 June 1987 on Artificial Fertilization. Norsk Lovtidend, Section I, 26 June 1987, No. 13, pp. 502–503. Norway," reprinted in *International Digest of Health Legislation* 38 (1987): 782–85.

55. "Swiss Academy," p. 348.

56. Robertson, "Technology and Motherhood," pp. 9–11. But see J. Kennard, dissenting in *Johnson v. Calvert*, 1993 Cal. LEXIS 2474 (1988).

57. *Davis v. Davis*, 1992 Tenn. LEXIS 400.

58. "Law No. 35/1988," p. 84; "Swiss Academy," p. 349.

59. "Instruction on Respect for Human Life in Its Origin and the Dignity of Procreation: Replies to Certain Questions of the Day." Doctrinal Statement of the Vatican, March 10, 1987, in *Ethical Issues in the New Reproductive Technologies*, ed. Richard T. Hull (Belmont, CA: Wadsworth Publishing Company, 1990), pp. 21–39; William E. Schmidt, "Birth to a 59-Year-Old Generates an Ethical Controversy in Britain," *New York Times*, December 29, 1993, p. A1.

60. Braverman, p. 1218.

61. American Fertility Society, "Guidelines," pp. 6S-7S.

62. Soules; Blackwell et al.

63. Martin Curie-Cohen et al., "Current Practice of Artificial Insemination by Donor in the United States," *New England Journal of Medicine* 300 (1979): 585–88.

64. Barry R. Furrow, Sandra H. Johnson, Timothy S. Jost, and Robert L. Schwartz, *Bioethics: Health Care Law and Ethics* (St. Paul, MN: West Publishing Co., 1991), p. 118.

65. Daniel Callahan, *What Kind of Life?: The Limits of Medical Progress* (New York: Touchstone, 1990), p. 160.

66. Lori B. Andrews and Nanette Elster, "Cross-Cultural Analysis of Policies regarding Embryo Research." Unpublished commissioned paper for the National Institutes of Health, Human Embryo Research Panel.

67. Mary Warnock, *A Question of Life: The Warnock Report on Human Fertilisation and Embryology* (Oxford: Basil Blackwell, 1985).

68. Royal Commission.

69. U.S. Congress, Office of Technology Assessment, p. 46. For a discussion of bioethics initiatives by 32 national governments, see ibid., pp. 43–52.

70. Ibid., p. 44.

71. Andrews and Elster, p. 14.

72. "Human Fertilisation and Embryology Act 1990," *International Digest of Health Legislation* 42 (1991): 69–85.

73. Andrews and Elster, p. 14.

74. Ethics Advisory Board, Department of Health, Education, and Welfare, *Appendix: HEW Support of Research Involving Human In Vitro Fertilization and Embryo Transfer*. Washington, DC: GPO. May 4, 1979.

75. Albert Gore, Jr., *Congressional Record* (November 17, 1983) 129, No. 160, Part II, 98th Congress, 1st Session H10292.

76. U.S. Congress, Office of Technology Assessment, p. 38.

77. NIH Revitalization Act of 1993 (P. L. 103–43, 107 Stat. 133).

78. Stephen Burd, "U.S. Won't Back Creation of Human Embryos for Research," *The Chronicle of Higher Education*, December 14, 1994, p. A32.

79. Fertility Clinic Success Rate and Certification Act of 1992. P. L. 102–493 (October 24, 1992).

80. "New FDA Rules for Donor Tissue," *American Medical News* 36 (December 27, 1993): p. 2.

81. Fracassini, p. 281.

82. "Bill Would Regulate Transplant Tissue," *American Medical News* 37 (January 10, 1994): p. 12.

83. Robert Pear, "Fertility Clinics Face Crackdown," *New York Times*, October 26, 1992, p. A7.

84. *Matter of Quinlan*, 355 A. 2d 647 (N.J. 1976).

85. Alan Meisel, "The Legal Consensus about Forgoing Life-Sustaining Treatment: Its Status and Prospects," *Kennedy Institute of Ethics Journal* 2 (1992): 309–45.

86. Patient Self-Determination Act of 1991. Sections 4206 and 4751 of the Omnibus Budget Reconciliation Act of 1990 (P. L. 101–508); *Cruzan v. Director, Missouri Health Department*, 111 L.Ed. 2d 224 (1990).

87. Royal Commission, p. 595.

88. B. M. Knoppers and S. LeBris, "Recent Advances in Medically Assisted Conception: Legal, Ethical and Society Issues," *American Journal of Law and Medicine* 27 (1991): 329–61; Derek Morgan and Linda Nielsen, "Prisoners of Progress or Hostages to Fortune?" *Journal of Law, Medicine, and Ethics* 21 (1993): 30–42.

89. Alan Riding, "French Government Proposes Ban on Pregnancies after Menopause," *New York Times*, January 5, 1994, p. A4.

90. Daniel Navot, Michael R. Drews, Paul A. Bergh, Ida Guzman et al., "Age-Related Decline in Female Fertility Is Not Due to Diminished Capacity of the Uterus to Sustain Embryo Implantation," *Fertility and Sterility* 61 (1994): 97–101.

TWELVE

LEGAL UNCERTAINTIES IN HUMAN EGG DONATION

John A. Robertson, J.D.

One of the fastest-growing areas of assisted reproduction is human egg donation. Over 137 *in vitro* fertilization (IVF) programs in the United States and Canada now offer the procedure,[1] and thousands of women suffering from ovarian dysfunction or advanced reproductive age are potential candidates. Egg donation raises several ethical and legal issues that need attention if it is to be used in a productive and beneficial way.

In egg donation, a woman's ovaries are stimulated with hormones, multiple eggs are removed, and the eggs are fertilized *in vitro* with the sperm of the partner of a woman who cannot herself produce viable eggs. The fertilized eggs or embryos are then placed in the uterus of the recipient (whose cycle has been synchronized with that of the donor) or cryopreserved for use by the recipient in a later cycle. If successful, the transferred embryos implant, and the recipient gives birth to a child that she and her husband then rear. Unless the egg donor is a friend or family member, the egg donor ordinarily has no contact with the recipient or offspring.

Medically, egg donation offers great hope to thousands of women who cannot themselves produce healthy or viable eggs. Many of these women have premature ovarian failure or are surgically castrate. Others are of advanced reproductive age and have a poor prognosis of fertility with other therapies. For example, women over 40 have a higher success rate with donor oocytes than with IVF using their own eggs.[2] Indeed, a recent report suggests that women in their late 40s or even early 50s can deliver children after egg donation.[3]

While the donor may be another woman going through IVF who donates extra eggs, the advent of cryopreservation of embryos has reduced the supply of donor eggs from this source. Increasingly egg donations come from friends or family members whom the recipient herself recruits, or from anonymous donors recruited by the center providing the service. In the latter case, the donors are extensively screened, and usually paid from $1,200 to $2,000 for their services.

Egg donation thus appears to be a medically safe and effective way to produce children for women who cannot themselves produce healthy eggs. It has a higher success rate for this group of patients than other therapies. It also replicates more closely than do donor sperm or surrogacy the biological ties that usually exist between parents and offspring. Egg donation enables each rearing parent to have a biologic connection with offspring, with only the female genetic connection missing.

Because egg donation is still relatively new, a full assessment of its effects on offspring, donors, infertile couples, and society must await further experience. Nevertheless, it is reasonable to assume that its net effects will be positive for most, if not all, participants. Given the existing acceptability of IVF and of donor insemination, the combination of IVF and gamete donation in the form of egg donation should also be ethically and legally acceptable.

Except in five states, however, there is no legislation or court decision that now directly addresses egg donation and thus clarifies whether the parties' intentions to exclude the egg donor from all rearing rights and duties in offspring will have legal effect. Some states also have laws against buying and selling human organs and tissue which could restrict buying and selling human oocytes. Nor is it clear whether donors who are injured in the course of donation must bear those costs or whether other parties can be held responsible. A variety of other legal questions arise, from the offspring's right to have information about her genetic mother to questions about whether egg donation to women who are past the normal age of childbearing can be banned.

While these uncertainties present no insuperable barrier to performing egg donation, they do require that physicians, hospitals, couples, donors, and others involved in egg donation pay careful attention to how they conduct the practice. The following discussion identifies the main legal issues that need attention and suggests reasonable steps to deal with current legal uncertainty. Until the law is clarified by legislation or judicial decision, egg donation programs that are conducted with full disclosure of existing risks and uncertainties should be legally acceptable, with the caveats discussed below.

REARING RIGHTS AND DUTIES

A major legal issue with egg donation concerns rearing rights and duties in offspring. In almost all instances, the intent of the parties is to have the sperm provider and the recipient be the rearing father and mother for all purposes, and for the donor to have no rearing rights and duties at all. This goal will exist even if friends or family members act as egg donors. Egg donation thus attempts to replicate the situation that ordinarily occurs with donor sperm to a married couple, in which the consenting husband is the legal father for all purposes, and an anonymous donor has no rearing rights or duties.

A problem, however, for recipients and donors at the present time is that only Oklahoma, Texas, Florida, North Dakota, and Virginia[4] have enacted legislation that specifically recognizes such intentions as legally determinative of rearing rights and duties in offspring. Until legislators or judges address this issue, participants in egg donation in other states will lack certainty that their preconception intentions will be legally binding. They must be fully informed of this uncertainty, and should execute consent forms and releases which clearly state their intentions and which acknowledge the uncertainty which they face.

The absence of legislation, however, does not mean that the express intentions of the parties will not be honored if a legal dispute arises over rearing rights and duties in children born of egg donation. In sperm donation, for example, the intention of the parties to exclude the sperm donor and assign all rearing rights and duties to the consenting husband is recognized by statute or court decisions in over 30 states.[5] A court faced with a dispute over rearing rights and duties in egg donation is likely to follow the donor sperm model, as do the egg donation laws enacted in Oklahoma, Texas, Florida, and Virginia.

DONOR ATTEMPTS TO REAR CHILD

Consider, for example, two types of disputes that could arise over rearing rights and duties with egg donation. One would be where the donor as genetic mother later attempts to assert some rearing rights in offspring. Since ordinarily a sperm donor would not have the legal right to play a parenting role, it is hard to see why an egg donor should have any greater claim. She explicitly waived or relinquished her parental rights in providing the egg, just as a sperm donor does, and a later change of mind should not give her any greater right of access to her genetic offspring than a sperm donor has. Although she did undergo ovarian stimulation and surgical retrieval to provide the eggs, she would not have had the experience of pregnancy and childbirth, which distinguishes the claim of surrogate mothers who in some states may retain rearing rights despite their promise to relinquish custody after birth. Fairness requires that the original intentions of the parties, on which all relied, be followed.

In the absence of a statute giving effect to agreements to exclude the genetic mother from rearing, it is reasonable to assume that courts, if faced with such a dispute, would side with the recipient couple and exclude the egg donor from any rearing role. Only a state that insisted on defining motherhood in genetic, but not gestational, terms might regard the matter differently. In *Calvert v. Johnson*, a case involving a gestational surrogate who wanted to play a rearing role after birth, the California Court of Appeals did hold that motherhood, like fatherhood, was to be determined on genetic grounds.[6] In that decision the court held that a gestational surrogate was not the "mother" of the child that she carried and gave birth to, because the egg was provided by another woman. If that rationale for the decision had been affirmed, an egg donor, like the woman providing the egg for surrogate gestation, would have been the "mother" under California law and thus have standing to seek visitation or custody of resulting children.

However, this rationale did not survive the California Supreme Court's affirmation of the court's decision awarding sole custody of the child to the hiring couple that had provided the embryo that the surrogate had gestated and brought to term.[7] That court excluded the gestational surrogate from any rearing role and awarded sole custody of the child to the contracting couple on grounds that would not give the egg donor in non-surrogacy situations a basis for claiming rearing rights in the offspring. This removed the potential legal barrier to egg donation that the Court of Appeals decision appeared to create.

Yet even under a purely genetic definition of motherhood, it would not follow that the egg donor—the genetic mother—would be entitled to visit the child or have any other rearing role when she had agreed at the time of donation to relinquish all rearing rights and duties in offspring born of her donated eggs. Doctrines of waiver and best interests of the child would still control. If she had not asserted her claim before or shortly after birth, she would most likely be found to have waived it, as unmarried fathers who do not assert any rearing right soon after birth are held to do.[8] Even if waiver doctrines did not apply and the case was decided solely in terms of the child's best interests, it will be difficult to show that the child's interests are best served by having a nongestational, genetic parent involved in rearing a child when the parties had reached a contrary agreement at the time at which the eggs were donated.

Ironically, the only reported case on custody issues arising out of egg donation involved a divorcing husband's attempts to gain sole custody of twins born as the result of an anonymous egg donation in New York, rather than a donor seeking visitation or custody.[9] The husband claimed that since the wife was the gestational but not the genetic mother of the twins, she was not their "natural" mother and therefore had no right to rear. The court's decision rejecting this claim, and awarding custody to the wife with visitation in the father, is not surprising. Having provided sperm for the insemination of donor eggs that were to be implanted in his wife, he had no basis for barring his wife (the gestational mother) from the rearing role agreed to by the parties. The principles underlying the court's decision would also bar a donor who had voluntarily relinquished her rearing rights and duties from any later rearing role.

In the final analysis, the resolution of disputes arising from donor claims to rear children born of egg donation will depend on society's view of the importance of genetic versus gestational motherhood and the importance of the parties' preconception intentions. In a state without egg donor legislation, a very risk-averse couple could have the donor terminate her parental rights after the child is born, and then have the recipient/gestational mother adopt her husband's child in a stepparent adoption. As a general rule, however, such steps are unnecessary until there are court decisions that give the egg donor the right to assert parental claims after birth. Given the original intentions of the parties, the gestational role of the recipient, and sperm donation practices, such court decisions are unlikely to occur.

DONOR'S LIABILITY FOR CHILD SUPPORT

A second type of dispute would arise if attempts were made to hold the egg donor liable after birth for child support or other rearing obligations toward her genetic child. Because egg donors ordinarily intend to be excluded from any rearing role, they will want legal protection from later duties to support or participate in rearing. One can imagine a scenario where the recipient dies after birth, or where the couple undergoes hardships that make it impossible for them to support the child. Either they or the state then seek to hold the donor as genetic mother responsible for child support.

Until state law makes clear that egg donors lose all rearing rights and duties, there is always some risk that such a duty could be imposed, but it is highly unlikely. The situation is unlike that of sperm donation to a single woman, where the donor has occasionally been held responsible for child support when no rearing father existed.[10] Here the donation is to a woman who intends to gestate, rear, and be completely responsible for the child's welfare. Holding the egg donor liable for support in this situation would deter egg donation to married and single women alike. Followed to its logical conclusion, it would also make doctors who assist reproduction by single women potentially liable for child support.

Although it is highly unlikely that such a duty would be imposed, the donor needs to be fully informed of this uncertainty. If she is very risk averse, she could demand that the recipient couple agree to hold her harmless for any financial obligation that might arise from the birth of such a child, but this guarantee would provide little assurance if they or the state need to turn to her for child support. Alternatively, she could terminate her parental rights at birth and have the recipient adopt the child to make clear that she has no parental obligations. Except for the most risk-averse donors, however, this step is unnecessary as a general rule until a court decision holds egg donors liable for later obligations. Judicial decisions that create duties contrary to the original intentions of the parties are as unlikely to occur as decisions that create rights in the donor contrary to the original agreement of the parties.

Questions about rearing rights and duties could also affect questions of inheritance. Donor sperm legislation usually makes the consenting husband the legal father for all purposes and the donor the father for none, so that devises to one's "children" or "heirs" or to children under intestacy statutes would, in the case of a deceased husband, go to the children born of sperm donation, while in the case of the deceased donor, they would not.[11] A similar result might be reached in states without donor sperm legislation, though the question has not yet arisen. Of course, either party could make specific bequests to make sure that certain individuals did or did not take from their estate.

A similar result would probably be reached in legislation establishing rearing rights and duties in offspring of egg donation. The child would be the "heir" or "child" of the recipient and not of the donor for all purposes, unless a specific bequest were made. Until such legislation is passed, however, it is unclear whether the offspring of egg donation are children of the donor, of the recipient, or of both under intestacy statutes or general devises to one's "children" or "heirs." To avoid problems and make sure that intentions are honored, both recipients and donors should specify in their wills by name or relation the persons whom they wish to share in their estate.

Finally, it should be noted that there may be instances of egg donation in which the donor and the recipient agree to share in parenting rights and duties.[12] While this will not be the usual case, and may not even be known to the physician providing the service, persons who plan such arrangements should execute agreements that make very clear what their mutual rights and obligations are. There is no guarantee that their agreements will be honored, and they should understand these limitations in proceeding.

RISKS TO DONORS

Egg donors face both psychosocial and physical risks of harm from participation in egg donation. The psychosocial risk is that they will wish more contact with resulting offspring than they are able to have, and thus feel cut off from their genetic offspring. There is also the risk that women who wish to have no contact with offspring may later be faced with offspring seeking them out or demands for child support. Donors should be fully informed that they might have different feelings about donation at a later point, and about the legal uncertainties that, in the absence of legislation or court decision, exist about determining rearing rights and duties by preconception agreement. As noted, the most likely scenario is that donors will be totally excluded from any contact or relationship with any offspring, no matter how much they later desire it, if they had so agreed at the time of donation. In addition, even though they cannot be guaranteed that they will not have unwanted contact or later obligations, the chances of that occurring appear to be very small.

Donors also face physical risks. Egg donors will have their ovaries stimulated with hormones to produce multiple eggs, which will then be surgically retrieved, either by transvaginal ultrasound-guided aspiration, or by laparoscopy. Several days of injections will also be necessary. Risks of complications or infection, while small, do exist. These include hyperstimulation syndrome, infection, and so on. They are the same risks that candidates for IVF undergo.

Although the complication rate with ovarian stimulation and egg retrieval is very small, it is possible that some egg donors will be injured in the process. An important legal question is to determine who will be responsible for the medical and other costs of such injuries. Potential donors need to be fully informed of the risks that they face, and also to be told who will bear responsibility for the costs of any injuries that occur.

One possibility would be to have the donor assume the costs of these risks. Just as human subjects of biomedical research bear the costs of any injuries sustained in the research process,[13] egg donors could also be asked to bear the cost. The risk of incurring these costs is part of what they are providing as egg donors. If so, it should be made clear to them that they are bearing that cost. However, the cost is limited to the cost of nonnegligently caused injuries, because they cannot waive their right to recover for negligence that causes their injuries.[14] If they clearly understand that they are bearing these costs, their assumption of that risk has a reasonable chance of protecting the program and recipient couple from liability for nonnegligently caused injuries that result from their participation as egg donors.

An alternative solution is to have the program assume all or some portion of the costs of any nonnegligently caused injuries to donors. Because such costs would ultimately be passed on to recipient couples, they should also be clearly informed of the extent, if any, to which they will be responsible for the donor's medical and other costs. The program cannot hold them liable unless they have specifically agreed to assume those costs. For their own protection they need to be informed of this risk, and set limits on their exposure.

The best solution to this problem would be to have the program that recruits the donor purchase a short-term health insurance policy to cover any medical costs that she incurs as a result of the donation. Programs that do not themselves recruit donors, but that retrieve eggs from donors identified by the recipient should also provide such insurance. The cost of this insurance would be paid by the program or the recipient, and would be the extent of their responsibility for nonnegligently caused injuries. Such a limitation should be clearly explained to potential donors and recipients, so that they are fully aware of their rights and responsibilities.

THE LEGALITY OF PAYING DONORS

Unless a couple seeking an egg donor has a friend or family member willing to donate, the main source of donor eggs is likely to be anonymous strangers recruited for that purpose. Although they will have mixed motives, including altruism and the desire to have genetic offspring without gestational or rearing burdens, women may be unwilling to donate unless they are paid for their efforts, which are not inconsiderable. Without payment to donors, many women may be denied access to egg donation.

While some ethicists have objected to paying women for their eggs on the ground that it is exploitive and commodifies offspring, there is no clear consensus that such payments are unethical. Since sperm donors are paid, it would be discriminatory to ban payment to egg donors, who undergo greater burdens. Nor is it clear that paying for eggs is exploitive or coercive of women. The amounts paid are not so large relative to the time and effort involved that they are likely to induce women to undergo unacceptable risks. Experience also indicates that most women who volunteer are not poor or members of minority groups. Finally, the transaction can be structured as paying for their physical services rather than for the eggs themselves, which reduces the risk that the transaction will be viewed as one involving the sale of children.

An important issue is whether federal and state laws which ban buying and selling organs for transplant also apply to paying egg donors. In response to fears that persons would sell living or cadaveric organs for transplant, the federal government and several states passed laws making it a crime (with penalties ranging from felony to misdemeanor) to buy or sell organs.[15] Although the intent of these laws was not to apply to sperm and egg donation, their language in some cases is drawn so broadly that the sale of eggs could be covered as prohibited.

The main threat here is from state law. The 1986 Federal Organ Transplant Act, which prohibits the acquisition, receipt, or transfer of "any human organ for valuable consideration for use in human transplantation," defines "human organ" in such a way that sperm and ova are clearly excluded.[16] Only Louisiana expressly prohibits "the sale of a human ovum."[17] However, prohibitions in Texas, Ohio, California, and several other states are less narrowly defined than the federal law and leave open the possibility that the sale of ova and even sperm is criminally banned.

The Texas statute, for example, defines human organ to include "the human kidney, liver, heart . . . or any other human organ or tissue, but does not include hair or blood, blood components (including plasma), blood derivatives, or blood reagents."[18] The question turns then on whether ova are "tissue." Under a standard dictionary definition of tissue—"a collection of similar cells and the intercellular substances surrounding them"[19]—the contents of one follicle would not be tissue, even if cumulus and follicular fluid is also aspirated, because only the egg is donated. On the other hand, the legislature failed to exclude sperm and ova as it did blood and blood products, and in a broad sense ova could be viewed as tissue. The Ohio statute raises similar issues.[20]

A law in Nevada bans the sale of specified organs and "any other part of the human body except blood."[21] Are oocytes a "part of the human body" or are they products of the body? Either interpretation is possible. Still other states follow the federal model and authorize the director of the state department of health to add other "organs" to the list specified in the law.[22]

Another kind of ambiguity arises in California[23] and South Dakota[24] statutes that make it a crime to receive, sell, transfer, or promote the transfer of "any human organ, for purposes of transplantation, for valuable consideration." Human organ is defined as "the human kidney, liver, heart . . . or any other human organ or nonrenewable or nonregenerative tissue except plasma and sperm." Because the statute explicitly excludes sperm and plasma but not ova, and ova, strictly speaking, are nonrenewable or nonregenerative, one could conclude that ova are included within the definition of "human organ." However, one could also reasonably argue that ova are not tissue, or that they are renewable tissue because a donor has a large supply of ova. One or more cycles of egg donation will not deplete the eggs available for the donor until she herself reaches menopause.

Finally, one can question whether California-type statutes ban payments to egg donors because egg donation is not for the purpose of "transplantation." Transplantation implies insertion of an organ or tissue in another person to replace a missing function. But eggs are not transplanted. Rather, they are fertilized *in vitro*, and then the cleaving embryo is placed in the uterus. Transfer of an embryo to the uterus followed by implantation and pregnancy is thus not "transplantation" of an organ or tissue. Indeed, in some cases, the donated eggs will not produce embryos, and all embryos may not be transferred to the uterus, much less successfully implant therein.

These examples of state statutes banning the sale of organs show that the definition of organ as "tissue" or "any other body part" opens the door to the possibility that sale of ova is included in the statutory ban, particularly when it is not included in certain exceptions. However, an arguably more persuasive reading of these laws would exclude sperm and ova from them. They were written with sale of solid organs in mind, sperm and ova (at least for a time) are sufficiently plentiful to be functionally renewable, and it is very doubtful that the donated ova and sperm are then "transplanted."

If they are fully cognizant of these uncertainties, physicians, couples, and donors in states with laws that could be interpreted to ban payment for egg donation might still reasonably proceed with paid egg donation when that is the only way to recruit suitable donors. While the risk of prosecution cannot be totally eliminated, it appears to be small. No prosecutions have yet been brought. If prosecution did occur, the participants would have a strong defense that the statute is unconstitutionally vague in that a reasonable person could not tell whether ova are included in the prohibition.[25] In addition, if they honestly believed that ova were not covered, they would also lack the specific intent to violate the law required in most cases for criminal liability. They could also attack the law as an unconstitutional interference with the right of infertile married couples to form a family with the help of an egg donor.[26] Since statutes are usually construed to avoid doubts about their constitutionality, they are likely to be found not to apply to egg donation.

To reduce the risks of prosecution even further, the relationship between the donor and the program or recipient should be structured as one in which they are paying for the services of the donor in undergoing the procedures necessary to produce the eggs, rather than the eggs themselves. Thus payment should depend on the number and kind of procedures undergone, and not be calibrated to the production of eggs or of any number of eggs. The agreement should state that payment is to compensate the donor for her time and services, and not for the eggs. It should also state that the donor is free to back out at any point, that she will be paid for any procedures undergone, including egg retrieval, even if she decides at the last minute not to relinquish her rights in retrieved eggs. Skillful writing of the contract/agreement with the donor will reduce the risk, which may already be small, that the participants will be prosecuted for, much less found guilty of, unlawful sale of organs or tissue under state law.

In any event, even if these laws do apply, there would still be room to pay donors their medical and other expenses. The statutes in question do allow for reimbursement of the donor's "expenses of travel, housing and lost wages."[27] Thus some fee to the donor would be possible if time off work were required, even if this did pose an upper limit. Also, such restrictions could be interpreted to permit one couple to pay the expenses of another couple going through IVF with the understanding that they would share the resulting eggs harvested. This practice is arguably the equivalent of paying of expenses necessary to produce the donation, and not a payment for the eggs themselves.

ISSUES OF OFFSPRING WELFARE

Egg donation, like other assisted reproductive techniques, raises questions about the impact on offspring. Legal duties aside, there is a strong ethical obligation to pay attention to how these procedures will affect the children who are produced as a result. Programs should be run and structured to minimize harm to offspring.

This duty creates a paradox, however. But for the assisted reproductive procedure in question, the child would never be born. Thus even if a procedure leads to a child with a novel set of parents, it is still not possible to say that the child is harmed by having two female parents because the child would not otherwise have been born, and the resulting parenting arrangement or confusion does not produce such dire consequences that the child would have been better off never having been born at all.

Even if one rejects this analysis generally, it is not easy to argue that egg donation creates such a confusing parenting situation that the child is clearly harmed irreparably just by being born in this way. After all, in the ordinary case the child will be reared by two biologic parents, which distinguishes egg donation from surrogacy and donor sperm. Of all collaborative reproductive arrangements, egg donation is closest to the norm of two parents contributing genes, gestation, and rearing. Indeed, a ban on egg donation on the ground that it harms offspring because it splits genetic and gestational parentage would not rise to the level of compelling interest necessary to justify infringing the fundamental right to procreate.[28]

This is true even if eggs are donated to an unmarried woman or to a woman who is past the normal outer limit of menopause—say to a woman in her 50s. Providing donor eggs to a single woman is no different from providing her with donor sperm, or indeed, from a single woman engaging in coital reproduction. In each case, a woman decides to conceive and give birth to a child knowing that there will not be a rearing male partner. Yet few people would now argue, particularly in the case of an economically stable woman, that birth to a single woman is such a detriment to the child that it should not have been born at all. Physicians treating infertility may decide not to participate in such situations, but they would not be acting unethically or illegally if they did. Indeed, a law that outlawed such assistance would be subject to attack on both equal protection and due process grounds, for it would deny an infertile unmarried woman the same rights that a married person has.

Similarly, the use of donor eggs with a woman past the normal age of childbearing is not clearly harmful to the child. Such cases will be relatively infrequent, but they will occur and may garner wide media attention when they do, as occurred with the 1993 birth of twins in Britain to a 59-year-old recipient of donor eggs.[29] Having an older mother does deviate from past practices and traditional views of motherhood, but men have been able to reproduce late in life. To deny women this opportunity when a technology permits it would seem to be discriminatory on gender grounds. Even if the child's mother dies at an earlier age than usual, the child is not so worse-off that it would have been better that it not be born at all. Again, individual programs or practitioners may choose not to offer egg donation to older recipients, but it would not be unethical to do so, and could not, given constitutional rights of equal protection and procreative liberty, legally be banned in the United States.

Even though egg donation cannot itself be banned to protect offspring, it should be conducted in ways that will respect their interests. The most important measure here is to keep confidential records about donor identity and characteristics so that offspring may later, if the law or changes in social policy permit, learn the identity of their genetic mother and even have contact with her if that can be arranged in a mutually satisfactory way. Recognition of the child's right to have information about or even learn the identity at some later point of its genetic mother does not also mean that the egg donor will have other rearing duties imposed against her wishes.

At present there is no law that requires that such records be kept or that enables offspring of sperm or egg donation to ever learn who their genetic parents are. While some state adoption laws allow the confidentiality of records to be pierced for good cause, there is no existing provision for offspring of gamete donation, and no records may be available if there were.[30] Whether and to what extent children should be informed of how they were born will have to depend on the families that raise them. Disclosure cannot and should not be legislated. But if state law does permit or require disclosure, or the parties otherwise agree to disclosure, it will be necessary to have records of donors and recipients available.

It is thus essential that donors be informed of the extent to which anonymity will be preserved, and records kept so that later contact or information, if mutually desired or otherwise required by state law, can be arranged.

CONCLUSION

Egg donation is a promising technique for treating a major source of infertility, but it now lacks the legal infrastructure necessary to provide the participants with certainty about the legal consequences of this collaborative form of assisted reproduction. Legislation, judicial decision, and standard practice will eventually cure these uncertainties.

In the meantime, interested parties need not refrain from participation in human egg donation, but they should be fully aware of the areas of uncertainty that exist and take steps to minimize undesired consequences. In the final analysis, full disclosure, free and informed consent, and respect for the interests of all parties will be the best protection for physicians, couples, and donors who participate in human egg donation.

NOTES

1. The American Fertility Society, Society for Assisted Reproduction, "Assisted Reproductive Technology in the United States and Canada: 1992 Results Generated from The American Fertility Society/Society for Assisted Reproductive Technology Registry," *Fertility and Sterility* 62 (1994): 1121–28.

2. M. V. Sauer, R. J. Paulson, R. A. Lobo, "Reversing the Natural Decline in Human Fertility: An Extended Clinical Trial of Oocyte Donation to Women of Advanced Reproductive Age," *Journal of the American Medical Association* 268 (1992): 1275–79.

3. Ibid.

4. Okla. Stat. Ann. Tit. 10, Sec. 544 (1991); Tex. S. B.512, 73rd Leg., R. S. (1993); S.2082, 1993 Reg.Sess., 1993 Florida Laws; Va. Code Ann. #20-158 (Miche Supp. 1994); N. D. Cent. Code #14-18-01 to #14-18-04 (1994).

5. U.S. Congress, Office of Technology Assessment, *Infertility: Medical and Social Choices* OTA-BA-358 (Washington, DC: U.S. Government Printing Office, 1988), pp. 242–49.

6. 286 Cal. Rptr. 369 (Cal.App. 4 Dist. 1991).

7. 822 P.2d 1317, 4 Cal. Rptr. 2nd 170 (1992).

8. *Lehr v. Robertson,* 463 U.S. 248 (1983).

9. *McDonald v. McDonald,* 196 A.D.2d 7; 608 N.Y. S. 2d 477 (1994).

10. *Jhordan C. v. Mary K.,* 179 Cal. App.3d 386; 224 Cal. Rptr. 530 (1986).

11. Tex. Fam. Code Ann. Sec. 12.03 (Vernon 1986).

12. John A. Robertson, "Ethical and Legal Issues in Human Egg Donation," *Fertility and Sterility* 52 (1989): 353–63.

13. President's Commission for the Study of Ethical Problems in Medicine and Biomedical and Behavioral Science Research, *Compensating for Research Injuries* (Washington, DC: U.S. Government Printing Office, 1982), pp. 81–98.

14. Ibid.

15. Note, "Regulating the Sale of Human Organs," *Virginia Law Review,* 71 (1985): 1015.

16. 42 U.S.C.A. # 274(e) Prohibition of Organ Purchases.

17. La. Civ. Code Ann. Art. 9: 122 (Supp. 1987).

18. Texas Health and Safety Code Ann., sec. 48.02 (West 1989).

19. Stedman's Medical Dictionary, 22nd Edition, 1972.

20. Ohio Rev. Code Ann. S.. 2108.11, 210812 (Baldwin 1980).

21. Nev. Rev. Stat. # 201.460 (1991).

22. New York Pub. Health Law, sec. 4307 (McKinney 1990).

23. Cal. Penal Code, #367f (West 1988).

24. S. D. Codified Laws Ann. S. 34–26–42.

25. *Margaret S. v. Edwards,* 794 F.2d 994 (5th Cir. 1986); *Lifchez v. Hartigan,* 735 F. Supp. 1361 (N.D. Ill. 1990).

26. John A. Robertson, "Technology and Motherhood: Ethical and Legal Issues in Human Egg Donation," *Case Western Reserve Law Review,* 39: (1989): 1–38.

27. Texas Health & Safety Code Ann. #48.02 (West 1989).

28. See notes 24 and 25 supra.

29. William Schmidt, "Birth to a 59-year-old Generates an Ethical Controversy in Britain," *New York Times,* Dec. 13, 1993, A1. See also Associated Press, "53-year-old Grandmother Gives Birth to Premature Test-tube Twins," *Austin American-Statesman,* Nov. 11, 1992, p. A18.

30. John A. Robertson, "Embryos, Families and Procreative Liberty: The Legal Structure of the New Reproduction," *Southern California Law Review,* 59 (1986): 942–1039; John A. Robertson, *Children of Choice: Freedom and the New Reproductive Technologies* (Princeton, NJ: Princeton University Press, 1994), pp. 123–25.

THIRTEEN

THE DIFFERENTIAL EFFECTS OF RACE, ETHNICITY, AND SOCIOECONOMIC STATUS ON INFERTILITY AND ITS TREATMENT

Ethical and Policy Issues for Oocyte Donation

Elizabeth Heitman, Ph.D., and
Mary Schlachtenhaufen, J.D.

The development of technologically assisted reproduction since the 1970s has coincided remarkably with three social forces that have shaped perspectives about technological intervention into procreation: the evolution of biomedical ethics and concern over the effects of technology on ethical values; the rise of a consciously feminist scholarship and attention to the treatment of women by medicine; and, more recently, the U.S. health care "crisis" and sociopolitical debate about the just distribution of society's health care resources. Thus, three themes have recurred in the social and ethical analysis of technologically assisted reproduction: (1) the commercialization of procreation and the "commodification" of women, children, and gametes in technological processes; (2) the more general mistreatment of women by physicians, medical researchers, and wealthy childless couples; and (3) the just distribution and appropriate funding of reproductive services.

For many ethicists, the full moral significance of any issue depends on the experience of the least powerful members of society, classically the poor and, in the contemporary United States, nonwhites. Consequently, one focus of the debate about reproductive services has been the impact on poor women and members of various ethnic groups. Typically, criticism has focused on their commodification or exploitation. This concern intensified in the controversy over contractual surrogacy, as criticism mounted that surrogacy was simply a modern, technological version of the rich buying children from the poor.

The recently developed practice of using nonspousal ova, typically known as "donor eggs," in *in vitro* fertilization (IVF) has revived many of the apprehensions raised by previous reproductive technologies. As outlined by the American Fertility Society,[1] the primary indication for oocyte donation (OD) is to redress premature ovarian failure, surgical removal of the ovaries, or impairment or destruction of ovarian function as a result of previous medical treatment. OD has also received considerable attention when used to overcome a woman's inability to reproduce using her own egg due to advancing age, including menopause.[2] Despite its limited indications, many infertility clinics expect that "consumer demand" for OD will outstrip the availability of eggs.[3] It has been suggested that the $1,500+ fees offered to egg donors may induce poor and/or ethnic minority women into procreative arrangements that may not be in their best interests. Because OD is possible only with IVF, and carries the additional cost of procuring an egg donor, the practice is also expected to be unavailable to all but the wealthy.

This paper explores the ethical questions and policy challenges raised by racial, cultural, and socioeconomic issues for the practice of OD. Its primary focus is an examination of problems raised by imprecise conceptual definitions and differences in cultural perspectives on fertility, motherhood, family, heritage, the role of women in society, and appropriate medical intervention in procreation. Many of these matters have not been well studied by relevant specialists in any field, and the lack of data prompts consideration of areas where in-depth research is needed.

Resolving many of these conceptual issues will be essential to understanding the appropriate role and potential benefits of OD for women of all races and classes. First, it is important to establish why and how racial, ethnic, and socioeconomic classification is significant for meaningful policy on OD, and how current classification schemes are inadequate. The difficulty of defining racial and ethnic groups meaningfully is a central problem both in the epidemiology of infertility and in social science research into the links between ethnicity and responses to infertility treatment. Moreover, because standard measures of poverty may not apply either to persons with limited access to infertility services or to those women who respond to financial incentives to donate ova, it is important to consider whether, why, and how economic factors might be important to policy governing these practices.

Any policy definition of the "appropriate use" of and "appropriate access" to OD will imply a definition of "appropriate demand" for the technology.

Thus it is especially important to distinguish the biological condition of infertility from both the perceived meaning of infertility and its effects, as well as from the demand for infertility services. As rates of infertility among the poor and nonwhites are reported to be high and their use of infertility services is negligible, the cultural and socioeconomic factors that affect these phenomena and their relationship should be examined with respect to the potential demand for and expectations of OD among specific groups.

Consideration of these conceptual questions and the nature of the current demand for donor eggs suggests that poor and nonwhite women—as these groups are usually understood—are unlikely to become the victims of commodification or more general exploitation from OD per se. Furthermore, increasing the demand of nonwhite and poor women for IVF and OD poses a significant dilemma. The increased use of IVF among nonwhite women would likely also subject them to the anxiety, depression, and sense of failure that is well documented among white IVF patients, and which some feminists have argued is an inherently oppressive feature of reproductive technologies.[4] Ironically, too, increased demand may create a greater perception of exclusion if services are not more widely available; yet access to "nonessential" reproductive technologies may actually shrink if the availability of and coverage for IVF services are reduced under current health care policies. Despite the ethical debate about the just distribution of health care resources and technological intervention in procreation, and despite current efforts to broaden access to medical services, the differential effect of OD on the poor and racial and ethnic minorities is likely to be a reinforcement and extension of current exclusionary practices. Whether this exclusion is an inherently or exclusively negative consequence, however, remains very much in question.

DEFINITIONS AND DEMOGRAPHICS: WHO COUNTS?

Infertility as a medical concept is typically defined as a couple's inability to conceive after one or more years of unprotected intercourse;[5] the broader category of *impaired fecundity* includes both infertility and the inability to carry a conceptus to live birth. *Primary infertility* refers to the inability to conceive a first child, *secondary infertility* to the inability to conceive additional children after one or more live births. For women, these definitions typically apply only during the normal reproductive years, roughly the midteens to the midforties. As a medical concept, the diagnosis of infertility implies that the individual or couple should be treated.

Differential treatment of poor and nonwhite women's infertility begins at an epidemiological level: There is little data available on the actual prevalence or causes of infertility among nonwhites and the poor.[6] In the United States and elsewhere in the industrialized world, the prevalence and causes of infertility have been measured primarily by researchers affiliated with infertility clinics with respect to the predominantly white upper-middle-class population seeking diagnosis and treatment.[7] This reliance on inferences from patient data is partly a methodological issue, as infertility is a medical diagnosis that can be established only after a thorough medical evaluation. However, although all current epidemiological methods are imprecise, the validity of such inferences for populations dissimilar from the majority of infertility patients is also methodologically suspect. The only direct, population-based study of infertility in the United States has been the National Survey of Family Growth (NSFG), conducted by the Center for Health Statistics in 1976, 1982, and 1988,[8] using methods from the 1965 National Fertility Study. The 1982 NSFG has been the basis for much of the U.S. literature in the epidemiology of infertility.[9] It is also the source of most of the data in the widely cited 1988 report on infertility by the U.S. Congress, Office of Technology Assessment (OTA).[10]

The sudden epidemiological interest in the demographics of infertility in the late 1970s and early 1980s is noteworthy, and its likely causes speak to the limited data on nonwhites and the poor. Since World War II, public health concern about reproductive health has focused on fertility as a *threat* to the health of women, their children, and their societies. Epidemiologists, health educators, and policymakers have sought to control women's fertility as a means of improving both their personal standard of living and that of their communities. Whether out of bigotry,[11] the desire to empower poor and nonwhite women to make "rational" choices about childbearing,[12] concern for the environment,[13] or a combination of these factors, publicly funded fertility control programs have focused attention on the social and medical problem of the *overfertility* of poor and nonwhite women.

The more recent epidemiological interest in infertility is not due to concern about the condition as a public health problem as much as to the marked increase in infertility consultations that began in 1972.[14] The surge in consultations is thought to have been the result of the intentionally delayed marriages and childbearing of the disproportionately large "baby-boom generation," which, when coupled with their higher rate of infertility and their typical desire for immediate results, created an unprecedented demand for medical services. In the late 1970s, this demand, the well-publicized technological advances in the treatment of infertility, and heightened public expectations of available treatment made reproductive services a lucrative medical specialty. The initiative for gathering demographic data on infertility was thus shaped significantly by the needs and interests of a population already seeking treatment, a population that was disproportionately white and middle class.

DEFINING RACIAL CATEGORIES: EXCLUSION BY DESIGN

The 1982 NSFG reported national rates of infertility based on interviews with 3,551 married[15] women between the ages of 15 and 44, divided into the categories of white and black according to the women's self-report. The advance summary of the more recent 1988 NSFG survey estimated rates of infertility based on 8,450 women, both married and unmarried, divided into the categories of white, black, and other. Although a later publication of NSFG data on the use of infertility services reported its statistics using the categories Hispanic, non-Hispanic white, and non-Hispanic black,[16] analysis of the more comprehensive findings is not yet available for racial and ethnic breakdowns.

Two- and three-group analysis such as that provided by the NSFG is typical of much of the literature on reproductive issues. Although these groupings may capture the vast majority of the U.S. population, their exclusive use ignores the diversity both within and outside those categories, as well as the variations between self-reported and observer-reported classification.[17] There is an unfortunate irony that analysts who seek to consider the diversity of experiences, attitudes, and responses among different racial groups are often compelled by the paucity of data to refer to blacks and "others" together as "nonwhite," with the misleading implication that "nonwhites" by definition have more in common with each other than they do with whites.

The NSFG's narrow perspective on race and ethnicity is not unique in the demographic analysis of health status. By the government's own admission, current principles used to determine race and ethnicity in federal health statistics were intended only to standardize the collection of data, and were neither scientific nor anthropological in origin.[18] In the past few years, the limitations of these guidelines and their problems in health surveillance have been the subject of a formal review by the Centers for Disease Control (CDC) and the National Institutes of Health (NIH).[19]

The OTA's 1988 report suggested that the federal government improve the collection of data on infertility by expanding the NSFG's sample and the frequency of follow-up surveys.[20] Others have called for standardizing definitions and methods in the epidemiology of infertility.[21] As with all epidemiological work, decisions about which racial and ethnic groups to include in an expanded study of infertility and how to identify their essential characteristics will be both a political and a public health issue, as the definition of "significant population" has both social or cultural and statistical meaning. The inclusion or exclusion of certain populations from demographic studies can determine how policy and social science define their roles and needs for many years;[22] moreover, respondents who are mistrustful of the public health and medical systems that they perceive to have excluded them or worked against their interests may refuse to provide information essential to accurate statistics.[23]

The new CDC and NIH guidelines on racial and ethnic classifications in health surveillance and research are an important beginning for studying infertility and its treatment among the poor and nonwhites. They suggest that *ethnicity*, as a matrix of racial (biological) and cultural (social and environmental) features is more accurate, more precise, and more flexible than any system that uses race alone.[24] They also call for greater issue-specific detail in descriptions of the meaning of ethnicity for the subject under study. Without clarity on such definitional matters, labels of race or ethnicity may obscure the real causes of impaired fertility and effective avenues for redressing them.

In expanding epidemiological studies of infertility, whether to assist family planning campaigns or the provision of reproductive technologies, the classification of race and ethnicity should consider several conceptual issues: What strictly biological/genetic factors appear to be important for fertility and its impairment, and how are these factors related to race or ethnicity? What are the cultural practices, such as diet or late marriage, that may have important biological consequences for fertility and that may correlate with race or ethnicity? What cultural beliefs and practices, such as a desire for large families or a preference for sons, have important consequences for the perception of infertility and the use of medical services for its treatment, including IVF and OD, among members of racial or ethnic groups?

SOCIOECONOMIC STATUS AND INFERTILITY:
HOW MEDICAL INDIGENCE REDEFINES THE QUESTION

Socioeconomic status is included in demographic data in recognition of the social context of illness, prevention, and treatment. However, socioeconomic status is almost as complex a phenomenon as race or ethnicity to distill into identifiable categories, which typically reflect educational background, occupation, and household income. Because nonwhites are statistically more likely to be poor and less well educated than whites, race is often used as a marker for socioeconomic factors as much as for inherent biological characteristics.[25] Where socioeconomic factors and their effects are not examined in detail, as in the NSFG, the effects of biological dimensions of race and ethnicity may be inappropriately weighted in describing differences among groups.

Socioeconomic status is a central factor in access to health services. Poverty, a standardized definition based on a level of household income that will provide subsistence living for a family of four, is associated with limited access to all types of health care, particularly specialized, technological interventions such as reproductive services.[26] In studying health services generally and infertility and its treatment specifically, the difficulty of defining socioeconomic status is compounded by the contemporary problem of "medical indigence." Even families living well above the poverty line may be unable to afford medical care if they are not covered by health insurance or if their coverage is inadequate to the problem. Thus a definition of high socioeconomic status that is meaningful for the epidemiology of infertility may not be useful for considerations of access to infertility treatment.

Many people may discover that their policies exclude treatment for infertility beyond a diagnostic work-up or perhaps surgical intervention to repair damaged reproductive organs.[27] Some couples in this circumstance sacrifice their financial stability to pay for infertility services themselves: with the cost of IVF at some $5,000 to $11,000 per cycle, the cost of preparing an egg donor around $7,000, and only a 10 to 20% chance per cycle of achieving pregnancy, it is easy for couples pursuing pregnancy through OD to spend a middle-class annual salary in the process.[28] For some women undergoing IVF, the process consumes so much time and attention that they are no longer able to hold a job, further reducing the household income.[29] Eight states now require insurance companies to cover or offer coverage for IVF with *spousal* gametes as part of any policy that includes pregnancy-related services;[30] however, many health insurance policies do not automatically cover pregnancy.[31] Thus the majority of even insured middle-class Americans may be unable to afford IVF, and fewer still OD.

Socioeconomic status is also a complex and potentially misleading factor in classification of egg donors. While there is concern that egg donors be adequately compensated for their effort and the risk that they assume, many worry that high fees—sometimes over $2,000 per cycle[32]—will induce poor women to donate eggs against their better judgment as a means to escape their poverty, or because they lack the sense of self to refuse such an apparently lucrative offer.[33] Some reports indicate that while altruism appears to be a primary motivation for donating eggs, money is a significant factor in women's decisions.[34] However, the background of the typical egg donor does not meet the standard definition of low socioeconomic status. Most donors appear to be educated, middle-class white women, who often accept the money offered to donors to pursue a middle-class lifestyle, for example, to reduce excessive credit-card debt or pay educational expenses. The ethical issue of financial inducement remains, but concerns about exploitation of women disempowered by a life of poverty appear to be unwarranted.

RATES, CAUSES, AND TREATMENT OF INFERTILITY AMONG NONWHITE AND POOR WOMEN

As analysts of the NSFG acknowledge, data on age-related rates and causes of infertility among poor and nonwhite women is important to the question of their potential use of reproductive services, including OD, and their role as egg donors.[35] Accurate, comprehensive data will be essential to policymakers at all levels—clinics, governmental and private funding agencies, researchers, and programs that train infertility specialists—if they are to plan effectively. Unfortunately, analysis of the data that are currently available can yield only some tentative conclusions.

As reported by the 1982 NSFG, the most recent data reported by race, there are significant differences in the rates of infertility among white and black women ages 15 to 44, and among members of different socioeconomic groups. The prevalence of infertility among married black women was found to be roughly 21%, 1.5 times greater than the rate of 13% reported among married white women.[36] Data from 1976 suggests that women with less than a high school education, a standard measure of lower socioeconomic status, were also more likely to be part of an infertile couple.[37]

Between the National Fertility Study in 1965 and the 1982 NSFG, rates of primary infertility doubled across all groups, compared with a 40% drop in secondary infertility during the same interval.[38] The number of women over age 35 with primary infertility rose markedly, in proportion to the large increase in the general population over age 35 during the period.[39] However, the rate of infertility among women ages 20 to 24 rose almost three-fold, from 3.6% in 1965 to 10.6% in 1982.[40] Much of the increase in infertility among young women has been attributed to an increased incidence of chlamydia and gonorrhea, leading to pelvic inflammatory disease (PID) and occlusion of the fallopian tubes.[41]

The 1982 NSFG found that black women were about twice as likely to have been treated for PID as white women, and both groups were more likely to have been treated than Hispanic women.[42] PID is widely suspected to be the primary cause of rising infertility rates among young black women.[43] These figures represent an instance in which race may be partly a marker for lower socioeconomic status; although the percentage of women treated for PID did not vary statistically with income, women with high school educations were more likely than college-educated women to have been treated. However, these data may also seriously underestimate the effects of PID on the fertility of black women, because a considerable proportion of women with PID do not seek treatment.[44]

The documented high prevalence of infertility among black women suggests that they should constitute a considerable proportion of women seeking infertility services. However, most women experiencing impaired fecundity do not seek treatment, and infertile nonwhite women seek reproductive services less often than their white counterparts.[45] Only some 30% of both black and Hispanic women with impaired fecundity interviewed in the 1988 NSFG had sought some form of infertility service, compared with 47% of white women.[46] The high percentage of infertility among black women attributed to PID suggests that those who are so diagnosed might be candidates for surgery or IVF due to blocked fallopian tubes. However, only 12.8% of black women in the NSFG sought specialized infertility services (including ovulatory drugs, artificial insemination, surgery or other intervention for blocked fallopian tubes, or IVF), compared with 17% of Hispanics and 27.2% of whites.

Again, statistics for race may be affected by socioeconomic status, as only

8% of poor women (0 to 149% of poverty level) had sought specialized fertility services, compared with 32% of affluent (400+% of poverty level).[47] Insurance coverage is an important socioeconomic factor, not measured by the NSFG, that influences the use of specialized reproductive services by nonwhites. Doctors who know of a woman's financial ineligibility may not provide referral information to fertility clinics, either in a conscious gate-keeper function, or out of unwillingness to add to the woman's sense of personal loss by informing her of options that are not open to her.[48] Women who depend on public health facilities will find almost nothing available for the treatment of infertility; although federal policies require that public facilities that provide family planning services also offer basic medical services to assist conception,[49] there are few public infertility clinics.[50]

Moreover, following the model of adoption, private clinics, and even clinics at state-funded medical schools, typically have treatment criteria for IVF that include such socioeconomic factors as a "stable" marriage, sufficient education to comply with treatment regimens, and often, sufficient financial resources to provide "adequately" for a child if conception and birth should occur. Although the legitimacy of such standards may be debated, each of these factors may weigh against nonwhite women, who are less likely to be formally married, and who may be perceived to be less likely to comply with medical orders and more likely to be at risk financially.[51]

Women's own knowledge about specialized reproductive services may give them more opportunity to seek a referral or to attempt to receive services on their own. Middle-class women, especially educated women, find their way into the system of infertility services in part because they know that such services are available. Poor women, especially those with little education, may not be familiar enough with even the overall medical system to know what technological interventions are possible or how to find them. Moreover, poor and nonwhite women who have not been well treated by medical professionals in the past, or who are suspicious of medical institutions in general, may be unwilling to submit themselves to medical treatment for something as personal as conception.[52]

WOMEN'S PERCEPTIONS OF INFERTILITY AND THEIR EFFECT ON ACCESS TO FERTILITY SERVICES

Even if treatment for infertility were more readily accessible to nonwhite and poor women, their use of such services would still depend on the extent to which they perceive infertility to be a medical problem. The use of preventive and treatment services generally is strongly correlated with the individual's belief in the medical constructs on which intervention is based, the perceived outcome of intervention, and the value that is assigned to the outcome.[53] In the field of obstetrics, where rates of prenatal care among blacks, Hispanics, and the poor are significantly lower than among middle-class whites, an important barrier to the use of prenatal services is the belief that pregnancy is not a medical condition and that prenatal care has little beneficial effect.[54] Are infertility and infertility treatment viewed similarly? Unfortunately, the experiences of nonwhite and poor women are rarely addressed.[55] Again, who gets studied is a function of who seeks treatment for infertility.[56] Because many studies are conducted at treatment centers, and with limited populations, researchers may also exclude nonwhites because a "relatively homogeneous group" permits researchers to conduct more sophisticated analyses with fewer subjects than would be possible otherwise.[57]

Middle-class white women are widely observed to experience infertility as a frustrating foreclosure of choice; they seek to regain personal control over their lives and bodies through medical intervention.[58] The predicted boom in the demand for OD is due to the willingness of such women to do almost anything until they have exhausted all other technological possibilities.[59] Their shame at having failed, first to conceive naturally, then with medical assistance, is compounded by ambiguity, anxiety, and confusion over the meaning of their loss of control.[60] For those poor and nonwhite women whose lives have not been oriented toward issues of control, infertility may be more readily interpretable in terms of the meaning of suffering and adversity generally. For many people, especially persons from traditional backgrounds, this meaning is fundamentally religious.[61] As infertile women struggle to find meaning in their condition, the medical view still competes with an ancient religious and cultural symbolism that often portrays infertility as a form of God's judgment.[62]

In traditional Judaism, a woman's primary duty to her husband is to bear children so that he may fulfill his religious duty to be fruitful.[63] Nonetheless, throughout Jewish writings fertility is portrayed as under divine, not human, control: God blesses the righteous with many children, while the childless woman has been judged unworthy. In some contexts, barren women are compared to the dead. In Talmudic teachings, a man could, and often was encouraged to, divorce an infertile wife and remarry. A woman's barrenness was often interpreted to be the result of her secret adultery, and a wife's infidelity was automatic grounds for divorce.

Traditional Christian teachings continue much of the Jewish view of children as a blessing and infertility as a judgment. However, Christianity links all human sexuality with interpretations of original sin and its sexual transmission. Pre-Reformation Christianity taught that only virginity and chastity were spiritually pure, but offered marriage and procreation to those who could not resist temptation as a means to redeem their inherently sinful activity.[64] Infertility was interpreted as a sign of God's disfavor and punishment, particularly for sexual transgressions, and an infertile woman needed to seek forgiveness before she could conceive.[65]

For women from non-Western societies where even in contemporary times motherhood is the chief role of women and procreation the primary motivation for marriage,[66] cultural and religious interpretations of infertility may be even more complex. Women from Asian countries influenced by the religious and cultural traditions of Confucianism may not only understand infertility to be a serious breach of the moral order, but may also define infertility to include the inability to bear sons.[67] For a Hindu woman, whose marriage is typically arranged by her family, infertility often means the loss of social, emotional, and even financial support from her husband and his family, as her status, too, is largely dependent upon her ability to bear sons.[68] Among African women of many tribal, religious, and national backgrounds, demonstrated fertility is essential to adulthood and social standing.[69] In Islam, where motherhood is the path to Allah for women, infertility implies Allah's disfavor and is grounds for the husband to take a second wife.[70] In each of these cultures and many others, a woman's infertility traditionally has been grounds for divorce, often leading to her abject poverty, prostitution, or death.

Among many women for whom motherhood is a woman's most important social role, infertility is exceptionally tragic because it also represents a loss of spiritual identity. For many poor and nonwhite women, the images of infertility as a religious, spiritual, or moral problem point to the need for a related response. If infertility is one in a series of negative, irreversible life events, it is more likely to be interpreted as fate or God's will, which no human intervention can redress.[71] Women who share this worldview would be unlikely to seek treatment under a system that focuses on medical/scientific questions to the exclusion of the spiritual and moral; however, the profound meaning of infertility for them and their families suggests that programs tailored to certain cultural perspectives might attract greater numbers of patients.

In the absence of accurate data on their responses to infertility treatments generally, predicting how infertile poor and nonwhite women in the United States might respond to the option of IVF with OD would be exceptionally difficult, particularly given the diversity of cultures, social backgrounds, and personal needs of women who might fall into that broad category. From the available statistics on the causes of infertility, the medical need for OD among black women would appear to be limited, as PID and tubal occlusion, rather than ovarian failure, is their primary cause of infertility. Most women for whom IVF might be indicated are likely to have healthy eggs that would be suitable for the procedure. Apart from international epidemiological data that also stresses the role of PID, information is simply not available for other groups.

Several factors that may figure prominently in poor and nonwhite women's response to OD warrant future study: women's understanding of the definition of family, the exclusivity of family relationships, and the extent to which children are "shared" among relatives or members of a community; the importance of family lineage and the value of maintaining clear records of family heritage; and views of embodiment and the essential nature of the human egg. Each of these culturally defined issues carries potentially conflicting influences on women's use of infertility services and acceptance of OD.

Despite many traditional cultures' harsh judgment of infertile women, these same cultures typically define families broadly, across generations and relationships. Children may live in several households while growing up, in the care of relatives and close family friends whose financial stability, proximity to schools, or need for extra hands for the family farm or business offer them a particular advantage. In such societies, formal and informal adoption extend a couple's ability to "have children."[72] Today, many middle-class white parents would balk at such arrangements. However, in previous generations among whites, and still in many poor and nonwhite communities, family relationships are not necessarily linear, and a child's primary family may not include his or her biological parents.[73] Emphasis on extended family relations and the sharing of children suggest that for infertile women of some ethnic backgrounds, OD by a female relative or close friend of the recipient might not be objectionable. Where concern about privacy prompts many white couples to seek an anonymous donation, women from more community-oriented cultures might not value donor anonymity.

But not all cultures that value extended families share children; for many it is essential to know not only the identity of the biological parents, but the entire family lineage. For some, the meaning of lineage, including the mother's family history, is essential to the individual's identity and place in the extended family. In such contexts, OD would likely be rejected as mixing bloodlines and confusing heritage, or possibly as a form of symbolic adultery, as has happened with sperm donation in some religious traditions.[74]

Finally, although much has been written through history about the significance and value of sperm as the "seed" that carries the family line, the egg is a relatively recent discovery with fewer symbolic meanings.[75] Little is known about women's perceptions of their eggs, and as eggs are never seen, it is likely that eggs and their role in procreation are both more idealized and less appreciated by women themselves. Eggs may be viewed as a piece of the woman from whom they come, as future children, as sparks of life, or as simple cells. Women's perceptions of their own embodiment, and that of the children that they conceive, varies greatly with culture,[76] and will have a significant influence on their willingness to donate or receive eggs.

COMMODIFICATION OF POOR AND ETHNIC MINORITY WOMEN, THEIR EGGS, AND THEIR CHILDREN

If a poor or nonwhite woman who might seek IVF with OD would likely bring a family member or friend as a donor, the possibilities for exploitation of such women by outsiders would appear to be limited. Two hypothetical scenarios, however, place young women at risk of coercion and their eggs at risk of commodification. In the first, poor women with blocked fallopian tubes but healthy ovaries might be induced to share their eggs with wealthier women willing to underwrite the expense of the IVF procedure. Such arrangements have been used in some facilities using OD, and are similar to the sharing of surplus eggs and embryos that has been a common feature of IVF and OD for many years.[77]

This kind of plan would likely require the services of a broker, potentially the IVF clinic itself, to present the offer to the potential egg donor and to coordinate the procedures. Such a dual role for the IVF team—both caregivers and egg procurers—poses a conflict of interest that may compromise the care of women with blocked fallopian tubes, should their eggs be sought by others.[78] Several economic factors argue against such arrangements. Because of the high cost of IVF, and because infertility services beyond the initial diagnostic work-up are neither covered by many insurance plans nor available in publicly funded health care systems, it is unlikely that many infertile women who are unable to pay for the service would get as far as an IVF facility. More importantly, many IVF centers that offer OD now have other arrangements for procuring donors, and although the fee to nonpatient donors can be as much as $2,500 per cycle, this sum is much less than the $7,000 to $10,000 that the patient-donor's IVF treatment would cost. Moreover, if the clinic pays donors on a per-retrieval basis, but charges each recipient that same fee per cycle of IVF with OD, there may be a financial incentive to procure paid donors if a single nonwhite donor can provide eggs for more than one nonwhite recipient.[79] While there is currently no clear indication that clinics make such a profit from their donors, policy on this issue is needed.

The second scenario involves a wealthy foreign couple who come to a U.S. IVF clinic with their "cousin" who wishes to serve as an egg donor. This situation is reminiscent of rich foreigners with kidney failure who occasionally create ethical controversy in U.S. hospitals by seeking a living-related-donor kidney transplant from an accompanying "relative" who is typically neither related nor a fully voluntary donor. Given the widespread use of both nonanonymous and paid egg donors in standard practice, this second scenario would create little stir in most clinics. The clinic's primary concern should be adequate informed consent for the donor—including professional translation where necessary—rather than the detection of deception. Following standard protocols for psychological screening and the full disclosure of risks is the surest, and perhaps the only way to determine whether the donor is being coerced. There is probably no way to ensure that the recipient honors any agreements, financial or otherwise, that she or her husband may have made with the donor.[80]

Generally, OD's commodifying practices work to the exclusion of eggs from poor and nonwhite women. Even if race or ethnicity were not an issue, there is little likelihood that poor women's eggs would be in demand. The uncertain genetic, behavioral, and environmental health of poor donors may create a perceived "product liability" risk that would make their eggs unattractive to both IVF clinics and prospective recipients. Doctors typically suspect that the poor lie about their medical histories and health-related behavior,[81] and the temptation to discount a potential donor's information would increase where doctors believed the donor's motives were purely financial. Currently, many clinics that offer OD are able to provide eggs for the majority of their patients from either known donors or anonymous middle-class donors.[82] The potential liability of brokering IVF labs would likely discourage recruitment among the poor, and encourage stiff screening criteria for donors. Additionally, because donors and recipients are typically matched by phenotype, there is little demand for eggs from nonwhite donors because there are so few nonwhite women seeking OD. But even if the number of nonwhite recipients were to grow, the large number of black and mixed-race children in foster care—224,000 of 450,000 foster children in America in 1993[83]—suggests that many infertile nonwhite couples may not want to raise "strangers' " children, and would be more likely to bring a friend or family member with them as an egg donor.

RACE AND ETHNICITY IN DONOR-RECIPIENT MATCHING: HERITAGE, PREJUDICE, AND THE VALUE OF CHILDREN

For nonwhite women who meet the medical criteria for OD and who do not have a known donor, the practice of matching anonymous donors by phenotype raises some intriguing questions about the social and existential meanings of race and ethnicity. Individuals of vastly different racial or ethnic background may have a similar appearance. Who determines the standards of resemblance and their role in matching? When clinic personnel know the differing racial and ethnic backgrounds of a potential donor and recipient, what role will this information play if the women's resemblance is strong? Would the recipient be told of the potential donor's racial or ethnic classification? Would the donor be told of the recipient's racial or ethnic classification?

The acceptability of phenotype-based matching versus more race-based matching will likely vary with the views of the donor and recipient concerning their own and others' heritage. Heritage, like ethnicity, is partly a function of the biological determinants of race, but historical definitions of heritage typically involve powerfully symbolic views of "us" and "others." In the past two decades, state laws and institutional policies on transracial adoption throughout the United States have created a great deal of controversy. The most outspoken proponent of a ban on transracial adoption has been the National Association of Black Social Workers, which claims that black children are the responsibility of the black community, and that the placement of black children into white families is a form of genocide.[84] Hispanics, too, have claimed that "their children" should not be adopted by white families, who will be unable to provide knowledge and experiences essential to the children's Hispanic heritage.[85]

The controversy over transracial adoption will likely have parallels in transracial OD, as some will almost certainly see eggs as belonging ultimately to the group. Although the extent of transracial OD from black donors to white recipients is unlikely to be at all significant, it is possible, given the unavailability of black donors, that a black woman would be given the eggs of a white donor. It was in just such a scenario that a mixed-race British woman received a white donor's egg in late 1993, after waiting four years for a black donor.[86] Before policy on transracial OD is established, the question of a child's heritage and its value remains a real one. Will a child raised by a nonbiological, gestational mother of a different race or ethnic group have a healthy and balanced self-image and appreciation of his or her ethnic origin? What do the self-images and experiences of mixed-race children conceived naturally imply for the creation of mixed-race children by technological intervention?

It is also easy to forget or ignore the prejudices and strife that may be common among groups with similar biological and cultural heritage. For example, an Iranian-American woman might accept an egg from a woman of Mexican or Filipino descent with a similar appearance much more readily than she would an egg from an Iraqi-American donor. One risk of intercultural egg donation is that the parents of the resulting infant may later feel estranged from the child, compounding the retrospective ambivalence toward the technological procedure. While it may be possible to screen for some of these unconscious responses during psychological testing, others may not appear until after the conception or birth of a child. Clinics that offer OD may not be able to resolve all of the issues of racial and ethnic bigotry that their patients and donors bring with them, but they should be prepared to address them as thoroughly as possible.

CREATING DEMAND AND DISAPPOINTMENT

Of all the considerations essential to meaningful policy on OD, an authoritative definition of its appropriate medical role is most important. In the United States, most technological advances in medicine are adopted into widespread practice long before they have been thoroughly assessed and their strengths and limits established scientifically.[87] IVF is one such widely diffused technology, where practice guidelines may be too late to have much effect on practice or growing public demand. Without attention to a medical definition of the appropriate use of OD, and practice guidelines that outline the limits of appropriate use, the growing consumer demand for OD that specialists already anticipate may far exceed what even they believe to be its medically justifiable application. OD has already received considerable publicity as a number of women in their late 50s and early 60s have become new mothers through the technique, although menopause was not originally included among the conditions for which OD was indicated.

Another pressing reason for clear practice guidelines in advance of adoption is that the establishment of limits after the creation of inappropriate demand leads to widespread disappointment and resentment among potential patients, and resentment and defection among practitioners. In Canada, where IVF has been used widely for a variety of indications, the recent report of the Royal Commission on New Reproductive Technologies has met with moral outrage from many who reject its recommendation that the application of IVF be sharply curtailed.[88]

While the United States does not have the nationalized system of health care that would make possible standardized definitions of appropriate treatment for all fertility clinics, current discussion of health care changes promises to make greater standardization a reality. Inasmuch as many private insurers already believe IVF to be not cost-effective, and many physicians and policymakers find it unjustifiable to extend infertility treatment to women covered by Medicaid or Medicare, it appears highly unlikely that IVF, and consequently OD, will be included in any package of essential services. The availability of reproductive technologies for poor women and nonwhite women is more likely to shrink than grow.

As evidenced in the debate about welfare reform, both policymakers and much of the public contend that the poor and nonwhites, typically viewed in this context as a single group, already have too many children at too great a burden to the public coffers. Whether the result of a potentially racist calculation of social costs or an assessment of the basis of the best interests of (future) children or parents still living in poverty, many conclude that greater public availability of infertility services would only increase the number of children dependent on the state. Careful, self-critical analysis of the motives behind limits on coverage for infertility treatment will be essential to ethical policy for the poor.

Many advocates of poor women's reproductive rights view the use of reproductive technology as a tragic medicalization of women's (and men's) personal experiences of procreation. Hence, proponents of women's choice are also likely to urge that IVF not be included in a standard health care package, provided that the "savings" are used to benefit women in other ways. The empowerment of poor and nonwhite women would not mean educating them to adopt a medical view of infertility, but rather educating them on the *causes* of infertility and providing support for behaviors that reduce the incidence of infertility-causing disease.

Two of the OTA's first recommendations on how Congress could address infertility were the establishment of a national data collection system to study chlamydia and PID, and the prevention of infertility through public education.[89] Neither of these options has been pursued. One of the unfortunate effects of technological advance in any area of treatment is the perception that it is easier to treat the condition than prevent it. In addition, education and prevention strategies often lack strong advocates. If debate on the allocation of resources in the area of fertility continues to focus on costly reproductive technologies, the prevention of infertility will likely receive even less attention, to the further detriment of poor and nonwhite women already excluded from treatment. A three-part preventive and primary care program, consisting of education, access to preventive services, and access to treatment for sexually transmitted diseases (STDs), could empower poor and nonwhite women to safeguard their own fertility and reproductive health.

Essential to the reduction of infertility is education about PID and the STDs that cause it. Currently, the primary focus of such public education is in the schools, where health education typically includes information on sexuality, reproduction, and STDs, including HIV. The increased rate of sexual activity among preteen girls in some groups means that educational campaigns are needed at the elementary as well as junior high school level. Educational programs for adolescents may make a more convincing case for abstinence and "safe sex" by stressing that unprotected intercourse *threatens* their ability to have babies.

Outside of the schools, especially in communities where fertility appears to be essential to a woman's identity, public health campaigns should emphasize that contraception with barrier methods protects future fertility as well as preventing unwanted pregnancy and the transmission of HIV. Greater access to preventive measures against PID-induced infertility, particularly barrier contraceptives, has been a fortunate side effect of campaigns against the spread of HIV. However, assumptions about poor and nonwhite women's compliance with birth control regimens often lead doctors and nurses to prescribe Norplant, Deprovera, or an IUD rather than forms of contraception that depend on a woman's own action.[90] Although the use of condoms may appear to be redundant, or may be difficult for women whose partners do not want them to use birth control, appeals to the protection of future fertility may add weight to current warnings about the dangers of HIV for both women and men. Again, programs to increase the availability of barrier contraceptives must acknowledge the early age at which many girls engage in sexual intercourse, even as such girls are taught the social and developmental skills necessary to postpone sexual activity.

Finally, easy access to diagnosis and treatment of infertility-causing STDs is both an essential element in any personal health care benefits package and integral to any meaningful public health system. The low-tech treatment of STDs through antibiotics for both men and women can significantly reduce the incidence of infertility from PID and the potential demand for high-tech reproductive services. Attention to the diagnosis and effective treatment of STDs, complemented by a culturally tailored message on the consequences of PID for fertility and the means for preventing it, offers a more just approach to allocation that respects individuals and the important differences among classes and ethnic groups.

NOTES

1. American Fertility Society, "Guidelines for Gamete Donation: 1993," *Fertility and Sterility* 59, Supp. 1 (1993): 5S.

2. Christine Gorman, "How Old Is Too Old?" *Time*, Sept. 30, 1991, p. 62; William E. Schmidt, "Birth to a 59-Year-Old Generates an Ethical Controversy in Britain," *New York Times* (National Ed.), Dec. 13, 1993, p. A1; Mark V. Sauer and Richard J. Paulson, "Understanding the Current Status of Oocyte Donation in the United States: What's Really Going On Out There?" *Fertility and Sterility* 58 (1992): 16–18; Mark V. Sauer, Richard J. Paulson, and Rogerio A. Lobo, "Reversing the Natural Decline in Human Fertility: An Extended Clinical Trial of Oocyte Donation to Women of Advanced Reproductive Age," *Journal of the American Medical Association* 268 (1992): 1275–79.

3. Paula Mergenhagen DeWitt, "In Pursuit of Pregnancy," *American Demographics* 15 (1993): 48–54; Martin M. Quigley, "The New Frontier of Reproductive Age (Editorial)," *Journal of the American Medical Association* 268 (1992): 1320–21.

4. See, for example, Elisabeth Beck-Gernsheim, "From the Pill to Test-Tube Babies: New Options, New Pressures in Reproductive Behavior," in *Healing Technology: Feminist Perspectives*, ed. Kathryn Strother Ratcliff et al. (Ann Arbor: University of Michigan Press, 1989), pp. 23–40; Gena Corea, "The Reproductive Brothel," in *Man-Made Women: How New Reproductive Technologies Affect Women*, ed. Gena Corea et al. (Bloomington: Indiana University Press, 1987), pp. 38–51; Gena Corea, "What the King Can Not See," in *Embryos, Ethics and Women's Rights: Exploring the New Reproductive Technologies*, ed. Elaine Hoffman et al. (London: Haworth Press, 1988), pp. 77–93; Judith Lorber, "In Vitro Fertilization and Gender Politics," in *Embryos, Ethics and Women's Rights: Exploring the New Reproductive Technologies*, ed. Elaine Hoffman et al. (London: Haworth Press, 1988), pp. 117–33; Barbara Katz Rothman, "The Meanings of Choice in Reproductive Technology," in *Test-Tube Women: What Future for Motherhood?* ed. Rita Arditti et al. (London: Pandora Press, 1984), pp. 23–33.

5. Ronald H. Gray, "Epidemiology of Infertility," *Current Opinion in Obstetrics and Gynecology* 2 (1990): 154–58; William D. Mosher and William F. Pratt, *Fecundity, Infertility, and Reproductive Health in the United States, 1982* (Hyattsville, MD: National Center for Health Statistics, 1987); U.S. Congress, Office of Technology Assessment, *Infertility: Medical and Social Choices* (Washington, DC: U.S. Government Printing Office, 1988).

6. OTA, *Infertility*, pp. 49–52.

7. Gray, "Epidemiology of Infertility"; Marilyn B. Hirsch and William D. Mosher, "Characteristics of Infertile Women in the United States and Their Use of Infertility Services," *Fertility and Sterility* 47 (1987): 618–25; Lynne Wilcox and William D. Mosher, "Use of Infertility Services in the United States," *Obstetrics and Gynecology* 82 (1993): 122–27.

8. Mosher and Pratt, *Fecundity, Infertility, and Reproductive Health*; William D.

Mosher and William F. Pratt, "Fecundity and Infertility in the United States, 1965–1988: Advance Data," *Vital and Health Statistics* (Hyattsville, MD: National Center for Health Statistics, 1990); William D. Mosher and William F. Pratt, "Fecundity and Infertility in the United States: Incidence and Trends," *Fertility and Sterility* S6 (1991): 192–93; Wilcox and Mosher, "Use of Infertility Services in the United States."

9. Gray, "Epidemiology of Infertility," 154–58; Hirsch and Mosher, "Characteristics of Infertile Women," 618–25. Advance data from the 1988 NSFG have been available since late 1990, but the survey's results are not yet reported in full and are much less well known.

10. OTA, *Infertility*, pp. 49–52.

11. Betsy Hartman, *Reproductive Rights and Wrongs* (New York: Harper & Row, 1987); Laurie Nsiah-Jefferson, "Reproductive Laws, Women of Color, and Low-Income Women," in *Reproductive Laws for the 1990s*, ed. Sherrill Cohen and Nadine Taub (Clifton, NJ: Humana Press, 1989), pp. 23–67, 46–49; Laurie Nsiah-Jefferson and Elaine J. Hall, "Reproductive Technology: Perspectives and Implications for Low-Income Women and Women of Color," in *Healing Technology: Feminist Perspectives,* ed. Kathryn Strother Ratcliff et al. (Ann Arbor: University of Michigan Press, 1989), pp. 93–117, 102–104; Thomas B. Littlewood, *The Politics of Population Control* (Notre Dame: University of Notre Dame Press, 1977); Dorothy E. Roberts, "The Future of Reproductive Choice for Poor Women and Women of Color," *Women's Rights Law Reporter* 12 (1990): 59–67.

12. Maggie Black, *Better Health for Women and Children through Family Planning* (New York: The Population Control Council, 1987); Kathleen Newland, "Women and Population Control: Choice beyond Childbearing, Worldwatch Paper 16" (Washington, DC: Worldwatch Institute, 1977).

13. Littlewood, *Politics of Population Control*; Hartman, *Reproductive Rights and Wrongs.*

14. Sevgi O. Aral and Willard Cates, Jr., "The Increasing Concern with Infertility: Why Now?" *Journal of the American Medical Association* 250 (1983): 2327–31; Mosher and Pratt, "Advance Data"; Mosher and Pratt, "Incidence and Trends"; Wilcox and Mosher, "Use of Infertility Services in the United States."

15. The NSGF recognizes both "formal" and "informal" marriage, although it appears not to include "informal" marriages between lesbian women, whose patterns and views of fertility are not specifically considered but who pose a number of ethical and policy challenges for reproductive services.

16. Wilcox and Mosher, "Use of Infertility Services in the United States."

17. Centers for Disease Control and Prevention, "Use of Race and Ethnicity in Public Health Surveillance: Summary of the CDC/ATSDR Workshop," *MMWR* 42/RR-10 (1993): 12; Nsiah-Jefferson, "Reproductive Laws, Women of Color, and Low-Income Women," pp. 23–67. Additionally, in its focus on married women, the NSFG disregards the prevalence of unmarried, sexually active women for whom impaired fertility may be a real concern. See Andrew J. Cherlin, *Marriage, Divorce, Remarriage* (Cambridge: Harvard University Press, 1992); Ellen Wright Clayton, "Women and Advances in Medical Technologies: The Legal Issues," in *Women and the New Reproductive Technologies: Medical, Psychosocial, Legal and Ethical Dilemmas,* ed. Judith Rodin and Aila Collins (Hillsdale, NJ: Lawrence Erlbaum Assoc., 1991), pp. 89–109, 91–92; Stephanie Coontz, *The Way We Never Were* (New York: Basic

Books, 1992), pp. 247–55; Nsiah-Jefferson and Hall, "Reproductive Technology," pp. 109–10.

18. Office of Management and Budget, "Directive No. 15: Race and Ethnic Standards for Federal Statistics and Administrative Reporting," in *Statistical Policy Handbook* (Washington, DC: U.S. Dept. of Commerce, Office of Federal Statistical Policy and Standards, 1978). Typically, demographic categories such as the NSFG's fail to define the distinguishing characteristics of race and ethnicity or account for mixed racial heritage. Reports of data seldom define how or why the definitions used are important to the questions under study. CDC, "Use of Race and Ethnicity," pp. 12–15. Variation in racial and ethnic taxonomies results in inconsistencies across databases; for example, information from the NSFG's three-category system does not merge well with U.S. Census data on patterns of fertility, which uses white, black, American Indian/Alaskan Native, Asian/Pacific Islander, and Spanish origin, all races. CDC, "Use of Race and Ethnicity," p. 7.

19. CDC, "Use of Race and Ethnicity"; Institute of Medicine, *Women and Health Research* (Washington, DC: National Academy Press, 1994), pp. 114–19.

20. OTA, *Infertility*, p. 16.

21. Gray, "The Epidemiology of Infertility."

22. CDC, "Use of Race and Ethnicity"; Richard Cooper and Richard David, "The Biological Concept of Race and Its Application to Health and Epidemiology," *Journal of Health Politics, Policy, and Law* 11 (1986): 97–116; Trevor A. Sheldon and Hilda Parker, "Race and Ethnicity in Health Research," *Journal of Public Health Medicine* 14 (1992): 104–10.

23. CDC, "Use of Race and Ethnicity," p. 5; IOM, *Women and Health Research,* pp. 118–19.

24. CDC, "Use of Race and Ethnicity," p. 5; IOM, *Women and Health Research,* pp. 114–15.

25. CDC, "Use of Race and Ethnicity," p. 10; Nsiah-Jefferson, "Reproductive Laws, Women of Color, and Low-Income Women," p. 23.

26. LuAnn Aday, *At Risk in America: The Health and Health Care Needs of Vulnerable Populations in the United States* (New York: Jossey-Bass, 1992), pp. 91–92, 181–85.

27. Clayton, "Legal Issues," pp. 91–92; OTA, *Infertility*, pp. 144–46.

28. DeWitt, "In Pursuit of Pregnancy," 48–54; Philip Elmer-DeWitt, "Making Babies," *Time* (Sept. 30, 1991), 56–63; Rebecca Dresser, "Social Justice in New Reproductive Techniques," in *Genetics and the Law III,* ed. Aubrey Milunsky and George J. Annas (New York: Plenum Press, 1984), pp. 159–74; Gina Kolata, "Young Women Offer to Sell Their Eggs to Infertile Couples," *New York Times* (National Ed.) (Nov. 10, 1991), Sec. A, p. 1; Sauer and Paulson, "Understanding the Current Status of Oocyte Donation."

29. Margarete Sandelowski and Christine Pollock, "Women's Experience of Infertility," *Image: Journal of Nursing Scholarship* 18 (1986): 140–44.

30. American Fertility Society, *State Laws on Infertility Insurance Coverage* (Washington, DC: AFS Office of Government Relations, 1992).

31. OTA, *Infertility*, pp. 149–55.

32. Kolata, "Young Women Offer to Sell Their Eggs"; Barbara Liebmann-Smith, "Medical Miracle ... or Baby Selling," *Redbook,* Nov. 1992, pp. 120–26; Barbara

Nevins, "The $2,000 Egg," *Redbook,* Nov. 1992): 119–26; Sauer and Paulson, "Understanding the Current Status of Oocyte Donation."

33. Gena Corea, "Egg Snatchers," in *Test-Tube Women: What Future for Motherhood?* ed. Rita Arditti et al. (London: Pandora Press, 1984), pp. 37–51; Gena Corea, *The Mother Machine* (New York: Harper & Row, 1985), pp. 232–34; Kolata, "Young Women Offer to Sell Their Eggs"; Julie Murphy, "Egg Farming and Women's Future," in *Test-Tube Women: What Future for Motherhood?* ed. Rita Arditti et al. (London: Pandora Press, 1984), pp. 68–75.

34. Elizabeth A. D. Kennard et al., "A Program for Matched, Anonymous Oocyte Donation," *Fertility and Sterility* 51 (1989): 655–60; Kolata, "Young Women Offer to Sell Their Eggs"; Liebmann-Smith, "Medical Miracle"; Nevins, "The $2,000 Egg"; Martin M. Quigley, "Establishment of an Oocyte Donor Program: Donor Screening and Selection," *Annals N.Y. Academy of Sciences* 626 (1991): 445–51; Mark V. Sauer and Richard J. Paulson, "Oocyte Donors: A Demographic Analysis of Women at the University of Southern California," *Human Reproduction* 7 (1992): 726–28; L. R. Schover et al., "The Personality and Motivation of Semen Donors: A Comparison with Oocyte Donors," *Human Reproduction* 7 (1992): 575–79; Roberta Lessor et al., "An Analysis of Social and Psychological Characteristics of Women Volunteering to Become Oocyte Donors," *Fertility and Sterility* 59 (1993): 65–72.

35. Mosher and Pratt, "Advance Data"; Wilcox and Mosher, "Use of Infertility Services in the United States."

36. Mosher and Pratt, *Fecundity, Infertility, and Reproductive Health.*

37. Aral and Cates, "The Increasing Concern with Infertility."

38. Gray, "Epidemiology of Infertility"; OTA, *Infertility,* pp. 50–52.

39. Gray, "Epidemiology of Infertility"; Wilcox and Mosher, "Use of Infertility Services in the United States."

40. Gray, "Epidemiology of Infertility."

41. Gray, "Epidemiology of Infertility"; Mosher and Pratt, *Fecundity, Infertility, and Reproductive Health,* pp. 16–17; OTA, *Infertility,* pp. 61–62.

42. Sevgi O. Aral, William D. Mosher, and William Cates, Jr., "Self-Reported Pelvic Inflammatory Disease in the U.S.," *American Journal of Public Health* 75 (1985): 1216–18; Mosher and Pratt, *Fecundity, Infertility, and Reproductive Health,* p. 16.

43. Gray, "Epidemiology of Infertility"; Mosher and Pratt, *Fecundity, Infertility, and Reproductive Health,* pp. 16–17; OTA, *Infertility,* pp. 61–62.

44. Gray, "Epidemiology of Infertility."

45. Clayton, "Legal Issues," p. 92; Nsiah-Jefferson, "Reproductive Laws, Women of Color, and Low-Income Women," pp. 48–52; Nsiah-Jefferson and Hall, "Reproductive Technology," pp. 107–11.

46. Mosher and Pratt, "Advance Data"; Wilcox and Mosher, "Use of Infertility Services in the United States."

47. Wilcox and Mosher, "Use of Infertility Services in the United States."

48. Corea, *The Mother Machine,* pp. 145–46; Kathryn Strother Ratcliff, "Health Technologies for Women: Whose Health? Whose Technology?" in *Healing Technology: Feminist Perspectives,* ed. Kathryn Strother Ratcliff et al. (Ann Arbor: University of Michigan Press, 1989), pp. 109–11.

49. Ratcliff, "Health Technologies for Women," pp. 109–11.

50. Those that do exist are likely to be teaching facilities that have a central goal of training medical specialists, not treating women's infertility. Moreover, where their budgets are based on tax revenue, they are very vulnerable to funding cuts whenever other obstetrical and gynecological services, such as prenatal care, need additional support.

51. Clayton, "Legal Issues," pp. 91–93; Corea, *The Mother Machine,* pp. 145–46; Nsiah-Jefferson, "Reproductive Laws, Women of Color, and Low-Income Women," pp. 50–51; Ratcliff, "Health Technologies for Women," pp. 109–11.

52. Nsiah-Jefferson, "Reproductive Laws, Women of Color, and Low-Income Women," pp. 51–52.

53. Irwin M. Rosenstock, "The Health Belief Model: Explaining Health Behavior through Expectancies," in *Health Behavior and Health Education: Theory, Research and Practice,* ed. K. Glanz, F. M. Lewis, and B. Rimer (San Francisco: Jossey-Bass, 1990), pp. 39–62.

54. Sarah S. Brown, ed., *Prenatal Care: Reaching Mothers, Reaching Infants* (Washington, DC: National Academy Press, 1988).

55. Nancy E. Adler, Susan Keys, and Patricia Robertson, "Psychological Issues in New Reproductive Technologies: Pregnancy-Inducing Technologies and Diagnostic Screening," in *Women and the New Reproductive Technologies: Medical, Psychosocial, Legal and Ethical Dilemmas,* ed. Judith Rodin and Aila Collins (Hillsdale, NJ: Lawrence Erlbaum Assoc., 1991), pp. 111–12; Nsiah-Jefferson, "Reproductive Laws, Women of Color, and Low-Income Women," pp. 51–52.

56. Adler, Keys, and Robertson, "Psychological Issues in New Reproductive Technologies"; Gray, "Epidemiology of Infertility"; Arthur L. Greil, *Not Yet Pregnant: Infertile Couples in Contemporary America* (New Brunswick, NJ: Rutgers University Press, 1991), pp. 20–21; L. Jill Halman, Antonia Abbey, and Frank M. Andrews, "Why Are Couples Satisfied with Infertility Treatment," *Fertility and Sterility* 59 (1993): 1046–54; Hirsch and Mosher, "Characteristics of Infertile Women"; Sandelowski and Pollock, "Women's Experience of Infertility."

57. Halman, Abbey, and Andrews, "Why Are Couples Satisfied with Infertility Treatment," p. 1047. Such a selection bias can seriously affect the validity of research questions as well as the hypothesis being tested. In this article on couples' satisfaction with infertility treatment, researchers claimed that they wanted to explore the factors that influenced couples' participation in treatment beyond the diagnosis of infertility. In fact, because they excluded those infertile couples who did not, or could not, continue past an infertility work-up, they studied only the reasons that married, white, middle-class couples with no previous children sought treatment.

58. Halman, Abbey, and Andrews, "Why Are Couples Satisfied with Infertility Treatment"; Rothman, "The Meanings of Choice in Reproductive Technology," pp. 23–33; Margarete Sandelowski, "The Color Gray: Ambiguity and Infertility," *Image: The Journal of Nursing Scholarship* 19 (1987): 70–74; Sandelowski and Pollock, "Women's Experience of Infertility"; OTA, *Infertility,* pp. 37–38; Wilcox and Mosher, "Use of Infertility Services in the United States."

59. Adler, Keys, and Robertson, "Psychological Issues in New Reproductive Technologies"; Greil, *Not Yet Pregnant,* pp. 4–5; Halman, Abbey, and Andrews, "Why Are Couples Satisfied with Infertility Treatment."

60. Adler, Keys, and Robertson, "Psychological Issues in New Reproductive Tech-

nologies"; Rothman, "The Meanings of Choice in Reproductive Technology," pp. 23–33; Sandelowski, "The Color Gray"; Sandelowski and Pollock, "Women's Experience of Infertility"; Wilcox and Mosher, "Use of Infertility Services in the United States."

61. H. Anderson, "After the Diagnosis: An Operational Theology for the Terminally Ill," *Journal of Pastoral Care* 43 (1989): 141–50; Elizabeth Heitman, "The Influence of Values and Culture in Responses to Suffering," in *The Hidden Dimension of Illness: Human Suffering*, ed. Patricia L. Starck and John P. McGovern (New York: National League for Nursing Press, 1992), pp. 81–103.

62. Greil, *Not Yet Pregnant*, pp. 10, 154–73.

63. Denise L. Carmody, "Judaism," in *Women in World Religions*, Arvind Sharma, ed. (Albany, NY: State University of New York Press, 1987), p. 187; David M. Feldman, *Marital Relations, Birth Control, and Abortion in Jewish Law* (New York: Schocken Books, 1974), pp. 49–56.

64. Feldman, *Marital Relations*, pp. 21–27; Elaine Pagels, *Adam, Eve, and the Serpent* (New York: Harper & Row, 1988), pp. 28–31; Geoffrey Parrinder, *Sex in the World Religions* (Oxford: Oxford University Press, 1980), pp. 218–35; Rosemary R. Ruether, "Christianity," in *Women in World Religions*, ed. Arvind Sharma (Albany, NY: State University of New York Press, 1987), pp. 209–15.

65. Kenneth Vaux, *Birth Ethics: Religious and Cultural Values in the Genesis of Life* (New York: Crossroad Publishing Co., 1989), pp. 121–22.

66. Katherine K. Young, "Introduction," in *Women in World Religions*, Arvind Sharma, ed. (Albany, NY: State University of New York Press, 1987), p. 20.

67. Greil, *Not Yet Pregnant*, pp. 7–8; Theresa Kelleher, "Confucianism," in *Women in World Religions*, Arvind Sharma, ed. (Albany, NY: State University of New York Press, 1987), p. 137; Parrinder, *Sex in the World Religions*, pp. 94–95.

68. Katherine K. Young, "Hinduism," in *Women in World Religions*, Arvind Sharma, ed. (Albany, NY: State University of New York Press, 1987), pp. 81–82; Parrinder, *Sex in the World Religions*, pp. 71–72.

69. Greil, *Not Yet Pregnant*, pp. 7–10; John S. Mbiti, *African Religions and Philosophies* (Garden City, NY: Anchor Doubleday, 1970), pp. 143–44; Parrinder, *Sex in the World Religions*, pp. 142–44. Thus, many African women with HIV infection continue to have children even when they understand that the child will likely die of the condition. To not bear children is to cut oneself off from life.

70. Parrinder, *Sex in the World Religions*, pp. 156–60; Aliah Schleifer, *Motherhood in Islam* (Cambridge: The Islamic Academy, 1986); Jane I. Smith, "Islam," in *Women in World Religions*, Arvind Sharma, ed. (Albany, NY: State University of New York Press, 1987), pp. 238–39.

71. Nsiah-Jefferson and Hall, "Reproductive Technology," p. 104; Sandelowski, "The Color Gray," p. 72.

72. Bonnie Thornton Dill, Maxine Baca Zinn, and Sandra Patton, "Feminism, Race, and the Politics of Family Values," Report from the Institute for Philosophy and Public Policy (School of Public Affairs, University of Maryland) 13/3 (1993): 13–18; Greil, *Not Yet Pregnant*, pp. 7–10; Nsiah-Jefferson, "Reproductive Laws, Women of Color, and Low Income Women," pp. 51–52.

73. Cherlin, *Marriage, Divorce, Remarriage*, pp. 107–19; Coontz, *The Way We Never Were*, pp. 207–31; Greil, *Not Yet Pregnant*, pp. 40–41; Nsiah-Jefferson, "Reproductive Laws, Women of Color, and Low Income Women," pp. 51–52.

74. OTA, *Infertility*, pp. 364–67.

75. Feldman, *Marital Relations*, pp. 132–43; Emily Martin, "The Egg and the Sperm: How Science Has Constructed a Romance Based on Stereotypical Male-Female Roles," *Journal of Women in Culture and Society* 16 (1991): 485–501.

76. Greil, *Not Yet Pregnant*, pp. 63–71; Ratcliff, "Health Technologies for Women," pp. 173–98.

77. Rene Frydman et al., "A Protocol for Satisfying the Ethical Issues Raised by Oocyte Donation: Free, Anonymous, and Fertile Donors," *Fertility and Sterility* 53 (1990): 666–72; Kennard et al., "A Program for Matched, Anonymous Oocyte Donation"; Kolata, "Young Women Offer to Sell Their Eggs"; Daniel Navot et al., "Poor Oocyte Quality Rather than Implantation Failure as a Cause of Age-Related Decline in Female Fertility," *Lancet* 337 (1991): 1375–77; Thordur Oskarsson et al., "Attitudes towards Gamete Donation among Couples Undergoing In Vitro Fertilization," *British Journal of Obstetrics and Gynaecology* 98 (1991): 351–56; John A. Robertson, "Technology and Motherhood: Legal and Ethical Issues in Human Egg Donation," *Case Western Reserve Law Review* 39 (1988): 23–25.

78. Such conflicts of interest between the role of caregiver and procurer is well recognized among specialists in the somewhat parallel field of organ transplantation; transplant surgeons do not care for a potential patient/donor or contact the patient's family about donation in order to avoid the appearance that the patient's caregivers are anything less than completely concerned with the patient's well-being.

79. Liebmann-Smith, "Medical Miracle"; Nevins, "The $2,000 Egg."

80. The typical use of standard psychological screening tests to screen egg donors and recipients may need to be reevaluated or supplemented where the woman being examined is of a significantly different cultural background. As the cultural contructs of these tests may not be intelligible to her, the appropriateness of her answers may not be a true indication of her mental health. See Walter J. Lonner and Fara A. Ibrahim, "Assessment in Cross-Cultural Counseling," in *Counseling Across Cultures*, 3rd ed., ed. Paul B. Pedersen (Honolulu: University of Hawaii Press, 1989), pp. 304–19.

81. Eric J. Cassell, *Talking with Patients, Vol. 1: The Theory of Doctor-Patient Communication* (Cambridge, MA: The MIT Press, 1985), pp. 120–23.

82. G. Horne et al., "The Recruitment of Oocyte Donors," *British Journal of Obstetrics and Gynaecology* 100 (1993): 877–78; Kennard et al., "A Program for Matched, Anonymous Oocyte Donation"; Kolata, "Young Women Offer to Sell Their Eggs"; Lessor et al., "An Analysis of Social and Psychological Characteristics"; Nevins, "The $2,000 Egg"; Quigley, "Establishment of an Oocyte Donor Program"; Sauer and Paulson, "Oocyte Donors."

83. Karima A. Haynes, "The Adoption Option," *Ebony* XLVIII August, 1993, p. 46.

84. National Association of Black Social Workers, *Preserving Black Families: Research and Action beyond Rhetoric* (1986).

85. Sarah Glazer, "Breaking Adoption Barriers: Texas Law Eases Same-Race Limits," *Houston Chronicle*, Jan. 2, 1994, p. 3D.

86. Michael Goldfarb, "U. K. Enacts Legislation to Control In Vitro Pregnancies," National Public Radio Morning Edition, Jan. 10, 1994, pp. 10–12 (transcript).

87. Ann L. Greer, "The State of the Art versus the State of the Science: The Diffusion of New Medical Technologies into Practice," *International Journal of Technology Assessment in Health Care* 4 (1988): 5–26.

88. Royal Commission on New Reproductive Technologies, *Proceed with Care:*

The Final Report of the Royal Commission on New Reproductive Technologies (Ottawa, ON: Canada Communications Group Publishing, 1993).

89. OTA, *Infertility*, p. 15–18.

90. Kim Yanoshik and Judy Norsigian, "Contraception, Control, and Choice: International Perspectives," in *Healing Technology: Feminist Perspectives*, ed. Kathryn Strother Ratcliff et al. (Ann Arbor: University of Michigan Press, 1989), pp. 61–92.

FOURTEEN

FUNDING NEW REPRO-
DUCTIVE TECHNOLOGIES

Should They Be Included in Health Insurance Benefit Packages?

Dan W. Brock, Ph.D.

I. INTRODUCTION

In 1952 the President's Commission on the Health Needs of the Nation declared that "access to the means for the attainment and preservation of health is a basic human right."[1] Thirty-one years later in 1983 the President's Commission for the Study of Ethical Problems in Medicine and Biomedical and Behavioral Research concluded that "society has an ethical obligation to ensure equitable access to health care for all." It defined equitable access as requiring "that all citizens be able to secure an adequate level of care without excessive burdens."[2] But such general endorsements of rights to health care or obligations to secure an adequate level of care leave open what care should be covered or included in the services available to all.

While at the present time, 1995, efforts for broad-ranging national health care reform have failed, the health care system is nevertheless undergoing fundamental change, driven largely by market forces. There will be no uniform basic benefit package of health care services guaranteed to all Americans in the foreseeable future, but decisions still will have to be made by insurers, employers, states, and others about what services particular health care plans will cover. The coverage of new reproductive technologies (NRTs) in health insurance plans is especially controversial. The recent priority-setting process in Oregon to determine what services would be covered in the state Medicaid program ranked infertility services well down on its list of services, thereby excluding them from coverage. The Clinton administration's ill-fated health care reform proposal also did not cover these services. Some states require coverage of these services, but most do not. These exclusions from coverage should not become embedded in public policy without critical scrutiny.

It is beyond the scope of this paper to present and evaluate either general or specific theories of justice in health care. I believe that nearly all such theories imply, whether explicitly or implicitly, that a comprehensive package of health care services should be available to all Americans, and I shall assume that here. Should NRTs such as oocyte donation be covered as part of that package and in private health insurance packages?

The health care system cannot make available to everyone every service they might want, no matter how small its likely benefit and how great its cost. There will inevitably and appropriately be some limits on what is covered. One ground for not covering these NRTs would be if the moral importance of the benefits of NRTs within a theory of justice in health care is sufficiently limited as not to warrant their costs. This issue concerns the relative moral priority of NRTs in comparison with other health care services. While I cannot fully evaluate here the place of NRTs in a comprehensive theory of justice in health care, in Section III below I shall sketch three different moral arguments, each of which supports assigning relatively high moral importance to NRTs in comparison with other health care services. If these arguments are sound, NRTs should be included in comprehensive health care benefit packages, whether public or private, packages which typically include services of significantly lower moral priority or importance.

However, even if the arguments in Section III are sound, there might be special features of NRTs which would justify excluding them from such coverage, despite their apparent moral importance. In Section IV, I shall consider and generally reject a number of such arguments. The overall conclusion of the paper will then be, with a qualification to be noted, that NRTs ought as a matter of justice to be included within comprehensive health care benefit packages that should be available to all.

Before proceeding to these arguments, however, I want to discuss briefly in the next section a different approach to these issues and indicate its relation to my argument in Sections III and IV. The moral issue of access to NRTs is often framed as a part of the general issue of reproductive freedom. More specifically, is there a moral right to reproductive freedom and, if so, what are the scope and limits of that right? In the next section I shall discuss several aspects of an overall right to reproductive freedom in order to show that access to NRTs is properly considered part of that right. But no substantive claims in the paper will turn on whether the language and concepts of rights provide the proper formulation of the issues. The argument can, but need not, be framed in terms of moral rights.

II. SHOULD INDIVIDUALS' REPRODUCTIVE FREEDOM INCLUDE ACCESS TO NEW REPRODUCTIVE TECHNOLOGIES?

John Robertson characterizes "procreative liberty," which I take here to be essentially equivalent to reproductive freedom, as "freedom in activities and choices related to procreation," but notes that "the term does not tell us what activities fall within its scope."[3] Moreover, if reproductive freedom is defined in the service of defending a moral claim to its protection, for example in defense of a moral right to reproductive freedom, then its characterization will be morally controversial. I will not attempt here to offer a full account of what reproductive freedom properly includes, but will only say enough to indicate why access to NRTs like oocyte donation should be included as part of reproductive freedom. Reproductive freedom includes both freedom to and freedom not to reproduce. New reproductive technologies are means of increasing the fertility of otherwise infertile individuals, while various forms of contraception, new and old, as well as abortion, are means of limiting fertility to prevent procreation.

A common distinction in moral and political philosophy is between negative and positive rights. Negative rights require that others *not* act in particular ways that would violate the right. For example, your right not to be killed morally requires that others not perform any action that would kill you. Positive rights require others *to* act in specific ways required by the right. For example, if you have a right not to be allowed to die from starvation, then someone is morally required to provide you with food when that is necessary to prevent you from starving. In moral and political discourse, as well as in the law, rights are often complex combinations of both negative and positive components—for example, the right to life is often understood to include both a negative right not to be killed and a positive right to at least some forms of aid necessary for life.

The right to reproductive freedom contains both positive and negative components. For example, it forbids the state to prevent access to means of contraception,[4] but it also requires that contraception be provided to women who would otherwise not have access to it. Every negative component of the right to reproductive freedom does not, however, necessarily have a positive correlate. For example, while it may be morally wrong to interfere with a woman's use of some very expensive new reproductive technology that she has secured with her own funds, it does not follow from this alone that this same reproductive technology must be made available at public expense to anyone who needs and wants it regardless of the cost. Distinct and different kinds of arguments are typically necessary to support the negative component—the claim against interference by others with what you are able and wish to do—and the positive component—the claim on the efforts and resources of others to make possible what you wish to do but otherwise are unable to do. The scope and extent of the positive components of the right to reproductive freedom are particularly controversial—what actions, services, positive aid, and circumstances specific persons or the state must secure for individuals as part of their right. An independent argument grounded in a conception of justice is needed. Here then are components of reproductive freedom that explicitly concern access to new reproductive technologies. What follows is explicitly not intended to describe the scope of reproductive freedom comprehensively.

THE CHOICE OF WHETHER TO PROCREATE, WITH WHOM, AND BY WHAT MEANS

Reproductive freedom involves, first, uncoerced choice about whether to procreate at all, or, more precisely, whether to participate in procreative activity with a willing partner. When the decision about procreation is positive, reproductive freedom includes the choice of whether to reproduce by coital or available noncoital means. In the case of coital means, it includes with whom to have intercourse among willing partners in order to reproduce. In the case of noncoital methods, it can include which available method and which other persons to involve in furnishing sperm, ova, uterus, or some other service. Reproductive freedom thus includes at least some access to new reproductive techniques.[5]

THE SOCIAL CONTEXT IN WHICH REPRODUCTION TAKES PLACE

Reproductive freedom also should include some control over and choices about the social context in which reproduction will take place, for example, in or out of marriage, in heterosexual or homosexual relationships, as a sole parent or with another who will share parenting, and so forth. Access to NRTs should not be based on conditions such as these. Put generally, reproductive freedom requires that reproduction not have to take place in circumstances in which it would result in unjust deprivations, or have other unjust impacts on those who choose to, or not to, reproduce; of course, whether a particular impact of a choice about reproduction is unjust will often be morally controversial.

THE CHOICE OF WHEN TO REPRODUCE

Modern methods of contraception and procreation have made the choice of when to reproduce an increasingly important component of reproductive freedom. New reproductive techniques make it possible for women to reproduce at times when it would have been either unlikely or impossible for them to do so in the past. Control over the timing of reproduction is important, for example, to enable women, and sometimes men as well, to work or pursue careers before they begin families. The timing of reproduction often has myriad, complex, and important impacts on a person's life over which reproductive freedom should provide some control.

We have then a very brief and preliminary sketch of the principal aspects of reproductive freedom that makes clear that the common understanding of reproductive freedom as essentially concerned with preventing pregnancy by contraception, or preventing procreation by abortion, is far too narrow. Merely broadening that understanding to include access to the means of enhancing or creating fertility by new reproductive techniques also remains too narrow because it still ignores many important effects on women's, and to a lesser extent men's, lives of reproductive choices which are plausibly considered a part of reproductive freedom. Of course, the extent to which a moral right to reproductive freedom ought to secure to individuals control over many of these aspects of reproductive freedom is morally controversial. I shall begin to address those issues in the next section of this essay.

III. THE MORAL BASES OF A RIGHT TO REPRODUCTIVE FREEDOM; THE RELATIVE MORAL IMPORTANCE OF THE BENEFITS OF NRTs

What moral arguments serve as the defense or basis of a right to reproductive freedom that includes access to the NRTs? I will sketch three alternative accounts or bases for securing that right. These three accounts can also be understood as addressing the relative moral importance of the benefits of NRTs. Is that moral importance sufficient that NRTs should be included within basic health care benefit packages in either public or private health insurance? I shall not note the differences in detail needed to apply these arguments to one or the other purpose when those differences do not affect the principal substance of the arguments.

Probably the most common argument for access to NRTs grounds that access in an individual right to, or interest in, self-determination. The second argument, most natural within, though not exclusive to, utilitarian or general consequentialist moral views, derives access to NRTs from the important contribution they typically make to individuals' good or well-being. The third argument grounds access to NRTs in a principle of equality; in the version I sketch here, specifically equality of expectations and opportunity. I emphasize that these three different moral arguments for access to NRTs are not mutually exclusive. Instead, I believe each captures something morally important about access to NRTs, so that a full account of the moral basis of that access must incorporate all three lines of argument.

SELF-DETERMINATION

By people's interest in self-determination, I mean their interest in making significant decisions about their own lives for themselves, according to their own values or conception of a good life, and having those decisions respected by others. John Rawls has characterized this as a highest-order interest, based on people's capacity to form, revise over time, and pursue a plan of life.[6] The idea is that because people have conceptions of themselves as beings who persist over time, they have the capacity to form more or less long-term plans, goals, and intentions for their lives. Other things being equal, the further into the future, the less detailed and fixed these plans will typically be.

In addition, persons have the capacity to form what Harry Frankfurt has called second-order desires, desires which take other desires, not first-order activities and experiences, as their object.[7] I prefer to put this point in terms of our capacity to value having particular desires or motivations. It is this capacity that makes it sensible to say that, unlike other animals, people have a conception of the good which is more than simply having desires and motivations, the feature we share with other animals.

By this second-order reflection about what we value doing, having, and being, we form and then act on a conception of our good, rather than simply being guided by instinct and environmental stimulus. Of course, none of this is to deny that people's social and natural environment deeply affects their values and conception of the good. But by having our choices respected by others, at least in the sense that they do not interfere within limits with those choices, even though they may disagree with them, we take control over and responsibility for our lives and for the kinds of persons we become.

In characterizing our autonomy or self-determination interest as a highest-order interest, Rawls meant in part that it is of a higher order of importance than the particular aims and values that give content to our conception of the good or plan of life at any point in time.[8] We know from our own and others' experience that these specific aims and values can and will change over time in both predictable and unpredictable ways. Our interest in self-determination is our interest in being valuing agents, able to guide our own lives in this way. Self-determination is a central condition of moral personhood, part of a moral ideal of the person, whose value does not lie only in maximizing the satisfaction of our other desires. Applied to decisions about reproduction, self-determination is not simply of instrumental value, resting only on individuals making the best or wisest decisions, but is also of intrinsic value, as part of an attractive moral ideal of the person.

The exercise of self-determination is also of more or less importance or value on different occasions and for different decisions. Perhaps the most important factor determining this differential importance or value is the nature of the decision in question. Other things being equal, the more central and far-reaching the impact a particular decision will have on an individual's life, the more substantial the individual's self-determination interest in making it. This is why self-determination is typically so important in most of the decisions or choices which compose reproductive freedom—specifically, choices about whether, with whom, when, how often, by what means, and in what circumstances to procreate. Few decisions that people make are more personal than these, in the sense that what is the best choice depends on people's own personal aims and values, or more far-reaching in their impact on people's lives.

The moral case for access to NRTs can thus be based on individuals' self-determination interest being of sufficient moral importance that decision-making authority regarding their use should in nearly all cases be left with those individuals. (I say "in nearly all cases" because I do not believe such a right is plausibly taken to be absolute or unlimited and never overridden by other moral considerations, although I cannot pursue these limits here.) Our moral right to or interest in self-determination is often interpreted as requiring only noninterference by others with relevant areas of behavior, that is as only a negative right. The ideal of the person that self-determination suggests can often ground moral claims on others to provide at least some necessary means to enable us to take control and responsibility for our lives. The importance of individual self-determination can ground at least some moral claim on others or the society at large to make NRTs available.

INDIVIDUAL GOOD OR WELL-BEING

A second line of argument in defense of access to NRTs appeals to the contribution they typically make to individuals' well-being or good. (Hereafter, I shall usually use only the notion of individual "good," though these concepts are not interchangeable in all contexts.) The precise form this argument takes will depend in part on the account of individual good employed. In the philosophical literature three main theories of the good for persons are commonly distinguished. Each is a theory of what is intrinsically good or valuable, that is, roughly, good independent of its consequences and relations to other things; many other things, of course, are instrumentally good because they lead to what is intrinsically good.

Conscious experience theories of the good hold that people's good is composed of certain kinds of positive conscious experiences, often characterized as pleasure or happiness (although on many theories of happiness, it is not fully reducible to any kind of conscious experience) and the absence of pain or unhappiness. Preference or desire satisfaction theories of the good hold that people's good consists of the satisfaction of their desires or preferences. Satisfying people's desires is different from, and should not be confused with, the satisfaction people normally experience when their desires are satisfied. A desire is satisfied when the object of that desire obtains; for example, my desire to be in Boston tomorrow is satisfied just in case I am in Boston tomorrow, independent of any conscious experience of satisfaction or enjoyment I may or may not experience when I am there. Finally, what I will call "objective good theories" deny that people's good consists only of positive conscious experiences or the satisfaction of their desires, but hold that some things are good for people even if they do not want them and will not obtain pleasure or happiness from them.[9] Different versions of objective good theories differ about what is objectively good for persons, but they typically appeal to the possession of certain virtues, for example, courage or trustworthiness, or ideals of the person, such as having deep personal relations like that between parent and child.

Many difficult and complex issues are involved in developing full and precise accounts of these alternative theories of the good for persons, and some of those issues have important implications for a defense of access to NRTs based on their promotion of individuals' good. Just to illustrate this point, for both NRTs and reproductive freedom more generally, desire satisfaction theories of the good for persons do not equate people's good simply with the satisfaction of their actual desires at any point in time. Rather, it is only the satisfaction of those desires which have been suitably corrected or "laundered" that can plausibly be held to be good for people.[10] People sometimes desire what will be bad for them due to misinformation about the objects of their desires, due to socialization that has shaped their desires in irrational ways, and due to the many other ways in which people's desires can be defective and not a reliable measure of their good.

When access to NRTs is defended as promoting people's good, what specific services, choices, and conditions should be provided will depend importantly on the details of the account of the good for persons employed. Nevertheless, it is clear that there is at least a broad connection between people's good and securing access to NRTs for them, as well as reproductive freedom more generally, on each of the three main accounts of that good. Securing access to NRTs for infertile individuals, like respecting other components of reproductive freedom, will generally contribute to people's happiness, satisfy people's desires concerning reproduction, and promote some typical objective components of the good such as the deep personal relations between parent and child. But it is important to this line of defense of access to NRTs, as well as of reproductive freedom more broadly, that each of these empirical claims is only plausible with the qualification "generally" that I have given it.

Securing access to NRTs for infertile individuals typically, but not always, provides them with a very substantial benefit, good, or contribution to their well-being. The claim is not that overcoming infertility is essential to human well-being, in the sense that it is necessary for mere survival or for a decent life. Infertile individuals can and often do compensate for this disability with other aims or pursuits, and so have a good life despite their infertility, just as people are able to do with other disabilities. The point is instead that for infertile individuals who want to overcome their infertility with the use of NRTs, being able to do so typically makes a substantial positive impact on their good or well-being. But in the case in which a person becomes resigned to being infertile and achieves a level of well-being from other pursuits comparable to what he or she would have obtained from parenting, there may still be a moral claim to access to NRTs to overcome infertility. The ground of that claim is likely the self-determination and/or the equality-of-opportunity argument, not the appeal to well-being.

Defending a moral right to access to NRTs, or to broader reproductive freedom, by their promotion of people's good comes up against the general problems of defending moral rights by appeal to the good consequences of respecting them—sometimes we believe that rights should be respected even when better consequences would be produced by violating them.[11] A distinctive feature of rights claims generally, and of a moral right to reproductive freedom in particular, is that the rights' possessor is morally entitled to make her own reproductive choices even when those choices may not produce the most good for all affected, or will not best promote her own good when others are not significantly affected. It is notoriously difficult to defend *moral* rights which have this nonutilitarian or nonconsequentialist character, as opposed to social or legal rights, within a general utilitarian or consequentialist moral framework of maximizing the good. The point is not that a consequentialist moral framework fails to make a moral right to reproductive freedom absolute, in the sense that it can never be overridden by other conflicting moral considerations. I do not believe any moral rights to reproductive freedom in general, or to access to NRTs in particular, are absolute in that sense. Instead, my point is that a moral right to reproductive freedom including access to NRTs that is nonabsolute, but nevertheless nonconsequentialist in its strength, is difficult or impossible to defend by appeal to the good consequences of having and respecting that right. However, this is only a problem for the formulation of the argument in terms of a moral right to reproductive freedom. It remains true that access to NRTs for infertile individuals does usually contribute substantially to their good.

EQUALITY OF EXPECTATIONS OR OPPORTUNITY

The third line of defense of reproductive freedom generally, and access to NRTs in particular, is based on a moral principle of equality. The equality defense is important in capturing a specific part of the case for securing access to NRTs on grounds of justice. I shall distinguish two different arguments that appeal to equality. The first sees reproductive freedom as important in preventing or mitigating unjust gender inequalities typically suffered by women. The second sees the opportunity for parenting as an important component of equality of opportunity that justice requires be secured to all members of society.

The first argument begins with the moral premise that gender, whether one is male or female, is a morally irrelevant property of persons for purposes of distributive justice. Gender should not be the source of substantial inequalities in people's social and economic expectations in life and in their opportunities to attain desired positions and benefits.[12] In this respect, gender is like race, and the premise about its moral irrelevance should be as morally uncontroversial as the analogous premise regarding race. This premise does not deny natural differences between the genders, since it is a banal truism that only women get pregnant. That is a natural fact of biology that it is not now possible to change and that by itself represents no unjust inequality between the genders. What are unjust gender inequalities, however, are straightforward gender discrimination, such as denying women access to desirable social or economic positions, and social arrangements in which natural gender differences, such as the fact that only women get pregnant, produce other systematic social and economic disadvantages for women. In the United States as well as most of the rest of the world, both of these kinds of gender discrimination against women are still common. A number of aspects of reproductive freedom then serve equality in two important ways: First, they can help mitigate gender disadvantages that women suffer that are specifically tied to reproduction; second, they can mitigate the effects of other gender discrimination against women that is not tied specifically to reproduction.

To illustrate this relation between reproductive freedom and equality, consider the three components of reproductive freedom for women of whether to procreate, when to do so, and how many children to have. Even with the best social supports and accommodations to pregnancy and childrearing, these choices typically have deep and far-reaching effects on women's lives. Childbearing and parenting are often deeply transforming, meaningful, and valuable experiences for both men and women, but they often have a disproportionate undesirable impact on women, such as reduced economic independence and disadvantages in the pursuit of careers. Gaining control over whether to procreate gives women the opportunity to decide whether the expected benefits outweigh the other disruptions and burdens of having children, at least to the extent these factors can be appreciated and weighed before having children. Control over the timing of procreation and the number of children they will have give women additional control over the nature and timing of the impact of reproduction on their lives. Serious and preventable disadvantages in opportunities and expectations often attend women's roles of childbearing and childrearing. In these circumstances, having the freedom to choose whether, when, how often, and with whom to procreate takes on commensurably greater moral importance by enabling women to mitigate the effects of these unjust gender-based inequalities on their lives.

The second argument focuses more specifically on how access to NRTs for infertile women or couples serves equality of opportunity. For many people, the opportunity to become a parent and raise a child is one of, if not the most important and valuable parts of their lives. It has deep, far reaching, and extended impacts on their lives. While infertility is not the only obstacle people face in attempting to have children, it is one of the most important and common. In what is the most developed account of justice in health care, Norman Daniels has argued that the importance of health care for justice lies most fundamentally in its securing and protecting for individuals access to the normal range of opportunities in their society.[13] Health care can often prevent, restore, or limit the loss of normal function that is the typical mark of disease. While we tend to associate equality of opportunity most commonly with education and work, it is not limited to those venues. NRTs often represent the means by which the opportunity to bear and raise children can be restored to infertile individuals. The moral importance — on grounds of equality of opportunity and justice — of doing so depends largely on the relative importance of parenting within the normal life plans of most people. This suggests that infertility is a disability whose alleviation by means such as NRTs has very high moral priority.

I have sketched three different accounts of the moral importance of the benefits of NRTs, or alternatively three bases or grounds of a moral right to reproductive freedom that includes access to NRTs. It bears repeating that these are not mutually exclusive accounts, but rather they each capture an important aspect of both the moral importance of the benefits of NRTs and of the moral bases of a right to reproductive freedom. Together, they form a strong case for inclusion of NRT services such as oocyte donation within any comprehensive package of health care services that purports to meet the requirements of justice. In the next section, I will examine a number of arguments that aim to rebut this case.

IV. SOME ARGUMENTS WHY NRTs SHOULD NOT BE INCLUDED WITHIN COMPREHENSIVE BENEFIT PACKAGES—CONSIDERED AND REJECTED

The arguments of the last section establish that NRTs have a moral importance greater than many other health care services that are included without question in virtually all comprehensive health care benefit packages. To cite just one example, chemotherapy for many forms of cancer in which the likelihood of even a few months of life extension is extremely small almost certainly produces less gain, evaluated in any of these three respects, than does access to new reproductive technologies such as oocyte donation that will have a greater rate of success and produce benefit of greater magnitude. Are there any objections to their coverage which overcome this moral importance?

Some opposition to covering use of NRTs such as oocyte donation in a comprehensive health care benefit package no doubt results from straightforward fiscal concerns to limit overall health care costs of those who fund health care services. New reproductive technologies may be seen as especially vulnerable to fiscal axes for at least two reasons. First, many people know they do and/or will not need these services either because they have already had children or because they do not want to have children; NRTs thus differ from treatments for most disease and illness which we may ourselves someday need or want. Second, because these services are relatively new and often not part of established health insurance coverage, most people have not already formed reasonable or legitimate expectations that access to the services will be available to them. Considerations such as these, however, may provide an explanation, but do not provide a justification, for the exclusion of new reproductive services from health care benefit packages. In the remainder of this chapter I shall consider and largely reject a number of arguments that might be thought to rebut the prima facie case for covering these services.

The first argument against funding expensive NRTs is that infertile couples can satisfy their desire and interest in parenting by adopting a child instead of using an expensive NRT. This would be a weak argument if made against funding *any* fertility treatment since the vast majority of fertility problems can be dealt with relatively inexpensively. But another difficulty with this argument is that the number of infertile persons far outruns the number of children available for adoption—"each year 2.3 million couples confront infertility, and less than 50,000 children are available for adoption."[14] Moreover, adoption can itself often be as or more expensive than NRTs. The main difficulty with this argument, however, is that many women have strong desires to experience pregnancy and many couples have strong desires to parent a child biologically related to at least one of them. If it is possible for them to do so by means of one or another form of NRT it is not at all obvious why this desire should be discounted as irrational or otherwise defective and not worthy of the respect of others. The desire to parent children is presumably deeply embedded biologically in humans, and the desire to have one's own biological children is probably inextricably psychologically enmeshed with the general desire to parent for many people. The strength and reasonableness of this desire forms part of the basis for the self-determination, well-being, and equality of opportunity arguments for its satisfaction.

The second argument against funding expensive NRTs is that infertility is not a disease or illness, and so use of NRTs to overcome it is not medical treatment. It is sometimes noted that NRTs typically do not correct the condition of infertility, but only enable persons or couples to have children in spite of their condition. Infertility, however, is properly understood as a disease; it is recognized as such by both the American College of Obstetricians and Gynecologists and the American Fertility Society. Very roughly, diseases are physical or mental conditions of an organism that result in deviations from normal species function.[15] Even those who argue that determinations of disease are not solely biological, but must unavoidably appeal to value judgments, do not deny the biological and functional component of our concept of disease. They typically want to add that to be a disease implies the value judgment that the deviation from normal species function is in normal conditions bad for those who suffer it, and to insist as well that whether a functional deviation is bad for individuals often depends on the social conditions in which they exist. Given the deep importance that parenting a biological child typically has for people, an importance that crosses most historical and cultural boundaries, it seems hard to deny that infertility is a deviation from normal species function that is bad for those who suffer it, certainly for those who want to parent biological children. One qualification that must be put on the claim that infertility is a disease because a deviation from normal species function is that this holds only for the normal period of childbearing years for women or men; for example, infertility is not a disease for a 70-year-old woman.

Finally, the fact that NRTs do not correct infertility, but only allow a person to overcome the functional deficit of the disease does not mean that their use is not medical treatment for a disease. Many medical and rehabilitative treatments, including many that are standardly covered by health care insurance, do not correct the underlying condition, but only correct for its attendant disability. For example, physical therapy and other rehabilitative services after strokes, accidents, and other disabling conditions often do not correct the underlying physical condition, but do restore at least limited function. More important, it is the seriousness of the disability responded to which gives health care its moral importance. This importance need not be affected by whether the underlying physical condition is altered or bypassed, so long as the bad impact of the disability for the individual is removed.

The third argument against funding expensive NRTs is related to the previous one, but requires separate treatment. It is that the need for treatment to overcome infertility is elective; it is a lifestyle choice, not a medical decision. Genuine medical treatment for disease, in contrast, is not elective in this way. There is a respect in which it is correct that infertility treatment is elective and a lifestyle choice, but it is no different in this respect from many other medical treatments whose coverage in health care benefit packages is not questioned. Surgical treatment of benign prostatic hypertrophy (BPH) is equally elective and a lifestyle choice. Many patients choose to pursue medical management of BPH and do not elect to have surgery for it. Moreover, the decision is in important respects a matter of how the two alternatives of medical management and surgery will affect one's lifestyle. Patients electing surgery typically do so in order to improve their quality of life. With either infertility or BPH, treatment is only elective to the extent that the person with the disease is prepared to continue to live with its attendant disability. The fact that some people are prepared to do so is hardly sufficient to establish that the condition is not a disease whose treatment should not be covered by health insurance plans for the patients who elect to pursue that treatment. Indeed, for almost any treatment for a medical condition, there are some people who decide not to pursue it. Treatment of every condition that is not directly life threatening is a lifestyle choice in the sense that it is intended to improve the quality of the patient's life.

A fourth argument for not funding NRTs, especially with public monies as opposed to private health insurance, is that some people have strong religious or moral objections to some or all forms of assisted reproduction. To fund these treatments in public programs is to force those with such objections to help to support the services financially, and so to implicate them coercively in the practices to which they object. This argument appears to have no force regarding private insurance plans which individuals are free to join or not, at least when there are reasonable alternative plans available which do not cover the service to which they object. But the argument fails for public insurance plans as well. When there are strong grounds, of the sort considered in Section III above, that a service should be available as a matter of justice or as a matter of right to those who need and want it, that service should not be excluded from coverage because some have religious or moral objections to it. This general issue is much too complex to be addressed fully here, but suffice it to say that the appropriate response to this disagreement is to leave individuals free to act according to their own conscience and to choose to utilize or forgo the controversial treatment or service. This is especially the case when the objection is essentially religious—public policy in a pluralistic, democratic society should not impose on all the sectarian religious beliefs of some that can be reasonably rejected.[16]

A fifth argument for not funding NRTs is that they have not met the conditions for standard therapy, but remain experimental; therefore they need not be covered in basic benefit packages. The assumption that if a therapy is experimental, it will not be covered for funding is questionable. An example to the contrary is provided by parallel-track programs of drug treatments for HIV-infected persons. These treatments, which are still experimental, have been funded. Although the rationale for this assumption and the criteria distinguishing experimental from validated treatment are often not adequately spelled out and defended, I shall not question them here. Instead, it is enough to note that the experience with and rates of success of most NRTs in use today appear to be well within the standards for validated treatments applied elsewhere in medicine. Since IVF was introduced in the United States in 1980, over 20,000 babies have been born using these procedures. The U.S. IVF Registry reports that in 1990, a total of 5,193 were born through assisted reproductive technologies. The overall delivery rate for IVF was 14% and for Gamete Intrafallopian Transfer 22%. In comparison, the reproductively normal couple has a 20% chance of achieving pregnancy in any given month and carrying it to term. These figures indicate that the principal forms of NRTs in use today, including oocyte donation, have passed the experimental point in their development. Consequently, there is no case for excluding NRTs generally from funding on the grounds that they remain experimental.

A sixth argument is that at a time in which world population is growing at an undesirable and insupportably high rate, it makes little sense for public policy to support expensive programs that will only exacerbate population problems. This argument can be disposed of quickly. First, the number of children born through the use of NRTs is so small in comparison with world population and population growth as to be completely inconsequential. But more important, even if that were not the case and policies needed to be imposed to limit future population growth, justice would require that those limits fall equally on persons with and without normal reproductive capacities. It would be unfair, indeed it would compound the disadvantage they already face, for infertile persons to bear disproportionately the brunt of population control policies.

A seventh argument against funding NRTs applies to cases in which women postpone pregnancy in order to pursue other interests until an age when the risk of infertility is substantially increased and learn at that time that they are infertile. It might be argued that these women have chosen other benefits, like pursuit of careers, knowing that this reduces their likelihood of being able to conceive later. Why should other persons, who have forgone those same or comparable benefits in order to start a family, have to bear some of the costs of use of NRTs by individuals who postponed childbearing?

There is some force to this argument, but it is a great deal more complicated than this simple statement of it supposes. The argument claims that funding NRTs in these cases would result in an unjust distribution of benefits and burdens between individuals or groups. But then we must take account of other factors affecting that distribution, such as the different and complex reasons for decisions to postpone childrearing, the other opportunities available to different women, and so forth. It is far from clear that not funding NRTs in these cases produces a more fair overall distribution of benefits and burdens. Moreover, making insurance coverage depend on these complex determinations of fairness would seriously compromise such values as personal privacy, especially if to be consistent we made other insurance coverage determinations on the same grounds. The moral costs of introducing such determinations into the health care system would almost certainly be unwarranted.

The eighth argument applies to the unlimited use of NRTs by individuals. Funding the use of NRTs for a first, and perhaps a second, child may be supported by self-determination, well-being, and equality, but these values do not ground a moral claim to use NRTs to have any number of children a person might want. The distinction is between the interests in becoming a parent or forming an average-sized family (which would be no more than two children in the United States at the present time), on the one hand, and having additional children beyond the norm for one's society, on the other. The former interests ground a stronger claim on social resources than do the latter. Thus, coverage for use of NRTs to produce a second child might be substantially reduced from the coverage for a first child, and coverage might be eliminated for any subsequent children beyond two. Of course, this policy would raise difficult issues of interpretation and application, such as a couple in which one or both of the parties have children from prior marriages, but who have none together. Despite such difficulties, this argument does identify a reasonable moral limit on insurance coverage for the use of NRTs.

The final argument against funding NRTs is for some the most persuasive. It is that the costs of these procedures are too high for the benefits they produce to warrant their funding through private or public health insurance programs. This argument does not apply to most treatment for infertility, which is accomplished without resort to NRTs and at relatively modest cost. The Centers for Disease Control reported that only 1.6% of infertile couples were treated with assisted reproductive technologies in 1990. In the aggregate, treatment of infertility is estimated to account for only 0.1% of the overall U.S. health care budget, and assisted reproductive technologies are estimated to account for roughly 0.03% of that budget. This latter figure is probably less than we spend on the care of patients in a persistent vegetative state, where there is arguably no benefit to the patient from care. Spread over a population, the costs of covering NRTs in insurance is small—the cost of comprehensive mandated coverage of infertility treatment in Massachusetts has most recently been estimated by the state's Division of Insurance as 4/10 of 1% of a family Blue Cross/Blue Shield premium.[17]

Nevertheless, in some individual cases, the cost of NRTs for a single pregnancy can mount into the thousands, or even tens of thousands, of dollars. Of course, many other treatments that improve people's quality of life, such as artificial hips and substance abuse treatment, have comparable costs, including treatments whose aggregate costs are much higher because of the much larger numbers of individuals treated. The aggregate cost data, combined with the data for annual live births from IVF, suggest, as an *extremely* rough estimate, a cost in the neighborhood of 40 to 45 thousand dollars per live birth from IVF. There is not space here to attempt detailed cost/benefit comparisons of various NRTs with other health care treatments and services, and there would be both methodological and moral difficulties in doing so; central among them would be how to measure the value to an infertile couple of being able to achieve pregnancy and give birth to a child. But the cost/benefit ratios of NRTs appear within the bounds of many other health care services. The burden should be on opponents of funding NRTs on grounds of their costs to show that those costs significantly exceed cost limits that we observe in other coverage decisions. I believe it is highly doubtful that this can be done.

V. CONCLUSION

The overall conclusion to my argument should be clear. Access to NRTs is properly understood to be part of reproductive freedom, including a moral right to reproductive freedom. Three central grounds—individual self-determination, individual well-being, and equality of opportunity—show the benefits of NRTs for infertile persons to be of sufficient moral importance that these services should be covered as part of any comprehensive package of health care benefits. Finally, while benefits need not cover use of NRTs by individuals to have an unlimited number of children, none of the arguments that I have considered in Section IV succeeds in defeating these general grounds for funding coverage.

NOTES

1. Quoted in the report of the President's Commission for the Study of Ethical Problems in Medicine and Biomedical and Behavioral Research, *Securing Access to Health Care* (Washington, DC: U.S. Government Printing Office, 1983), p. 4.

2. Ibid.

3. John A. Robertson, "Embryos, Families, and Procreative Liberty: The Legal Structure of the New Reproduction," *Southern California Law Review* 59 (1986): 955.

4. *Griswold v. Connecticut*, 381 US 479 (1965).

5. I use "new reproductive techniques" here instead of the more common "new reproductive technologies" since some noncoital means of reproducing hardly qualify as technology.

6. John Rawls, *A Theory of Justice* (Cambridge: Harvard University Press, 1971).

7. Harry Frankfurt, "Freedom of the Will and the Concept of a Person," *Journal of Philosophy* 68 (1971): 5–20.

8. John Rawls, "Kantian Constructivism in Moral Theory," *Journal of Philosophy* 77 (1980): 515–72.

9. I have discussed all three of these theories at much greater length in "Quality of Life Measures in Health Care and Medical Ethics," in *The Quality of Life,* ed. A. Sen and M. Nussbaum (Oxford: Oxford University Press, 1993). There I called objective good theories "ideal theories" because they typically posit some ideal of the person as what is objectively good. One of the best recent treatments of these alternative theories is James Griffin, *Well-Being* (Oxford: Oxford University Press, 1986).

10. See Robert Goodin, "Laundering Preferences," in *Foundations of Social Choice Theory,* ed. J. Elster and A. Hylland (Cambridge: Cambridge University Press, 1986).

11. Much of the very large literature on this problem is within the framework of giving a utilitarian or general consequentialist account of moral rights. See, for example, Thomas Scanlon, "Rights, Goals, and Fairness," in *Public and Private Morality,* ed. S. Hampshire (Cambridge: Cambridge University Press, 1978) and Raymond Frey, ed., *Utility and Rights* (Minneapolis: University of Minnesota Press, 1984).

12. There is a substantial philosophical debate about what should be the object of egalitarians' concern. The principal alternative positions include equality of welfare, of resources, of opportunities, and of capabilities and functionings. My appeal here to "expectations" in the equality defense of reproductive freedom and of funding NRTs aims to be neutral between these different positions, though of course a full specifica-

tion of the appeal to equality would have to spell out the specific conception of equality employed.

13. Norman Daniels, *Just Health Care* (Cambridge: Cambridge University Press, 1985).

14. Cited in "Talking Points for the Inclusion of Infertility Treatment in a Health Care Benefits Package," issued by Resolve, 1310 Broadway, Somerville, MA 02144.

15. Christopher Boorse, "Health as a Theoretical Concept," *Philosophy of Science* 44 (1977) and "On the Distinction between Disease and Illness," *Philosophy and Public Affairs* 5 (1975): 49–68.

16. For the development of this general contractualist moral principle, see T. M. Scanlon, "Contractualism and Utilitarianism," in *Utilitarianism and Beyond,* ed. Amartya Sen and Bernard Williams (Cambridge: Cambridge University Press, 1982).

17. Data provided by Susan L. Crockin in personal correspondence.

PART C

Report and Recommendations
on Oocyte Donation by the
National Advisory Board on
Ethics in Reproduction (NABER)

INTRODUCTION

In 1884, Dr. William Pancoast of Jefferson College of Medicine in Philadelphia impregnated a woman whose husband was infertile with sperm donated by "the best looking medical student" in his class. This first successful donor insemination was shrouded in utmost secrecy because Pancoast feared adverse responses. (Indeed, even the husband and wife were at first kept in the dark!) When it was reported 25 years later, the controversy the Philadelphia physician had anticipated broke out. Many physicians, clergy and public figures spoke out against making babies "by test tube," and condemned it as nothing more than mechanical adultery, equivalent to rape and clearly contrary to the laws of God.[1] Although artificial insemination has received a larger measure of acceptance since then, moral objections continue to be raised to it.

The most dramatic innovation in the last 50 years— fertilization of the human embryo *in vitro* and implantation of the resulting zygote into the uterus of a woman who carried the pregnancy to term—raised a similar storm of controversy.[2] Yet the procedure has now become part of accepted medical practice, although some of its spin-offs, such as the disposition of frozen embryos, raise heightened moral questions.

Each new development in medically assisted reproduction seems to echo the Pancoast episode. Technical advances that allow for unprecedented manipulation of the reproductive process are introduced with little moral or legal caution. The states, which largely control law regulating the use of assisted reproductive technologies, have passed only limited legislation. The judicial gloss in this area remains insubstantial. Consequently, these new reproductive methods have stimulated not only amazement, but moral and legal doubt and confusion.

In vitro fertilization is the centerpiece of an array of reproductive technologies now available to those seeking to conceive a child. These range from the medically simple, such as advice about timing of intercourse and modification of the reproductive cycle by means of drugs, to complex manipulation of reproductive endocrinology and gametes. The ethical questions that surround them vary with the nature of the particular method. Today little objection is raised to artificial insemination by spouse (except, notably, by Roman Catholic moral theology), anxiety over the risks of *in vitro* fertilization to the conceptus have lessened, and freezing of sperm causes little concern. Freezing of embryos, however, still troubles some consciences and can raise complex legal problems and surrogacy arrangements remain ethically and legally perplexing, to the point that some jurisdictions have outlawed them in their commercial form. Ethical evaluation of assisted reproduction ranges from almost total condemnation by Roman Catholic teaching to almost exceptionless approval by libertarian thinkers.

Oocyte or egg donation, a relatively new procedure, enables women who cannot produce or utilize their own eggs to use those provided by other women to bear children. Donated eggs are fertilized *in vitro*, usually with the sperm of the recipient's partner and, if this is successful, the resultant embryo is transferred to the recipient's uterus to be carried to term. The use of oocyte donation has increased rapidly since its introduction in 1984. In 1987, this technique was reported available at 17 programs in the United States.[3] By 1991, the number of oocyte donation programs reported to exist in the United States and Canada had grown to 75.[4]

Oocyte donation is dramatically altering human reproductive potential. The procedure is creating questions about whether to expand age boundaries for reproduction beyond menopause, potentially allowing women of any age to become pregnant. It is transforming intergenerational relations, as daughters donate eggs to mothers who give birth to their own children-grandchildren and their daughters' siblings-children.[5] A treatise on the ethical aspects of oocyte donation becomes, in effect, a compendium of the ethics of the use of the new reproductive technologies. It is for this reason that the ethical issues raised by oocyte donation were chosen as the focus of this report.

It might be asked why oocyte donation should be treated any differently than sperm donation, since both involve the provision of donor gametes to those who are infertile. There are notable similarities in questions raised by these two techniques. Both lead us to wonder how significant the genetic relationship should be to parenthood; whether biological cooperation in conceiving, bearing and rearing children should be undertaken only by spouses and partners in long-term stable relationships; whether widespread use of these techniques will change the very meaning of family; whether those involved in their use should be protected by a veil of secrecy; whether it is ethically acceptable to pay donors; for what characteristics, if any, donors and recipients should be screened.

Oocyte and semen donation, however, differ in significant respects. In oocyte donation, the recipient has a gestational relation with the child, whereas in sperm donation, there can be no similar biological connection between the male rearing parent and the child. Further, oocyte donation involves a procedure that is medically more complicated for the donor and the recipient than sperm donation. Oocytes are relatively inaccessible and therefore more difficult to obtain. Moreover, there is a need to synchronize the ovulatory process in the donor with endometrial maturation in the recipient,[6] which requires drug regimens and an intrusive oocyte recovery procedure. These place the donor at some medical risk and considerable discomfort and raise questions about risk for the recipient. Sperm donation, in contrast, involves no comparable medical procedure, risks, or inconvenience. Finally, because oocytes are less accessible than sperm, they currently constitute a scarce resource relative to demand.

Oocyte donation, consequently, raises distinctive ethical and policy questions of its own. These include how significant the gestational relation is to motherhood, whether donors should receive special protection from the greater risks to which they are exposed, whether women of advanced reproductive age should have access to this technique, and whether considerations of justice should enter decisions about access to the limited supply of oocytes. It raises unique questions about the welfare of women and children and about their possible objectification and commodification. Since these questions do not arise in the same kind or degree in sperm donation, oocyte donation should be considered as a separate technique in need of distinct ethical and policy guidelines.

The National Advisory Board on Ethics in Reproduction (NABER), which developed this report, is a broadly based multi-disciplinary panel in the private sector many of whose members have served on national bioethics commissions.* It was established in the absence of any government-sponsored body to address the profound ethical and policy questions raised by

---

*Members of NABER at the time this report was developed were Albert R. Jonsen, Ph.D., Professor and Chair, Medical History and Ethics, University of Washington, Seattle, WA, Chair; Ruth Macklin, Ph.D., Professor of Bioethics, Albert Einstein College of Medicine, Bronx, NY, Vice Chair; Ezra Davidson, Jr., M.D., Professor and Chair, Department of Obstetrics and Gynecology, King-Drew Medical Center, Los Angeles, CA, Treasurer; Lisa Sowle Cahill, Ph.D., Professor of Theology, Boston College, Boston, MA; Thomas E. Elkins, M.D., Professor and Chair, Department of Obstetrics and Gynecology, Louisiana State University, New Orleans, LA; Clifford Grobstein, Ph.D., Professor Emeritus in Science, Technology, and Public Affairs, University of California School of Medicine, San Diego, CA; John S. Hoff, J.D., Swidler and Berlin, Chartered, Washington, DC; Patricia King, J.D., Professor of Law, Georgetown Law Center, Washington, DC; Mildred T. Stahlman, M.D., Professor of Pediatrics and Pathology, Vanderbilt University School of Medicine, Nashville, TN; Moses Tendler, Ph.D., Professor of Biology, Talmudic Law, and Jewish Medical Ethics, Yeshiva University, New York, NY; and Walter J.

rapid growth in the reproductive sciences and technology. It is funded by respected private foundations,** after having received initial funding from the American College of Obstetricians and Gynecologists (ACOG) and the American Fertility Society (AFS), and is independent of those physician organizations.

As NABER discussed the issues related to oocyte donation, we often found ourselves in agreement about the definition of the problems and the most reasonable resolutions. Yet this was not always the case. Indeed, the very name of the procedure used in the title of this Report, "oocyte donation," some argued, was inappropriate, since providing eggs is becoming more an act of paid labor, rather than altruism. Other members argued that the practice of financially compensating some donors for their time and inconvenience does not necessarily nullify their generous intent. In the end, it was decided to retain the term "oocyte donation" to refer to this form of assisted reproduction, as that is the label under which the procedure has firmly entered the public and professional vocabulary. Yet NABER agreed that the ethical hazards raised by donor compensation should also be analyzed.

It probably remains true for most board members that not all of their own views are equally represented by every part of this Report. Even so, there are significant moral issues surrounding egg donation about which NABER members were able to reach consensus, even though they disagreed about the weight of the moral values involved. The Report's contents are not designed to give legal guidance, although they take account of current legal findings and scholarship. Our broader goal is to lay the foundations for an ethical framework that can be brought to bear on issues raised by the entire gamut of reproductive technologies.

Consequently, we have tried in this Report to present the arguments on both sides of these issues, to indicate those arguments that seem most plausible, and to build a consensus about them that reflects a broad societal consensus whenever possible. We are aware that readers may disagree with our conclusions. We invite them to formulate their views so that they can be used to challenge, broaden, and deepen ours. We hope that our views and debate that they stimulate will contribute to a broad social agreement about the innovative practices of reproductive medicine.

Wadlington, LL.B., Professor, University of Virginia School of Law, Charlottesville, VA; Cynthia B. Cohen, Ph.D., J.D., Executive Director.

We are grateful to Valerie Hurt, Elizabeth Leibold McCloskey, M.Th., and Elise Ayers, M.P.H., for their invaluable research and writing assistance.

**The Ford Foundation, the Greenwall Foundation, the Walter and Elise Haas Fund, the Josiah Macy, Jr. Foundation, and the Rockefeller Foundation.

SECTION I

ETHICAL QUESTIONS RAISED BY OOCYTE DONATION AND VALUES INFORMING THIS REPORT

Oocyte donation is already established practice. Yet having been introduced and established over only a brief ten-year span, many of the most fundamental questions about its moral acceptability have been bypassed. Thus, it is important to consider the underlying question of whether this practice is ethically unobjectionable in principle and to inquire how it affects, for good or ill, our cultural and religious understandings of procreation, marriage, parenthood, children, and women. The issues raised by reproductive technologies, including oocyte donation, are broader than those of safety and consent, which have provided the primary focus of ethical and policy deliberations. What is at stake is "the idea of the humanness of our human life and the meaning of our embodiment, our sexual being, and our relation to ancestors and descendants."[1] Much of the following discussion is based on objections to the practice of gamete donation in general or is analogized from objections to sperm donation. Some unique concerns arise, however, in the special context of oocyte donation.

As frequently happens in ethical debate, the arguments about the ethical status of oocyte donation fall into two categories. The first asserts that the practice itself is unethical for some fundamental reason, such as that it is contrary to the normative meaning of parenting a child or to marital integrity and fidelity. Arguments of this sort are sometimes called "essentialist" or "deontological." The second category of argument examines the consequences of the practice for the resulting children, or for the donors, or for the parenting function, and finds them either acceptable or unacceptable. This sort of argument may be designated "consequentialist."

Essentialist arguments are difficult to counter. They are advanced on the basis of profound ethical commitments and global views of morality. Those who do not share the commitments and views in which such positions are grounded may advance their own, but rarely can they directly refute the former. Those who follow the debate may consider the contrasting views and choose the approach that seems most appropriate. In this section of the Report, we present some of the major essentialist arguments against the practice of oocyte donation (and many other reproductive technologies), as well as some consequentialist concerns. Several of our members are especially attuned to these essentialist positions. Thus, we present them as fairly as possible and add the critical comments of respondents that, to most of our members, seem appropriate. In the remainder of the Report, attention will be paid both to certain central ethical values that we outline at the end of this section and to the issues of appropriate use and abuse that consequentialist considerations raise for practice and policy. NABER members who are sympathetic to these essentialist positions recognize the necessity of bringing additional considerations to bear in the formation of public policy.

A. PROCREATION

The use of assisted reproduction is rejected by those who believe that bringing a child into the world in this way fundamentally alters and injures our understanding of what it means to create human life. The Roman Catholic Church rejects assisted reproduction that would replace sexual intercourse between a married couple. It understands the unitive and procreative aspects of human sexual intercourse to be morally inseparable in every sexual act. The creation of a child is seen as the convergence of the spiritual and physical love of the parents, and thus fertilization outside the body is seen as "deprived of the meanings and the values which are expressed in the language of the body and in the union of human persons."[2] When a third party enters the reproductive scene, the unity of body and spirit in the procreative process is further eroded. The argument from Catholic doctrine is that a procreative act devoid of full personal and bodily communion would not be completely human.[3] The child created is an actual physical embodiment of the love and union of the parents; "the parents find in their child a confirmation and completion of their reciprocal self-giving: The child is the living image of their love, the permanent sign of their conjugal union, the living and indissoluble concrete expression of their paternity and maternity."[4] When a donor egg is used, the procreative process is stripped of its essential nature.

This argument—or an argument similar to it—is not unique to the Roman Catholic Church. Leon Kass[5] and Paul Ramsey[6] have also maintained that moving procreation into the laboratory is dangerous because it suppresses the biological, sexual, bodily meaning of marital love. As Leon Kass argues, "To be human means not only to have human form and powers; it means also to have a human context and to be humanly connected."[7] Creating life by sundering the bodily and spiritual unity of husband and wife, Ramsey argues, "Means a refusal of the image of God's creation in our own."[8] What is at stake, according to Oliver O'Donovan, is the image people have of themselves and of their children in relation to nature and to their own powers of mastery over nature.[9] When we regard ourselves—mistakenly, according to O'Donovan—as over and above nature, then we will also regard our children—mistakenly and disastrously—as products, as "made" rather than "begotten."

These essentialist views present proponents of reproductive technologies with a thought-provoking challenge. They force serious reflection about the nature of human reproduction and the way in which children should be created. Still, proponents would respond, these views are not invulnerable to criticism. Some would argue that the claim that there must be an inseparable connection between procreation and sexual intercourse has insufficient warrant and backing. Lauritzen, for instance, maintains that it is to assume "a narrowly physicalist, act-oriented natural law methodology. . . . "[10] While perceiving an important relation between reproduction and sexual love, they claim that the unitive purpose of sexuality—its capacity to express love—is fundamental.[11] Many who believe that biological cooperation in conceiving a child should be undertaken only by spouses accept that conception will not always take place through sexual intercourse. It is sufficient that love and procreation are held together within the whole marital relationship, not necessarily in each act of sexual intercourse. When nature makes reproduction through sex impossible, these proponents maintain, it is not necessarily morally wrong to separate the two and to procreate in other ways.[12] Yet the concern raised by critics about the objectification of persons, about their conversion into products to be produced through a technical, mechanistic joining of oocytes, remains significant.

B. MARRIAGE

Marriage, with its vows of covenant fidelity, is the appropriate context for both intercourse and procreation, according to some critics of sperm and ovum donation. When procreative acts take place in a context other than marital fidelity, they are—according to this position—diminished and distorted, reduced to mere physiology or to contract, to a marketable reproductive capacity, or to a technology for producing children without a commitment to care for them. Such an argument would permit the use of artificial insemination and *in vitro* fertilization within marriage, but it would caution against acts and practices which reduce acts of begetting to mere physiology and to consent, and it would understand the donation of sperm or ova to be such acts.[13]

By bringing a third party into the procreative life of married parties, some have argued, the use of donated gametes fundamentally violates the unity of the couple. It raises concerns about adultery, since the total dedication to one's partner is disrupted by using another's body to achieve conception, these critics maintain. Use of a third party to create a child "is violative of the marriage covenant wherein exclusive, nontransferable, inalienable rights to each other's person and generative acts are exchanged."[14] Others who question the moral value of using donor gametes argue from the positive nature of the marriage bond, rather than from outer boundaries that might be violated. They maintain that the unity of a couple is expressed sexually and in their shared relation with the child they conceive. When one partner undertakes a biological procreative relationship with a donor, this infringes on the unity of the marriage and introduces an asymmetry into the parental relationship.

Those who favor the use of gamete donation observe that there is a distinction between accepting a gamete contributed by a third party in order to have a child and adultery. Gamete donation need not involve any sexual contact between the woman and the donor. Indeed, it need not involve any personal relation between them at all. Usually the procedure is undertaken with full knowledge and consent of the other partner in the marriage. A couple may undertake gamete donation out of a strong commitment to their marriage, rather than with any intention of unfaithfulness.[15] To some, the introduction of a third party into the procreative process is analogous to an adoptive process that begins at the time of zygote formation and that does not diminish the relationship between the adopting couple.[16] The desire of the husband for a child and the wife for the gestational experience and the ensuing maternal bonding with a child is to be viewed with compassion. Therefore, when only one parent can contribute genetically to the procreation of a child, but both can nourish and nurture a child, respondents maintain, it is ethically acceptable for them to seek to have a child by means of third-party donation.

C. PARENTHOOD

Those who challenge the use of donated gametes also point to the confused notions of parenthood that might emerge from this arrangement. Parenthood is traditionally understood as a unity of genetic, sexual, gestational (in the case of a mother), and rearing components. Although there are well-established and well-accepted arrangements that divide these components, such as adoption, step-parenting, and extended kin relationships, these divisions are generally not intended when conception occurs. When donor eggs or sperm are used, a child is created with the deliberate intention of separating these components. The two interrelated moral questions this creates are whether the deliberate separation of genetic kinship and nurturance severely damages our notion of parenthood and whether biological parenting bears some moral responsibility for the well-being of children that result from the use of one's gametes.[17]

Critics of gamete donation answer, "Yes," to both questions. They observe that "[i]n third party methods, the parties act as though there were no morally important relation of genetic reproduction either to a marital or a parental personal relation."[18] Biologically parenting a child, they hold, imposes claims on a person.[19] According to one version of this position, acts of begetting are "essentially parental, entailing obligations for nurturing the child."[20] When biological parents care for a child born to them, they simply keep obligations that belong to a relationship already established in the act of begetting. This version of the basic argument does not prohibit the use of technologically assisted reproduction to prospective parents, but it does prohibit donors from treating the donation of ova or sperm as though a biological relationship carries no obligation to support and nurture the children who are born.

Some have argued forcefully that sperm donation is a practice that has institutionalized the socially problematic phenomenon of paternal abandonment.[21] While it is generally assumed that a man who impregnates a woman through natural conception should take responsibility for the resulting child, sperm donation sanctions a complete severance of the man's relationship to his biological child. There is no historical analogy of women abandoning their genetic child, since the possibility of implanting one's fertilized egg in another woman's womb did not previously exist. Now that this possibility can be realized, some argue, oocyte donation presents the same problem of genetic and parental irresponsibility as sperm donation.

Those in the opposite camp argue that while the genetic connection is important, it is not an essential requirement of parenthood. Instead, nurturing and raising a child is of greater significance. When the genetic and rearing relation between parent and child cannot be combined, as is the case for those who are unable to have a child using their own ova, it is not wrong for them to have a child who is not related to them genetically. Further, those who donate eggs for this purpose have an obligation to ensure that parenting responsibilities for the resulting child are fulfilled. They need not do so themselves, but should seek assurance that those to whom they provide their gametes will take responsibility for the social and rearing parentage of the resulting child.

D. CHILDREN

Critics of egg donation argue not only that the practice injures our ideal of parenthood, but that it may have harmful consequences for children. Their major concern is that children born of this procedure will have no firm grounding in an identity because they have multiple parents. By purposefully breaking the link between begetting and rearing, egg donation puts children in the position of being denied a kinship bond with their genetic mother. While the gestational mother may make the decision that a genetic connection to her child is not ultimately important to her, some argue that this denies the child major dimensions of significant relationships that biological kinship creates. The question that emerges is how significant the tie is to one's genetic parent. Couples who seek some genetic connection to their child by using the husband's sperm and a donated egg seem to be affirming the importance of some genetic tie. Yet since half of the conceived child's genetic parentage will be unknown to the child, this seems to trivialize the genetic tie. If a genetic connection is important enough to warrant extensive technological aid to conceive a child, some argue, "then it is undesirable deliberately to produce children who will be denied one genetic parent."[22] Thus, a major argument against the use of oocyte donation is that it will harm the child by obscuring its identity within a family lineage. The argument is, in effect, not a consequentialist one, but a logical one in that it points out that both the importance and the insignificance of the genetic tie are contradictorily asserted by those who favor oocyte donation.

Others argue, however, that the child born of oocyte donation will have some likeness to one parent, a sense of belonging to a family over a period of time, and a place within the heritage and kinship of a family, at least on one side. In addition, the woman of the infertile couple carries the child through pregnancy, thereby establishing a powerful mothering bond that is at least as compelling as genetic connection. According to one report, "[R]ecipients perceive their offspring as immediately, fully and permanently theirs. Exchanges between mother and fetus during pregnancy, childbirth and early mother-infant bonding make these oocyte donation children the true offspring of the women who carried, gave birth to and nursed them, regardless of the source of the oocytes from which they developed. Biology takes over from genetics and emotional ties are based on the privileged period of pregnancy."[23]

Unlike adoption, in oocyte donation the child usually has a biological tie with both parents—with the mother, through pregnancy, and with the father through a genetic tie if the husband's sperm is used. Indeed, when relatives serve as oocyte donors, this gives the couple a child who is not only genetically related to the husband, but also to the wife. Some argue that this arrangement makes egg donation an optimal reproductive possibility for infertile couples because it "creates a more stable rearing and family situation than exists in other collaborative reproductive arrangements . . . and has the least risk of blurring or confusing offspring lineage."[24]

E. WOMEN

Special concerns regarding the welfare of women fuel the argument that the practice of egg donation reinforces sexist notions. Some feminist literature suggests that an underlying and unacceptable premise of egg donation assigns exaggerated weight to the importance of women actually bearing a child, rather than rearing and nurturing a child. The intense desire to bear a child is at least in part socially constructed, according to this view. Women seeking parenthood are influenced by notions that parenthood is an essential part of marriage and family formation and necessary to the female gender role, and that having children is natural and instinctive.[25] Women are taught that their identities are wrapped up in fertility, pregnancy, childbirth, and mothering.[26] The cultural imperative to have a child drives women to undergo financially, physically, and emotionally costly treatment in pursuit of that child.[27] Egg donation is yet a further step in what some perceive to be a nearly endless quest to make reproduction possible for infertile couples, the very premise of which is a limited definition of womanhood.

Some who would urge a halt to the practice of using donated eggs for reproduction also point to the splintered notion of womanhood that this practice encourages, both with respect to the woman who donates and the woman who receives an ovum. Separating the physical component of reproduction (the egg) from the psycho-spiritual dimension of reproduction, represents a disembodied dualism that violates what it means to be a whole person. In addition to challenging a dualistic notion of the person, this argument points to the danger of commodification when a woman sells her procreative capabilities and a part from herself.[28] Some feminists have argued that assisted reproduction uses women as "living laboratories" whose body parts are manipulated in various ways, although little is known about the consequences of these maneuvers to these women.[29]

Others claim that the practice of oocyte donation has positive consequences for women that justify its use. One argument in favor of third-party donation of eggs is that, regardless of its origin, whether cultural, natural, or other, the desire to bear and raise children is basic and can appropriately be satisfied by egg donation because of the real bond that is formed when a woman carries a child during pregnancy. Donated ova enable women to establish a biological tie with their children, even when no genetic tie is possible. In addition, women benefit from any expansion of reproductive technologies because this provides them with greater reproductive options[30] and enhances their reproductive freedom.

F. ADOPTION AS AN ALTERNATIVE

Some critics of such new reproductive technologies as oocyte donation hold out adoption as a morally preferable alternative for those who are infertile. This is because adoption allows a childless couple to provide a home and family for an already existing parentless child in need of assistance. These critics find it difficult to justify the use of new reproductive technologies to bring additional children into the world when there are hundreds of thousands of children already born around the world in need of assistance and care.

Many of those who are infertile contemplate adoption as an alternative should methods of assisted reproduction prove unsuccessful. One study of 200 couples applying for IVF treatment indicated that more than two-thirds of them were positive or neutral toward adoption.[31] About one-third would continue to consider adoption if their IVF efforts were unsuccessful. However, many infertile couples prefer to use methods of assisted reproduction first. This is due, in part, to the declining number of children available for adoption. In 1970, 89,200 adoptions took place. Since the mid-1970s, the number of adoptions has lessened, remaining fairly stable at about 50,000 a year.[32] As a result, those considering adoption find that they must endure a long and emotionally draining wait for a child. Infertile couples, who may be in their thirties by the time they discover their problem and undergo treatment for it, are disinclined to go through a long waiting period for adoption. They fear that they may be too old to be allowed to adopt by the time they reach the top of the list.

Moreover, adoption can be very expensive. The legal adoption of infants costs between $6,900 and $14,900 and up, depending on whether a public or private agency is used, and whether it is a domestic or international adoption.[33] This makes adoption seem more like buying a product than assuming responsibility for raising and nurturing a child to some who are infertile. Further, those considering adoption must work through a difficult and often frustrating system. Prospective parents tend to see the application procedures as complex and the screening measures as intrusive. They feel they have little control over how the process is conducted.

While the use of assisted reproduction presents some of the same drawbacks as adoption, it provides a possibility for those who are infertile that adoption does not—it may enable them to have a child who is biologically related to at least one of them. Many people attach great importance to having children who are genetically theirs. The desire to reproduce through lines of kinship and to connect to future generations through one's genes exerts a powerful and pervasive influence on members of our society.[34] The range of fulfilling experiences associated with pregnancy and childbirth are also viewed as significant and desirable. "Infertility is a problem, in part, because being pregnant and giving birth can become elements of personal history that give shape to one's subsequent life, contribute to one's understanding of oneself, and create bonds with the rest of the community, especially with other women."[35] Assisted reproduction represents the first choice of many who are infertile, as it offers them the possibility of having a genetically related child and the experience of pregnancy and birth.

The impetus to have children and a family that is experienced by many in our society should be treated sympathetically. Some may consider the degree of invasiveness and expense of methods of assisted reproduction too great and decide to attempt adoption. Others may weigh the implications of adoption for family relationships and opt for intrafamilial gamete donation. Still others may consider the social consequences of their situation of infertility and elect to find a confidential gamete donor. Those who are infertile and seek the good of having children to love and nurture need to weigh the arguments and choose that method of having children—whether it be adoption or the use of assisted reproduction—that best accords with their values, beliefs, and life plans.

G. CONCLUSION AND VALUES INFORMING THIS REPORT

These major arguments against the use of egg donation mingle essentialist and consequentialist considerations. This is not unusual. Such mingling occurs often and arises in at least three different ways. It may be asserted that 1) a practice is essentially acceptable ethically, but it may have some unacceptable consequences; 2) a practice is essentially unacceptable ethically, but for reasons that cannot provide the basis for public policy in a pluralistic society, and therefore the question of social consequences must be independently examined; and 3) a practice may be ambiguous, questionable, or still under moral discussion, but its social consequences must be addressed to avoid obviously unacceptable outcomes. This Report of the National Advisory Board on Ethics in Reproduction (NABER) takes an approach that is compatible with all of these ways of interweaving essentialist and consequentialist considerations in that it focuses on avoiding or minimizing potentially deleterious consequences of the practice of oocyte donation.

While NABER accepts as public policy the use of third party donation when it is carried out with certain ethical safeguards, we recognize troubling aspects of the practice. Oocyte donation raises serious ethical concerns, such as those about the relation between the genetic and social bases of parenthood, the connection between procreation and an ongoing committed relation to one's co-procreator, the role and obligations of third parties who contribute materially to the creation of a child, possible confusion of the child's identity and genetic inheritance, and the stereotyping and commodification of women. Although appeals to individual liberty and procreative rights are often the primary focus of those who defend such reproductive technologies as oocyte donation, we maintain that this practice should also be examined through the lens of certain additional central ethical values. NABER's acceptance of the practice of oocyte donation is limited by the requirement to recognize and apply a framework of moral values to it.

Human reproduction has, from time immemorial, been surrounded by powerful emotions and social conventions. Ethical imperatives, while differing from society to society, have ever been present and through history debates can be heard about the values that should guide reproductive choices. NABER, conscious of the complexity of these questions and of the diversity of views in a pluralistic society, suggests that contemporary debate about reproductive technologies should reflect at least the following values: respect for personal autonomy, support of individual and family privacy, promotion of the well-being of participants, concern for the interests and welfare of children, acknowledgment of the requirements of professional ethics, recognition of basic values that tie us together as a community such as the importance of procreation and the family, and the orderly introduction of social innovation. Aware that the process of creating life is relational in nature, we give special priority and concern to assuring that those relationships created by methods of assisted reproduction are protected and flourish. This list, while perhaps not yet as full and rich as the values of particular communities with traditions about begetting, is nevertheless richer than maximizing preference satisfaction and liberty.

Respect for personal autonomy is a central value of modern ethics. While we do not believe that it is the only value, it is unquestionably a fundamental one. In reproductive matters, the choices and preferences of individuals deserve respect; that is, they should not be interfered with without strong justification. Informed consent of those receiving treatment and of those donating gametes is essential for ensuring respect for their personal autonomy and for avoiding coercion. Privacy is a concomitant value: persons other than parents and those whom they invite into their private domain should not intrude into their reproductive behaviors without serious cause. It is essential to promote the well-being of participants in the procedures of the new reproductive technologies. The bodily health and the psychological, intellectual, social, and spiritual dimensions of the well-being of recipients of these procedures, as well as of donors, must be given consideration and support. Moreover, decisions to reproduce mean that the interests of the resulting children must be of primary concern. Children must be assured that there will be persons responsible for caring for them and providing for their safety and flourishing. The ethical traditions of the various health care professions must also figure in decisions made concerning the use of the new reproductive technologies. The professional obligations to relieve suffering and illness and to provide treatment that is efficacious are especially relevant in this area. Professional standards governing who may offer infertility treatments and assessments of new techniques by institutional review boards that include experts in the area provide ways of minimizing physical and psychological risks to patients while protecting their well-being.

Certain basic values important to our life as a community, such as non-commodification of human beings and their bodies, the moral significance of the family as a basic social unit, equal respect and concern for all human beings, and the fair and appropriate distribution of societal resources must also enter into deliberations about the new reproductive technologies. We suggest that a value not usually discussed in ethics is important when assessing novel technologies, namely, the careful introduction of social innovations. Technologies are not merely techniques; they effect a variety of social changes, some of which may be unexpected and undesirable. Thus, the potential of novel technologies must be carefully assessed and cautiously applied. While it is beyond the scope of this report to present and evaluate broad or specific theories of justice, questions related to justice inevitably surface when issues of costs and access to the new reproductive technologies enter into our discussion in this Report.

We emphasize the relevance of this framework of values in connection with the special questions that are raised by the technique of oocyte donation. Application of this framework will require weighing and balancing values against one another when they conflict and prioritizing them. We will investigate the way in which these values apply to the use of other techniques of assisted reproduction in future reports. Ultimately, we plan to develop a comprehensive ethical framework that can be used to guide the development of current and future reproductive technologies that is grounded in careful case studies of several reproductive technologies. We believe that more discussion is needed not only among NABER members, but within our society, before that significant step is taken.

We would encourage participants in any reproductive technology, whether as donors, recipients, medical professionals, nurses, social workers, or counselors, to understand and discuss their own values, beliefs, and life plans before entering this area. Should they decide to participate in the practice of oocyte donation, they need to receive accurate information and helpful ethical guidance. It is to this task that this Report turns in its next few sections. In its final section, the Report addresses related matters of public policy that are of special concern to policy makers and government officials.

SECTION II

ETHICAL AND POLICY ISSUES RELATED TO OOCYTE RECIPIENTS IN THE CLINICAL SETTING

A. BACKGROUND CONTEXT

I. WHO ARE OOCYTE RECIPIENTS?

Oocyte donation has been used to assist women to become pregnant who are without ovaries or whose ovaries are not functional due to chemotherapy, radiation treatment, or surgical removal. It has also been employed for those at risk of transmitting significant genetic disease to their offspring and women who have not responded to other forms of infertility treatment.[1] The most common use of the procedure is for women who experience premature menopause.[2] The technique is also being used for women of advanced reproductive age who no longer produce their own eggs.[3]

Until recently, many clinics set an upper age limit of 40 for women undergoing any form of assisted reproduction.[4] This was presumably because female fertility decreases with age in both natural and assisted reproductive systems, beginning at approximately 35 years of age.[5] However, the development of oocyte donation in the 1980s made it possible for women of advanced reproductive age to become pregnant using eggs derived from younger women;[6] hence treatment is now provided to women beyond the age of 40 in many programs.[7] A 1992 survey of American oocyte donation programs indicated that the average upper limit of the age of oocyte recipients was 55 years.[8] In 27% of the oocyte donation programs, no upper age limit at all was set for recipients.[9]

Those most likely to obtain specialized infertility services such as egg donation at present are older, white, college-educated, married women of higher socioeconomic status.[10] A 1991 survey of oocyte donation centers found that expenses to recipients per retrieval ranged from $2,500 to $15,000.[11] This appears to indicate that oocyte recipients must either have health care insurance coverage for the procedure or independent means to cover these costs. Those who are generally without access to goods and services, therefore, are not likely to have access to new reproductive technologies such as oocyte donation.[12]

2. HOW POTENTIAL RECIPIENTS LEARN ABOUT OOCYTE DONATION

Some women and their partners learn about oocyte donation when they are referred to infertility centers by their gynecologists or other physicians. Articles in newspapers about the procedure lead some potential recipients to contact local infertility programs.[13] Others learn of it through public presentations of information concerning a variety of infertility treatments, including oocyte donation, offered by local infertility programs.[14] Still others are told about the technique by relatives and friends. Resolve, a group in the private sector formed to offer support to those with reproductive difficulties, informs couples about the availability of various kinds of treatments for infertility, such as oocyte donation, and about alternatives, such as adoption.

3. WHY POTENTIAL RECIPIENTS SEEK DONATED OOCYTES

Little is known about the specific motivations of those interested in receiving donated eggs other than that they want to have babies. The theme of desperation and willingness to try almost anything occurs again and again in the literature. A 1991 study of those who received ova from a relative or close friend found that their primary motives were a) to have children, b) to experience pregnancy, c) to provide the spouse with genetic offspring, and d) to have genetically related offspring.[15]

4. MEDICAL PROCEDURES USED TO PROVIDE OOCYTES TO RECIPIENTS

Medical treatment of oocyte recipients involves inducing artificial menstrual cycles to create a receptive endometrial environment.[16] Hormones are administered to the recipient in coordination with the administration of human chorionic gonadotropin to the donor in order to synchronize their cycles. Eggs are removed from the donor, fertilized *in vitro* with the sperm of the partner of the woman without viable eggs or with donor sperm and transferred to the recipient approximately two days after recovery. The recipient receives a steroid supplement until approximately the ninth week of gestation to maintain an optimal endometrial environment.[17] Thereafter, if the procedure proceeds successfully, the recipient goes through pregnancy and gives birth to a child.

Pregnancy rates for recipients of donated eggs are markedly higher than those from other methods of assisted reproduction.[18] A 1988 American survey indicated that of 130 women who underwent 158 oocyte donation procedures, 32% experienced clinical pregnancies and 23% live births.[19] This contrasted with the 12% live-birth rate in that year for those who underwent *in vitro* fertilization using their own ova. A 1991 report indicated that 31.4% of 1,045 egg retrieval procedures resulted in clinical pregnancies and 25.6% deliveries per retrieval.[20] It should be noted, however, that the success rates for oocyte donation vary from center to center. One center, for instance, reported a live birth rate of nearly 50% per embryo transfer in its donor oocyte program in 1990.[21] This may be due to differences in patient populations, as well as such other factors as differences in medical techniques and degree of experience.

A high rate of multiple births has been reported in women receiving donated oocytes because typically several embryos are transferred after *in vitro* fertilization.[22] A recent study suggests that recipients with multiple births experienced an increased incidence of maternal complications, although they generally delivered healthy babies.[23] Other recent reports suggest that use of fertility drugs, particularly clomiphene, may increase the risk of ovarian cancer.[24] To assess whether the link between these drugs and ovarian cancer is causal and, if so, to determine the magnitude of the risks, the National Institutes of Health has funded expansion of a 1994 study and is planning another.[25] It has been suggested that in the present uncertain situation about risks to recipients and the resulting children, it seems prudent to limit exposure to fertility drugs by avoiding more than a few cycles of stimulation.[26]

Multiple births also carry a relative increased risk for severe handicap of 1.7 for twins and 2.9 for triplets when compared to single births.[27] Serafini et al. observe that "Preterm labor, hospitalizations during pregnancy, the necessity of using neonatal intensive care facilities, an increased number of surgical deliveries, and associated rearing difficulties are among some of the immense hardships caused by multiple pregnancies."[28]

B. OOCYTE RECIPIENTS IN THE CLINICAL SETTING

I. ENABLING POTENTIAL RECIPIENTS TO MAKE AN INFORMED CHOICE ABOUT WHETHER TO BEGIN SCREENING PROCEDURES

Those receiving treatment for infertility indicate that they needed to be better informed about their options and alternative treatment plans.[29] Participants in one study, when asked to give advice to their physicians anonymously, observed that they wanted to know the probable long-term plan at the beginning of treatment for infertility and also what alternatives were available, including adoption.[30] The obligations to respect the autonomy of potential egg recipients and to promote their well-being and that of any children that may result from treatment require that physicians adequately apprise recipients of the options available to them. This should be done in a comprehensive manner, rather than incrementally when various treatment efforts fail. At some centers, such as the one at Montefiore Medical Center/Albert Einstein College of Medicine, ethics committees assist in developing the information given to recipient candidates.[31]

Therefore, in the interest of promoting well-informed and deliberate decisions, NABER recommends that before potential oocyte recipients undergo testing and screening at an infertility center, they be provided with full and accurate information about the procedure of oocyte donation. This should include information about its physical and psychological risks and side effects. We further recommend that potential oocyte recipients be provided with information about the pregnancy and delivery rates for those of their age group undergoing oocyte donation throughout the country, at the center at which they are considering receiving treatment, and at other available centers in the area.[32] They should be apprised of factors affecting these rates, such as the number of recipients who have been treated at the relevant centers, their diagnoses, and the period of time that the quoted rates cover. In addition, we recommend that potential oocyte recipients be given the opportunity to discuss and compare other alternatives for their infertility (including adoption) with medical practitioners and also with skilled counselors independent of the practitioner who would perform the procedure and with other advisors, such as clergy.

2. THE ETHICAL IMPORTANCE OF SEPARATING RECIPIENT SCREENING FROM COUNSELING

Potential oocyte recipients should be evaluated and counseled before they are accepted into programs. This is necessary to ascertain whether they are appropriate candidates for the program, provide them with important information, and assist them to address medical, psychological, or social questions they may have. Why should those seeking access to egg donation programs have to undergo screening when those who can conceive and bear children coitally need not? This is appropriate because the situation changes ethically when others are involved in assisting procreation. Health care professionals must be involved and this, in turn, introduces the special responsibilities they have to patients. They have an ethical obligation to screen and counsel potential recipients, out of concern for the welfare of those recipients and the children born of the procedure. They also have an obligation to assess that recipients are choosing to enter the program voluntarily and competently, out of concern for the integrity of their autonomy. Such evaluation and counseling recognizes the value we ascribe to the physical, psychological, social, and spiritual dimensions of the well-being of potential egg recipients and to their self-determination. It also recognizes that innovative technologies such as oocyte donation must be cautiously applied until they have been fully evaluated.

At some centers, potential oocyte recipients are seen not only by physicians who conduct initial medical screening procedures, but by a variety of other health care professionals for medical, psychological, and social screening.[33] Trained counselors with backgrounds in psychology, social work, or related fields evaluate potential recipients and their partners and offer them counseling. A number of pre-admission interviews are often required of recipient candidates with different health care professionals because it takes considerable time to discuss the complex situation presented by an infertility technique involving a third party.[34] According to a 1991–92 survey, potential recipients are interviewed by physicians for an average of 1.45 hours, nurses for 2 hours, and mental health professionals for 1.45 hours.[35]

When the same interviews are conducted both to screen candidates and to counsel them about issues of special personal concern, potential recipients are placed in an ambiguous position. Instead of seeing this series of required interviews as a form of emotional support carried out for their own welfare, some perceive it as a mechanism that may be used arbitrarily to prevent them from undergoing egg donation.[36] They perceive interviewers as gatekeepers who may judge them "crazy" and deny them admission to the program.[37] Some potential recipients, consequently, may not feel free to discuss pressing individual concerns during their screening evaluation. A delicate balance must be maintained between screening and counseling, since each of these processes has different purposes. They cannot, however, be kept totally separate. When they overlap, this is not ethically objectionable unless the recipient is led to believe that screening sessions are directed solely toward counseling and is not informed that she is being assessed for acceptance or rejection.

We recommend that pre-treatment screening of potential oocyte recipients be kept distinct from pre-treatment counseling as far as possible. While screening and counseling may be difficult to separate in practice, it is important to attempt to keep them apart so that recipient candidates will speak freely during counseling about any difficulties they may have. We further recommend that potential recipients be informed about the purpose of both screening and counseling interviews. In addition, we recommend that non-medical aspects of screening and counseling be carried out by skilled professionals especially trained for this purpose who function independently of the physician who would carry out the procedure.

3. PRE-ADMISSION SCREENING OF POTENTIAL RECIPIENTS: SEEKING ETHICALLY APPROPRIATE GOALS AND MEANS

By what standards should providers screen women and/or their partners? Any society has a concern about the welfare of parents and of children who live in it. The value we ascribe to personal autonomy, to the well-being of individuals, to nurturing children, to the family as a basic social unit, and to the fair and appropriate distribution of societal resources requires that certain kinds of screening of potential recipients of donated eggs be performed. Yet our society has formulated few criteria by which to address these values and concerns. Unfortunately, we cannot use current practices as the basis for developing global screening measures for potential recipients, as little has been published about them. Indeed, many oocyte donation programs have no stated criteria for determining who will be selected for oocyte donation and on what grounds.[38]

We recommend that detailed inter-center guidelines for medical, psychological, and social screening of potential oocyte recipients be developed across oocyte donation programs in the country by a task force of physicians, nurses, and counselors who are experienced in the provision of this procedure, as well as consumers, patient representatives, ethicists, lawyers, and other relevant persons from outside the clinical setting. (See Section IV.) This task force should be established through a cooperative effort by those oocyte donation programs. Guidelines should be developed by those who have experience in the clinical setting with the assistance of experts and laypeople from outside that setting to ensure that they have a foundation in clinical realities and yet reflect significant ethical and social values. We believe that recommendations made below will provide a starting point for such guidelines.

Until guidelines are developed and adopted across the board by oocyte donation programs, medical, psychological, and social criteria used by individual fertility centers and professionals for screening potential recipients should be set out in writing so that candidates for oocyte donation can know of these in advance. The majority of oocyte donation programs surveyed in 1991–92 had available some form of ethics committee or internal ethics advisory board that could assist individual institutions and professionals in developing screening guidelines.[39] Such ethics advisory groups should be involved in developing and advising individual oocyte donation programs about screening and matching criteria and procedures.[40]

We recommend that medical practitioners and trained counselors screen potential oocyte recipients, actively involving them, to ensure as far as possible that their health and that of any child born of this oocyte donation will not be damaged by the procedure. Potential recipients should also be interviewed to ascertain that they are entering the program voluntarily and competently. The final decision about admission to an oocyte donation program should be taken mutually by health care professionals and recipient candidates, rather than unilaterally by physicians, nurses, and counselors. We recognize, however, that there are circumstances in which providers, informed by professional ethics and personal conscience, may elect to decline their services to potential oocyte recipients; such decisions should be respected.

a. Medical screening of recipients and partners

A systematic approach should be taken to the evaluation of infertility, first using noninvasive procedures and proceeding to the more invasive and specialized ones only as needed, leading infertility specialists recommend.[41] Patients should not be exposed unnecessarily to extensive batteries of screening tests. Moreover, these specialists note, they should be given a reasonable amount of time for pregnancy to occur independent of treatment, rather than offered premature treatment.

Several oocyte donation program directors have described standards and requirements in force for medical screening of recipients and their partners at their centers. These can provide a starting point for the development of inter-center standards for medical screening for oocyte donation. Rosenwaks at Cornell University in New York, to give one example, maintains that potential oocyte recipients should have a normal uterus and their condition should provide no contraindications for pregnancy.[42] To ascertain the latter, they should have a medical work-up that includes a baseline hormonal study; karyotyping; hysterosalpingography (to assess the uterus and tubes); cardiopulmonary assessment; blood chemistry and hematologic profile; rubella antibody test; screening for hepatitis, venereal disease and HIV; and HLA-antibody typing. Preparatory menstrual cycles should be evaluated to assess the adequacy of the natural or artificially induced endometrial cycle.[43] The American Fertility Society maintains that women over the age of 40 should undergo more extensive tests than those carried out for younger oocyte recipients before they are approved to receive donated oocytes. These tests include cardiovascular screening and high-risk obstetrical consultation.[44] (See Section II. B.6., "Special Ethical Considerations Related to Older Women Who Seek Donated Oocytes.")

The woman's partner should also be screened medically.[45] It has been recommended that he have an adequate spermatogram and undergo HIV screening, HLA antibody typing and, if indicated, Tay-Sachs or other genetic tests.[46] As new information about the human genome is developed and genetic testing capabilities increase, new questions will arise about whether the partners of recipients of donated eggs should be tested more extensively for genetically transmitted characteristics.[47]

We recommend that medical screening measures for potential oocyte recipients currently in use be analyzed for adequacy and effectiveness. Inter-center guidelines for medical screening of potential oocyte recipients should be among those developed by the inter-center task force recommended above. Such inter-center guidelines should take into account the health and well-being of recipients, their partners, and any children who might result from the procedure of oocyte donation. Consideration should be given to testing for genetic conditions that are incompatible with life or that are of such severity as to force life into a narrow focus on disease and its treatment.

b. Screening recipients for decisionmaking capacity

Respect for the autonomy of potential oocyte recipients means that health care professionals should consider whether potential oocyte recipients have the capacity to make decisions related to the procedure. Candidates should be able to understand the relevant information concerning oocyte donation, consider it in light of their values and goals, and communicate their thoughts and concerns with those who are involved in providing the treatment to them.

Potential recipients should be presumed to have the capacity to make relevant decisions concerning the reception of oocytes unless a question about this is raised and a determination is made by qualified health care professionals that they lack adequate capacity. Should it be considered necessary to conduct an assessment of the decisionmaking capacity of a potential recipient, it is the responsibility of the recipient's physician to ensure that this is carried out properly.

We recommend that programs develop policies for assessing decisionmaking capacity. They should notify those applying for admission that they have such policies.

c. Screening recipients for voluntariness and freedom from coercion

Concern for the autonomy and well-being of potential oocyte recipients also requires consideration of whether they are choosing to enter an oocyte donation program voluntarily and without coercion. For instance, family values and expectations, while not overtly coercive, may be so strong as to override a woman's personal choice.[48] A careful review of the social history and current situation of potential recipients may bring this to light and allow couples the opportunity to reconsider.

Some feminist critics maintain that it is not just individual families, but pervasive social structures in which infertile women find themselves embedded that undermine the voluntariness of their choices and reproductive autonomy.[49] If a "true" choice is "an uncoerced selection of one course of action over another and the ability to follow one's chosen course,"[50] the social framework that structures reproduction, they declare, renders it impossible for women to make such a choice. Other feminists view women as active agents freely pursuing their goal of overcoming infertility, rather than as victims of a coercive social structure.[51] Indeed, some feminists maintain that reproductive technologies hold out to women the promise of increasing their own reproductive freedom.[52] Without control over reproduction "women cannot gain access to or participate effectively in the political and social processes which shape their lives."[53]

In light of these feminist concerns, we recommend that professionals meeting with potential oocyte recipients ascertain that they understand what is involved in oocyte donation and are choosing to engage in this procedure of their own volition. To enhance their control over the decision, potential recipients should be counseled about other alternatives, such as adoption, by persons who have no vested interest in carrying out oocyte donation.

d. Psychological screening of recipients and partners

Some centers, such as that at the University of Washington, perform no psychological testing of recipients unless specific psychiatric disorders are suspected.[54] Other centers routinely require potential oocyte recipients and their partners to undergo psychological evaluation before they can be approved to receive oocytes.[55] At Huntington Reproductive Center, tests include the Minnesota Multiphasic Personality Inventory, and, at times, the Thematic Apperception Test and Wechsler Adult Intelligence Scale.[56] Additional tests such as psychiatric assessment through the life events checklist, Perceived Stress Scale, and the Hopkins Symptom Checklist-90 are also used for both recipients and donors. Psychological screening is distinct from, albeit related to, screening for decisionmaking capacity. The latter focuses on whether the individual has the ability to make a decision about the specific treatment being considered, whereas the former covers a broad range of considerations about the mental health of potential recipients. It has been observed of current forms of psychological screening that "it is unclear what the purpose of the screening is and what criteria are being established for the information gathered."[57]

Several justifications have been given for performing psychological screening. The first centers on the need to ascertain that potential recipients are able to make decisions autonomously and in light of their own well-being and life plans. Many infertile couples, on learning of their situation, endure a personal and family crisis that may, in some instances, exacerbate pre-existing psychological difficulties.[58] Some have been through a long period of treatment for infertility that has been both physically and psychologically taxing and that may have created extravagant expectations of the child. The non-contributing partner may feel alienated and this could impair the relationship between husband and wife and between parents and child. Psychological assessments assist in identifying those who might have serious difficulty in coping with the stress of oocyte donation.

Other justifications offered for psychological screening focus not only on the autonomy and well-being of recipients, but on the well-being of children who might be born of the procedure. This is the case, for example, when psychological tests are used at some centers to evaluate the couple's motivations, the stability of their marriage, their capacity for parenthood, whether their expectations are realistic, and the degree of social support available to them.[59] Unfortunately, those carrying out these tests do not specify which recipient motivations are acceptable and unacceptable, which characteristics indicate that recipients do or do not have a capacity for parenthood, or how to assess whether recipient expectations are realistic. Moreover, such screening tends to merge psychological with social assessment of potential recipients. These should be kept distinct from one another. (See II. B.3.e., "Social screening of recipients and partners" below.)

Psychological screening can be biased and prejudicial. The ability to discern by psychological means good from bad motives or to assess the capacity to parent well, except in the most egregious cases, such as serious personality disorders, is limited. Therefore, we have reservations about the validity of using psychological screening for anything other than assessing emotional stability relative to the stressful process of infertility treatment and for serious personality disorders such that providers could reliably predict parental harm to the child.

We recommend that psychological screening measures for oocyte recipients that are currently in use be analyzed for adequacy and effectiveness and that inter-center guidelines for psychological screening of potential oocyte recipients be included among those developed by the inter-center task force recommended above. Such guidelines should be geared to assisting potential oocyte recipients to choose autonomously and to protecting their well-being and that of any children born of the procedure. Insofar as possible, clear psychological criteria for exclusion from oocyte donation programs should be developed.

e. Social screening of recipients and partners

The goals of the social evaluation[60] of potential recipients stated at some centers include: to assess whether they would make suitable parents, to gauge the stability of their marriages, and to determine the degree of social support available to them.[61] In at least one program, an assessment is made of the stability of the incomes of potential recipient couples.[62] Such goals open wide the door to discrimination. Women with disabilities, for instance, have reported that they have been denied access to reproductive technologies on social grounds.[63] The value of equal respect and concern requires that we refrain from making stereotyped prejudgments about the ability of individuals to bear children.

There is considerable disagreement about whether it is possible to screen out those who would be unsuitable parents. Hollinger, for instance, maintains that we have no accepted standard of parental fitness nor any empirically validated criteria for determining who would be good parents.[64] She argues that "the small number of unworthies who might be detected and weeded out by fitness screening hardly justifies the financial and social costs of trying to devise reliable tests." Yet the capacity of individuals for parenthood is among the fundamental concerns any society must have about its current and future citizens.[65] We must take into account not only the deep desires of couples to have children, but the welfare of those children themselves. Concern for the interests of children requires that consideration be given to whether children born of oocyte donation would be brought into a supportive environment in which serious physical and mental harm is not an obvious danger.

We recommend that screening for parental suitability should be carried out at oocyte donation centers, but that criteria for such screening should be generous. Only the most obviously questionable candidates for oocyte donation should be denied access because of their probable inability to care for a child adequately. Consideration of the well-being of oocyte recipient candidates and of the children who might result means that fair consideration should also be given to the stability of the couple's relationship and to whether they have adequate social support to raise and nurture a child without placing that child at risk of serious physical or mental harm.

f. Rejection of recipient candidates

Those carrying out the screening of potential oocyte recipients should not turn away candidates for reception of donated oocytes for arbitrary or irrelevant reasons. It is ethically appropriate for providers to decline to provide service on a showing of medical inadvisability, insufficient decisionmaking capacity, lack of voluntariness, or manifest psychological or social pathology. Providers should, however, make strenuous efforts to avoid making such decisions on the basis of bias or beliefs for which there is little evidence.

We recommend that those who are denied access to an oocyte donation program be given an indication of the reasons for this denial and that counseling be offered to them to help them address the deep personal loss that such a decision creates.

4. THE NEED FOR POST-SCREENING RECIPIENT EDUCATION AND COUNSELING PRIOR TO SOLICITING INFORMED CONSENT

Providers have an ethical obligation to attempt to make the assisted reproduction situation less technical and more humane. Patients need to assimilate the technical and medical into the emotional and attitudinal features that surround the conception and bearing of children. Counseling can provide those pursuing oocyte donation with the opportunity to discuss benefits, risks, and success rates frankly and to address special considerations.[66] Sessions with counselors can encompass discussions of how recipients might react to procedures that will be intrusive, painful, embarrassing, and, perhaps unsuccessful, and ways in which they can address these reactions. At this stage, counseling may help recipients to begin to address personal and marital difficulties that may have arisen in connection with their growing awareness of infertility. Information derived from earlier medical, psychological, and decisionmaking evaluations can be of assistance during such counseling.[67]

Informed consent should not be solicited from potential recipients until a point after they have been counseled about issues relevant to their situation and have made a decision to enter the program. To ask them to consent to the reception of donated eggs during the screening process creates an incorrect presumption that they have been admitted to the program and does not allow time for counseling.

Recipients should be encouraged to address some of the overarching questions of special importance to them, such as what to tell the child about his or her origins, whether to use a known donor or one whose identity remains confidential, how to address the reality that several "parents" will be involved in bringing the child into the world, and how to cope with social attitudes toward the use of donor gametes.[68] Support groups that permit networking of recipient couples can be of assistance in such efforts.[69]

Therefore, we recommend that potential oocyte recipients and their partners who successfully complete the pre-treatment screening evaluation receive additional education and counseling before they make a final commitment to receive donated oocytes. Although additional education and counseling take time and mean that the efforts of couples to have a child will be delayed, studies indicate that allowing a period of several months to elapse between the suggestion of the use of oocyte donation and implementation of the procedure is associated with better adjustment to the process.[70]

We further recommend that informed consent be sought from oocyte recipients entering the program after discussions have been held on such matters as the risks and benefits of treatment; what is involved in ovulation induction, uterine preparation, egg retrieval and egg transfer;[71] and what expectations they have of the child that might result from treatment. The rights and responsibilities of all involved should be clarified during discussions, including those of the institution, medical and mental health teams, donor and partner, recipient and partner, and children born of the procedure. Moreover, confidentiality, donor compensation (if any), responsibility for disposition of oocytes and embryos, responsibility for risks incidental to donation, and responsibility for children born of the procedure should be agreed upon beforehand and should be outlined in a separate document.

5. THE NEED FOR CONTINUING POST-ADMISSION RECIPIENT EDUCATION AND COUNSELING

Not surprisingly, those who had received infertility treatment indicated in one study that they were more satisfied with their care when they were included in decisions about when to begin a treatment or which treatment to use.[72] Yet oocyte donation programs vary in the degree to which recipients are involved in such decisions. Some provide recipients with no option to choose known or confidential donors, as they use only donors whose identity is kept confidential.[73] Others require recipients to bring their own donors.[74] Recipients may be involved in the process of matching with donors in some programs and not in others. Recipients going through diagnostic and therapeutic procedures—the preparation phase, start of the cycle, daily callbacks, and intake of medication—need technical and supportive explanations. The timing of tests and sexual relations is critical to their treatment.[75]

The majority of those who undergo oocyte donation will not meet their goal of delivering a child. Greenfeld et al. have described disruptive "grief reactions" experienced by some women following the failure of *in vitro* fertilization.[76] Such reactions may also be experienced by those for whom oocyte donation is unsuccessful. Some who undergo infertility treatment find it difficult to end it even after numerous failed attempts at becoming pregnant. They may go through a whole series of devastating disappointments.

Therefore, we recommend that oocyte recipients be offered on-going education and support during the work-up and the process of receiving donated oocytes and that they be actively involved in decisions about their treatment as it evolves.[77] We also recommend that when treatment is unsuccessful, short-term counseling be offered to disappointed patients.[78] Counseling and discussion of other options can be especially helpful to couples who are reluctant to stop treatment despite repeated attempts to conceive and carry a child to term.[79]

6. SPECIAL ETHICAL CONSIDERATIONS RELATED TO OLDER WOMEN WHO SEEK DONATED OOCYTES

Women of advanced reproductive age may seek to have a child by means of donated eggs for a number of reasons. Some have married late and now want to start a family. Others have been married for years without having had children, but, upon learning of oocyte donation, become interested in the prospect. In some instances, women have remarried and want to have children with their new husbands. In others, they have suffered the tragic death of a grown child and hope to have another. One study indicated that women over 40 who applied for oocyte donation were more apt to have undergone cosmetic surgery; its authors speculated that their desire to reproduce might be a further attempt to challenge their chronologic age.[80] In a few cases, women offer to act as surrogate gestational carriers for their daughters or daughters-in-law who can produce eggs, but lack a uterus. All of these potential oocyte donation recipients hope to counter the aging process and go through pregnancy and childbirth.

A 1991 survey of oocyte donation programs in the United States found that over 70% had age-based criteria for oocyte recipients ranging from 35 to 55 years.[81] In 31% of the programs, recipients over 40 years of age were excluded. In programs that accept older women, clinicians screen potential oocyte recipients and exclude those with preexisting medical conditions. At the University of Washington, for instance, an extensive physical and laboratory testing regimen is used to assess the general health status of older women. Patients are counseled and decisions are made on an individualized basis.[82] In the egg donation program at IVF America, women over 40 receive special screening and counseling regarding significant contraindications to pregnancy; all women aged 45 to 50 receive special review from the Medical Director.[83] Even with careful screening, however, oocyte recipients still have to run the increased obstetric risks associated with pregnancy at an advanced reproductive age.

The use of donated oocytes to achieve pregnancies in women of advanced reproductive age raises concerns about the well-being of these women and the resulting children.[84] Little is known about the effects of pregnancy on older women or on their fetuses. It is clear that pregnancy exposes older women to physical risks not confronted in the same degree and kind by those who are younger.[85] It places their organ systems, particularly their cardiopulmonary system, under major stress at a time when these systems are decreasing in functional reserve.[86] Studies indicate that older women who go through pregnancy and childbirth have a greater degree of gestational hypertension and antepartum hemorrhage than younger ones and that they are more likely to need an operative delivery.[87] They have increased maternal mortality rates.[88] Women aged 40 or more in one study had a maternal mortality rate of 53.9 per 100,000 pregnancies as opposed to a rate of 5.3 in women aged 20 to 24.[89] There may also be increased developmental risks to children born to older women, although current data about the condition of children born to older women who undergo oocyte donation do not appear to indicate that there is a generalizable pattern of such risk.[90] Further studies are needed about this question.

Some physicians have conscientious objections to providing older women with donated eggs; they view the risk to these women as too high and consider it contrary to their professional ethic to expose patients to such risk. Physicians may also be concerned about legal liability and the stigma of a malpractice action should an oocyte recipient suffer an untoward event. Others maintain, however, that older women should make the decision about whether to receive donated oocytes after they have been adequately informed and appropriately counseled. They should be provided with an account of what is not known, as well as what is known about the risks that pregnancy and childbirth present to women of their age. On this second view, the autonomy of women should prevail.

The phenomenon of women of advanced reproductive age seeking pregnancy, some critics maintain, involves the misuse of reproductive technology to solve social issues or personal misfortune. Methods of assisted reproduction are not designed to correct a malfunctioning organ system or disease, they note, but to reverse part of the normal aging process. They believe this exemplifies a refusal to confront the rhythms of the human life cycle, especially aging and death, and exhibits how social images of youth and femininity can pressure women into reproductive choices that may be unwise.

The welfare of the children who might be born is also of concern. A major argument against access to oocyte donation for older women is that the resulting children will run a higher risk of being orphaned at a crucially important young age. This concern, however, needs to be undergirded by evidence about the life expectancy of women in good health today in the United States. The age and life expectancy of the father are also relevant to the question, since he might stand a good chance of surviving to care for the child should the mother die. Another factor is whether there would be a family support system that could care for the child should one or both parents die.

Some express concern that children born to older women will be neglected because their mothers will not have the stamina to keep up with them. Although they might be able to care for a baby while they are in their fifties, it would be more difficult for them to provide supervision and emotional support for a teenager fifteen years later. Moreover, their health might deteriorate during the aging process, making it difficult for them to carry out their parental role.[91] Although there can be little control over such events when they happen unexpectedly to younger people, it is ethically questionable, they maintain, deliberately to bring children into the world by egg donation knowing they may face such a disadvantage.

Others respond that even if older women have a lower energy level, those attempting oocyte donation are likely to be reasonably well off and to have help in caring for their children. Those who are not well-to-do may have a strong family system to assist them in raising the child. They point out that although childrearing can be taxing, grandmothers are raising their daughters' children today because of the latter's employment situation, divorce, or young age[92] and there is little indication that this practice has had a major detrimental effect on the rearing grandmothers or the children. The decision should not depend solely on age, but should take other factors into account as well. The particular circumstances of older women who are potential oocyte recipients, they argue, need to be addressed.

The question whether it is a good use of a scarce resource to allow older women to resort to egg donation is also significant. Oocytes given to older women may have a greater likelihood of being wasted, since they may have a lower probability of implanting in these women; further, if they do, the resulting pregnancy may have a higher likelihood of not going to term. This is a legitimate concern and one that led the Canadian Royal Commission on New Reproductive Technologies to recommend against allowing post-menopausal women access to donated eggs.[93] One way in which it could be addressed would be to require older women to bring their own known donor.

This would ensure that the existing supply of donor eggs would not be diminished. There are many other questions to ask besides those related to age when considering whether to allow women access to scarce eggs. Should a woman with a past history of miscarriages be given this scarce resource, since she has a higher likelihood of not being able to carry the pregnancy through to term? Should a couple using frozen sperm because of male factor infertility, have access to donated oocytes, since freezing sperm lessens by half the chances of fertilization? To bar women access to donated eggs on the basis of age to the exclusion of other relevant considerations could lead to inappropriate discrimination on account of age. Questions of gender discrimination would also arise were older women barred from access to donated eggs while older men were not prohibited from becoming fathers.

We find especially serious the concerns that have been raised about the health of women of advanced reproductive age who are candidates for oocyte donation and the children who might be born to them. Unfortunately, there is a general lack of information about pregnancy and childbirth in older women and about its effects on children. If evidence were amassed indicating that pregnancy had previously unenvisaged negative effects on older women and on children born to them, it would be highly appropriate to limit their access to oocyte donation. However, in the absence of such evidence, older women and physicians have to grapple with reasonable probabilities, asking such questions as whether the cardiovascular system of the woman is likely to withstand the strain of pregnancy and childbirth. Circumstances that fall at the margins of probable scenarios involving women of advanced reproductive age should not be taken to apply to the entire range of such scenarios. The health of women who are 52 to 55 may be wholly different from that of those who are 60 and may provide greater justification for granting them access to donated oocytes. Therefore, whether egg donation would have detrimental effects on the health of older women cannot be determined in the abstract.

After careful consideration of the issue, we are left with major reservations about the use of oocyte donation in women of relatively advanced reproductive age. The higher risks to these candidates, the taxing effect of childrearing on older persons, and concerns about the well-being of the children lead us to conclude that this practice should be pursued only with extreme caution. We recommend that women of advanced reproductive age who are candidates for oocyte donation undergo thorough screening and evaluation of their general physical status, as well as screening for conditions that could adversely affect them during pregnancy, including those associated with age.[94] Guidelines of the American Fertility Society propose that recipients over the age of 40 should receive special psychological assessment, cardiovascular screening, and high-risk obstetrical consultation.[95] We concur and add that they should also be given counseling and education. Whenever possible, the final decision about oocyte donation for women of advanced reproductive age should be taken mutually by caregivers and recipient candidates, rather than unilaterally by health care professionals. However, we recognize that the situation in which women of advanced reproductive age request access to oocyte donation represents one in which providers may decide that they must, in good conscience, refuse to provide this procedure. In such instances, they may assist in identifying a referral.

7. SPECIAL ETHICAL CONSIDERATIONS RELATED TO SINGLE WOMEN WHO SEEK DONATED OOCYTES

The new reproductive technologies were initially developed almost exclusively for infertile heterosexual couples in traditional marriages—although the technique of artificial insemination certainly was used by single women. Thus, in 1973, one author stated definitively, "Most practitioners . . . dismiss the possibility of using [AID] for unmarried women."[96] However, as these techniques have been developed and as social and cultural practices regarding marriage and sexuality have changed, the question has been raised whether the desire of single women to bear children and to avail themselves of medical assistance in order to do so, should be accommodated. Concerns have been expressed, not only about the rights of individuals who wish to have a child by means of the new reproductive technologies, but also about the future of the traditional nuclear family and the welfare of the children born outside such families. The literature addressing whether single women should have access to assisted reproduction deals primarily with their access to artificial insemination by donor (AID). Since both AID and oocyte donation involve third-party gamete donation, similar ethical and policy questions are raised by each. Yet certain distinctive questions related to oocyte donation and the single woman must also be considered.

Little is known about policies governing the admission of single women to oocyte donation programs in the United States. A 1991 survey indicated that most of them have no stated exclusion criteria for recipients other than those related to their choice about donor anonymity.[97] Some, however, do restrict access to married women.[98] It appears that as a matter of practice, it is primarily married couples or those in a long-term stable relationship who are admitted to gamete donation programs.[99] Such decisions are usually made by physicians.[100] A 1987 OTA survey of physicians who provided AID indicated that 52% rejected women on grounds that they were unmarried and that an additional 15% rejected women because they were homosexual.[101]

Concerns about whether single women should have access to such reproductive measures as oocyte donation tend to focus on two different, albeit related issues: 1) Should those who are not married be given access to these techniques? and 2) Can single women provide an adequate support system for children born to them by means of the new reproductive technologies?

Several religious bodies are among those groups and individuals who consider it morally wrong for those who are unmarried to have children. They maintain that childbearing should take place within the covenantal commitment of marriage and hold that procreative acts outside this context of marital fidelity are diminished and distorted. (See Section I, "Ethical Questions Raised by Oocyte Donation.") Those within these religious traditions and some outside them share a further concern that allowing single women to procreate by means of alternative reproductive techniques will have a detrimental effect on the family.[102] The significant role of the family in protecting basic social goods and values could be weakened and ultimately destroyed, they maintain, if single motherhood were to become an accepted part of our social structure.

Those who favor providing access to new reproductive techniques such as oocyte donation to single women tend to focus on the effect of changing social values on the meaning and composition of the family. They note that the family in the United States is moving away from a traditional two-parent format because of divorce, remarriage, and single motherhood through natural reproduction. In 1970, traditional nuclear families composed of two married parents with children comprised 40% of all households. By 1990, their numbers had declined to 26%.[103] This does not necessarily indicate that the functions performed by the family are being weakened, defenders of access to single women claim. Single women often can rely on extended families and a network of friends for support that traditionally has been provided by the family. Moreover, these proponents maintain, the number of single women requesting oocyte donation and other forms of assisted reproduction is so small that it is unlikely they will have a significant impact on the structure of the family.

Some critics of providing oocyte donation to single women ask: Should egg donation be used in conjunction with sperm donation for the sole purpose of enabling single women to go through the experience of pregnancy? The single woman who cannot produce her own eggs must use the gametes of two other unrelated people to conceive a child *in vitro*. The question is whether the degree of procreative anomaly for all three persons, as well as the child, can be justified by the value of the experience of pregnancy for the single woman. Critics contend that it cannot and that this use of egg donation strays so far from the paradigm case of the infertile heterosexual couple that it should not be allowed.

Those who favor the use of oocyte donation for single women observe that the situation parallels that of adoption by single women. In both cases, a child is raised by a woman with whom he or she has no genetic connection. If we allow adoption, there is no reason to disallow oocyte donation. Indeed, the woman in oocyte donation has a closer relation to the child than in adoption, as she has a biological tie with the child conferred by having carried him or her through nine months of pregnancy and giving birth. Therefore, these respondents maintain, single women should not be denied access to oocyte donation.

A related argument given by opponents of the use of new reproductive technologies for single women is that it is ethically suspect to have a child in order to satisfy one's personal desire for parenthood. Children should be brought into the world for their own sake.[104] On this view, use of alternative reproductive technologies such as oocyte donation for single women transmutes the child into an object created solely for the personal pleasure of the woman and endangers the child's dignity as a valuable individual. "Why should a child, at its creation, be treated as a property, a product, or a means to satisfy the wishes of adults?"[105]

Respondents claim that the child born to a single woman is no more or less the product of adult needs and desires than the child born to a married couple. They complain that no reasons have been presented to explain why single parenthood brought about by assisted reproductive techniques is more likely to lead to the objectification of children than married parenthood brought about by such means. Some women, they argue, are single by chance, not by choice, and should not be discriminated against because of the arbitrariness of fate.

Some opposed to giving single women access to the new reproductive techniques argue that this would threaten the welfare of the children by depriving them of a male role model.[106] The Warnock Report concluded that "the interests of the child dictate that it should be born into a home where there is a loving, stable, heterosexual relationship and that, therefore, the deliberate creation of a child for a woman who is not a partner in such a relationship is morally wrong."[107] Those concerned about the well-being of the children point to studies indicating that fathers play a greater role in the moral, social, and sexual-identity development of children than has heretofore been realized[108] and maintain that children need fathers for healthy psychological development. The lack of a male sex-role model may have a negative effect on children's acquisition of appropriate sex-role behavior and traits,[109] they indicate. Further, studies show that the decreased time in child-adult interactions when there is only one parent in the household has an adverse impact on the social and cognitive development of children.[110] Two-parent families have the added practical advantage that arrangements usually can be made to have one parent attend to the needs of the child if the other must be unavailable. Moreover, in two-parent families, one parent is usually available to buffer the child from the anger or extravagant expectations of the other.

Proponents of access for single women cite studies indicating that the greater likelihood that children in female-headed families will have emotional problems is not necessarily the consequence of being raised in a fatherless family.[111] Poverty, isolation, economic hardship, and the family discord that can precede separation, and the lack of support that can follow it, negatively influence the development of these children. After reviewing several empirical studies, Golombok and Rust concluded that there would not be any "unforeseen special problems" for children brought up in such families.[112] Others maintain that no correlation has been found between the absence of a father and inappropriate sex-role behavior in children.[113] Children in fatherless families learn sex roles from a variety of sources, including extended family members, peers, literature, and the media.[114]

The concern that children of single women spend less time interacting with adults and consequently have poor cognitive and social development, proponents of access for single women maintain, is not clearly supported by the empirical literature. Studies suggest that children from female-headed households have cognitive abilities comparable to those from two-parent households.[115] Daughters in such families are independent, have high self esteem, and are more achievement-oriented.[116] Furthermore, mothers and children seem to have a closer family relationship in nontraditional households.

Proponents further argue that a double standard is at play when single women are denied access to new forms of assisted reproduction because of fears about the welfare of children. They maintain that the traditional nuclear family does not provide any guarantee that children will be raised in a loving, stable relationship. Large numbers of children have been physically and psychologically damaged within the family circle.[117] Given the degree of child abuse that occurs in our traditional system, those responding claim, it is hypocritical to deny single women the opportunity to have children by means of assisted reproductive techniques.

Another argument presented by some opposed to providing new reproductive techniques for single women is that they may not be able to provide adequately for their families and may contribute to the welfare burden.[118] Allowing them to have access to reproductive techniques such as oocyte donation, consequently, will have an adverse impact on their children and society. The costs of child care and health insurance also raise the question whether single women will be able to provide for children.

Although women tend to have lower salaries than men in our society, proponents of access to single women respond, this does not provide grounds for denying all such women access to oocyte donation and other alternative reproductive technologies. A single woman's financial situation may be more than adequate to meet the needs of a child.

Lesbian women are among the single women who seek donated eggs.[119] Critics of their participation in egg donation hypothesize that their children will have difficulty developing gender identity, sexual orientation, and sex-role behavior, since their mothers do not present "normal" role models.[120] These children, they claim, will experience more adjustment difficulties and exhibit greater behavior problems than those born to heterosexual parents.[121] They are also concerned that these children may be rejected and stigmatized by their peers.[122] Some courts have denied custody to lesbian mothers on such grounds.[123]

Those who favor giving lesbian women access to new reproductive techniques such as egg donation point to evidence indicating that the sexual orientation of parents does not determine that of their children.[124] They also note that children in lesbian households do not differ markedly in their sexual identity from children raised in heterosexual households in which the father is absent[125] and that children of lesbian mothers are not especially confused about their gender identity, sex-role behavior, or sexual orientation.[126] Evidence suggests that their development is comparable to that of children raised in non-lesbian families.[127] Proponents of access for lesbians acknowledge that little is known about the effect of such social disapprobation on these children. The applicability of the few studies that have been carried out on children born to lesbian women is unclear.[128]

The law in the United States appears to acquiesce in, but not to endorse, the use of reproductive technologies for single women.[129] For instance, a Texas law that protects the parental rights of rearing parents if they have given written consent to oocyte donation before it is carried out covers only married couples. However, it does not explicitly bar single women from access to the procedure.[130] Similarly, state laws that have addressed the issue of AID have covered only married couples, but have not made it illegal for unmarried women to have access to AID.[131] Indeed, the Ohio and Oregon statutes governing AID specifically acknowledge that a single woman might use donor sperm.[132] Moreover, single person adoptions have been in effect for some 20 years.[133]

A clinic policy that excluded single women and lesbian women might be viewed as legally discriminatory in the United States.[134] A single woman who is denied AID at a clinic affiliated with a state or federal institution might claim that her privacy right to make procreative decisions and her equal protection right to access to the same procedures as married women are violated by such policies. In one case settled out of court (and that consequently has no legal status), a clinic affiliated with a state university agreed to drop the marriage requirement for recipients of AID and to consider a single woman for insemination.[135]

Although we favor the two-parent heterosexual family as the structure most likely to protect and nurture children, we recognize that single women historically have had to care for and support children when they have been widowed or divorced. They have been accepted as capable of providing a suitable environment for children in these and in certain adoptive circumstances. Moreover, today many single women cannot be successfully barred from procreating children by means of reproductive technologies, since techniques of artificial insemination by donor can be self-administered.[136]

Therefore, we recommend that single women who are potential oocyte recipients undergo the screening procedures recommended above for the

receipt of oocytes. We suggest that it is wise for such single women to review their situation with the assistance of qualified counselors and to address special considerations that may arise because they are single. Since a sperm donor will be needed to fertilize the donated egg, the child born of this arrangement will be in a position similar to that of an adopted child. Has the potential oocyte recipient considered adoption as an alternative to egg donation? Will she have adequate emotional and social support in raising a child?[137] Is an extended family or other support system available? Will male role models be available? The possible legal problems that might arise for the single woman who bears children from an egg donated by another also need to be taken into consideration. Whenever possible, the final decision should be taken mutually by caregivers and recipient candidates, rather than unilaterally by health care professionals. However, we recognize that the situation in which single women request access to oocyte donation represents one in which some providers may decide that they must, in good conscience, refuse to provide oocyte donation. In such instances, they may assist in identifying a referral.

SECTION III

ETHICAL AND POLICY ISSUES RELATED TO OOCYTE DONORS IN THE CLINICAL SETTING

A. BACKGROUND CONTEXT

I. WHO ARE OOCYTE DONORS?

A major challenge for oocyte donation programs has been to find sufficient numbers of women willing to provide oocytes for others. The discomfort, pain, and time involved, as well as the risks, have apparently discouraged many from volunteering.[1] Even so, women in three different sorts of circumstances have agreed to give oocytes to others.

1) Until recently, some women who produced more oocytes than could be used during *in vitro* fertilization were willing to give their extra oocytes to others. With the increasing availability of embryo cryopreservation, however, most such women and their partners now prefer to have their surplus oocytes fertilized and frozen for their own future use.[2] Consequently, those seeking donated oocytes have become increasingly dependent on other sources.

2) Some women having pelvic or abdominal procedures have been willing to undergo ovarian hyperstimulation and oocyte recovery, in addition to procedures integral to their surgery, in order to donate oocytes to infertile couples.[3] Relatively few donors have been available from this source, however, as it can be difficult to time donor surgery to correspond to the cyclical readiness of recipients for the oocytes.

3) Women who are not themselves undergoing a medical procedure have agreed to go through ovulation induction and oocyte recovery solely for the purpose of donating eggs to others.[4]

Donors range in age from 18 to 41 years.[5] Some centers look for women who are married and have children. Others seek out college students who are young, healthy, and are able to follow instructions well. No general survey has been carried out to determine the social and economic backgrounds of donors. A few studies indicate that they tend to come from middle-class backgrounds and do not appear to be in financial need.[6] No indication has been given of the socioeconomic status of college students who donate eggs.[7] Since those seeking eggs are primarily white, and since donors and recipients are matched phenotypically, there does not appear to be a strong demand for donor eggs from women who are not white. It has been speculated that the perceived uncertain environmental and genetic health of eggs from donors classified as poor makes them less likely to be sought as donors.[8]

2. HOW DONORS LEARN OF THE POSSIBILITY OF DONATING

Potential donors find out about oocyte donation programs in several different ways. Some learn about them by word of mouth[9] or through "human interest" stories in the media. Others are apprised of them through advertisements placed in newspapers by oocyte donation programs.[10] Still others are contacted by relatives and friends in need of eggs.[11] Recipients who choose family members do so for such reasons as that they want a known donor, wish to have a genetic tie with the child, are in a cultural tradition that places strong emphasis on family relations, want to reduce expenses by having a donor who does not expect compensation,[12] and/or the oocyte donation center at which they are being treated requires recipients to provide their own donor. Children have donated gametes to a parent in 37.5% of 82 oocyte donation programs in the United States, a 1991–92 survey indicates, and parents to a child in 28.6%.[13]

3. WHY DONORS PROVIDE OOCYTES

Financial compensation is often viewed as the primary incentive for women to donate eggs. A 1991 survey revealed that those who received compensation were paid from $500 to $2,000 per retrieval.[14] Average compensation for oocyte donors in a 1992 survey was $1,548 with a range of $750 to $3,500.[15] It has been suggested that if oocyte donors were compensated at the same $25 rate per hour as many sperm donors, they would receive $1,400 for their time.[16] This would not, however, compensate them for a greater amount of lost work time, inconvenience, and risk.

Centers that use paid donors report that they can obtain adequate numbers of donors.[17] This seems to confirm the hypothesis that financial reward is a major factor motivating donors. Yet donors were not paid for their assistance in 15% of 83 ovum donation programs surveyed in 1992.[18] Donors report that their motives center around assisting others, rather than receiving money.[19] A 1990–92 American study of 95 women who had donated oocytes with a guarantee of confidentiality revealed that they wanted to make possible for others experiences they had enjoyed of giving birth and rearing children.[20] Of these, only 5 to 10% reported that their primary motivation was financial. In another study of confidential donors, the most frequent reported motive was to help an infertile couple have a child; this was followed by empathy with an infertile friend or relative.[21] In this study, 27% of respondents indicated that they had volunteered to donate oocytes primarily for financial reasons. An English report indicates that 90% of 35 confidential donors who received no compensation gave their oocytes to assist other women to have children.[22] Moreover, 80% of them felt that no payment was necessary. A study of 16 known donors who did not receive payment revealed that their reasons for donating eggs included a) a desire to give a gift of eggs that would otherwise be wasted (94%); b) a desire to respond to being asked (50%); c) a desire to atone for a prior voluntary abortion (33%); and d) a way to test their own genetic make-up (12%).[23] Donors apparently have several motives for donating that center on an altruistic desire to help others and that also include a desire to work out past reproductive losses and a desire to earn money.

4. MEDICAL PROCEDURES FOR COLLECTING OOCYTES FROM DONORS

Donating oocytes is invasive, physically demanding, and often painful. Since oocytes are not readily accessible, a surgical procedure is required to extract several at a time. Donors are required to receive daily injections of drugs[24] that induce ovarian hyperstimulation (the ovaries are caused to produce several eggs at a time).[25] For three weeks donors must go to the infertility center every morning so that physicians can monitor egg development and take blood samples to ascertain hormone levels indicating egg growth. Approximately 34 hours before egg extraction, donors receive an injection of human chorionic gonadotropin to trigger ovulation and they begin to take antibiotics to ward off infection.

Until recently, laparoscopy, an invasive surgical procedure requiring a general anesthetic, was employed to retrieve eggs. Eggs are now usually recovered by less invasive ultrasound-directed procedures.[26] In transvaginal ultrasonography-directed follicle aspiration, a probe is inserted into the vagina and an attached tube guides a suctioning needle into the ovary where the follicles are flushed out and the eggs removed from the donor.[27] Ultrasound-guided oocyte retrieval has recognized advantages over laparoscopy, including the use of local anesthesia or sedation for the donor, its speed and ease, and the rapid postoperative recovery for the donor.[28]

The extraction of eggs from donors is accompanied by certain medical risks, such as injury to structures adjacent to the ovary and iatrogenic pelvic infection.[29] These occur infrequently. A study of 674 infertile women who underwent transvaginal oocyte retrieval found that 1.5% required hospitalization secondary to perioperative complications.[30] Ovarian hyperstimulation syndrome, a dangerous but treatable condition, occurs in 3% of cycles in which human chorionic gonadotropin is used.[31] Drugs given to suppress normal ovarian function can cause temporary menopause-like symptoms, such as hot flashes and vaginal dryness. Hormones can create a feeling of swelling, pressure and tension in the area of the ovaries.[32] Donors at some centers must not drink, smoke, or take drugs,[33] which they may find an inconvenience, especially if urine tests are given to ascertain their compliance. At some centers, donors must abstain from sex for their own protection.[34] At others, they are required to discontinue oral contraceptive pills and are told to use barrier methods of contraception should they have sex. The most common complication in one study of 110 donors was that 7% experienced unintentional pregnancy between donation cycles.[35]

Little is known about the long-term risks of oocyte retrieval for donors.[36] A recent report suggesting that use of fertility drugs may increase the risk of ovarian cancer appears to apply to women who receive such drugs for a year or more.[37] Since most egg donors do not remain on these drugs for a great length of time, they may be at less risk. In 1993 the Royal Commission on New Reproductive Technologies of Canada recommended prohibition of the donation of eggs, stating that "the Commission does not believe that it is ethical to permit such an invasive surgical procedure, with its attendant risks, on an otherwise healthy woman for the benefit of someone else, particularly in the absence of information about the long-term effects of these procedures."[38] Current opinion among infertility specialists is that while the risks to donors are not insignificant, they do not appear so serious as to warrant forgoing oocyte donation.[39]

5. DEGREES OF DONOR SATISFACTION

Many donors are content with their experience. At one center, for instance, 91% of women who were donors indicated that they were moderately to extremely satisfied with the process; 74% stated that they would donate again.[40] Several other studies have found that a majority of donors would participate in a program again.[41] Some centers, however, have reported that donors have found treatment difficult and stressful.[42] There are several possible explanations for these disparities. They may reflect responses to different procedures used at different oocyte donation programs or they may express the reactions of differing donor populations. Overall, however, reports appear to indicate that many donors do not feel that they have been maltreated or misused and that they state they have had a satisfying experience.

6. DONORS' VIEWS OF THE ETHICAL ACCEPTABILITY OF DONATION

Do donors consider their act of donation ethical? The few statements in the literature from those who have donated eggs do not reveal that they had ethical reservations about doing so. One donor maintained that since her oocytes would have "died naturally" had they not been used, she had no qualms about donating them to others.[43] Some donors acknowledge that their view of the morality of the use of reproductive technologies differs from that of their church, but they believe their stance is ethically tenable.[44] In one program, donors were told by those administering the program that they had no responsibility to the couples who received their gametes or to the children born of them.[45] These donors did *not* comment upon or object to this statement on grounds that they had obligations to children who resulted from their gametes.

Yet some who have been asked to donate eggs have refused on ethical grounds. In one study, 88% of candidates for tubal ligation who were asked to donate ova and were informed that oocyte retrieval added little risk to the procedure refused to donate.[46] The most common reason they gave was the belief that "the resulting pregnancy would be partly theirs." They appeared to have a sense of parenthood and responsibility toward children born of their gametes and therefore were reluctant to provide eggs to create children whose care they could not oversee.

B. OOCYTE DONORS IN THE CLINICAL SETTING

I. THE ETHICAL IMPORTANCE OF SEPARATING SCREENING FROM COUNSELING

Those administering oocyte donation programs have an ethical and legal obligation to screen potential donors to protect the welfare of the donors, recipients, and children born of their oocytes. Donors should also be given counseling to help them decide whether they wish to serve in this capacity, to bring to their attention significant factors of which they may be unaware, and to address their concerns about the procedure. Some programs employ professionals who have special training in counseling to carry out these services.[47]

As noted in the case of oocyte recipients, a delicate balance must be maintained between screening and counseling, since each of these processes has different purposes. The two should not be conflated—but they cannot be kept wholly apart. For instance, those who carry out screening must assess whether a potential donor is free from undue pressure. Should a donor reveal a background situation that borders on the coercive, screening will inevitably lead to counseling, and information revealed in counseling may cause the potential donor to be rejected or to withdraw. The overlap of screening and counseling in such instances cannot be avoided and is ethically appropriate. The merger of screening and counseling becomes objectionable when the donor is led to believe that she is receiving assistance but, in reality, she is also being evaluated with an eye toward possible rejection.

We recommend that the screening process for potential oocyte donors be distinguished from the counseling process and that the two be carried out

separately as far as possible. During the screening process, it should be made clear to potential donors that the information they provide during interviews may be used to bar them from donating oocytes. We further recommend that, to avoid a conflict of interest on the part of physicians who wish to have sufficient donors for potential recipients, those carrying out counseling of potential donors be skilled, trained professionals independent of the physician involved in the oocyte donation procedure.

2. DONOR SCREENING: SEEKING ETHICALLY APPROPRIATE GOALS AND MEANS

Most oocyte donors, except for those who are undergoing *in vitro* fertilization, put themselves at a risk to which they would not otherwise be exposed. Precautions should be taken to ensure that they are in sufficiently good health to undergo the physical demands of oocyte donation.[48] Concern for the well-being of recipients and children provides additional ethical grounds for screening donors. It is also important to ascertain that donors have chosen to donate autonomously and would be entering the program voluntarily and competently.[49]

A 1991–92 survey revealed great variation in the criteria used for donor screening by oocyte donation programs across the country.[50] Moreover, this survey indicated that the kind of screening performed in many oocyte donation programs is very limited. Some form of medical and psychological screening was performed at most programs; implicit social evaluations were also carried out at some.

We recommend that before potential donors undergo testing and screening at an infertility center, they be given detailed information about the nature of the procedure of oocyte donation. They should also receive information about its physical and psychological risks, side effects, and the degree of discomfort associated with it so that they can make an informed choice about whether to become candidates for admission.

We further recommend that detailed inter-center guidelines for medical, psychological, and social screening of potential oocyte donors be developed across oocyte donation programs in the country by the inter-center task force recommended in Sections II and IV. Guidelines should be developed by those who have experience in the clinical setting with the assistance of experts and laypeople from outside that setting to ensure that such guidelines have a foundation in clinical realities and reflect significant ethical and social values. We believe that recommendations made below will provide a starting point for the development of such guidelines.

Until guidelines are developed and adopted across the board by oocyte donation programs, medical, psychological, and social criteria currently used by individual fertility centers and professionals for screening potential oocyte donors should be set out in writing so that donors can know of these in advance. An institutional ethics committee or internal ethics advisory board should be involved in developing and advising those in charge of oocyte donation programs about donor screening criteria and procedures.

a. Medical screening of donors

Included among the tests performed by the vast majority of oocyte donation programs surveyed in 1991–92 were the following: HIV, hepatitis, physical exam, rapid plasma reagin/Venereal Disease Research Laboratory, chlamydia, and gonococcal. Among the tests performed by the minority of programs surveyed were tests for blood groups and Rh factor, cytomegalovirus, T-mycoplasma, Pap, rubella, complete blood count, FSH level, genetic screening, drug screening, and toxoplasmosis. It is significant and troubling that some programs surveyed did not carry out HIV or drug testing or even physical examinations on donors. Recipients, and children born of oocyte donation, should be given the protection that such testing and exams provide. Guidelines of the American Fertility Society (AFS) recommend that donors be disqualified if they exhibit risk factors for HIV infection; test positive for syphilis, hepatitis B and C, or HIV I-II; or test positive for genetically transmitted traits prevalent in the donor's background.[51] They also indicate that donors should not carry any major mendelian disorder, should not be heterozygous for an autosomal recessive gene prevalent in the donor's ethnic background, should not have a major malformation such as spina bifida or heart malformation, should not have any family disease with a major genetic component, and should not carry a chromosomal rearrangement that might result in unbalanced gametes.

The guidelines cited above are primarily directed toward the well-being of the recipient and any child born of the procedure. The well-being of the donor also needs to be protected more specifically, since oocyte donation is a physically demanding procedure that carries some risk. Individual practitioners at oocyte donation programs around the country indicate that they currently carry out stringent medical evaluation measures to protect donors.[52] However, standard medical screening criteria for donors need to be established across programs.

We recommend that medical screening measures for oocyte donors that are currently in use be analyzed for adequacy and effectiveness by the inter-center task force described above and the results used in developing inter-center guidelines. Such guidelines should take into account not only the health and well-being of recipients and children born of the procedure, but of oocyte donors as well. We recommend, in addition, that oocyte donors receive pretest counseling for HIV and post-test counseling should they test positive for HIV. We further recommend that, as the number and kinds of tests for hereditary disorders and diseases increase, oocyte donors be screened only for those generally regarded as sufficiently serious to constitute a reason not to procreate.

b. Screening donors for decisionmaking capacity

Potential oocyte donors should have adequate decisionmaking capacity to participate. That is, they should be able to understand information about the procedure, to review this in light of their beliefs and values, and to communicate their thoughts and concerns to those involved in carrying it out. Unless there is some reason to consider their judgment impaired, oocyte donors should be presumed to have adequate decisionmaking capacity.

c. Screening donors for voluntariness and freedom from coercion

Donors should be free from manipulative and coercive influences exerted by others and should make a voluntary decision to participate.[53] There are degrees of influence others can have, ranging from simple requests, to persuasion, enticement, manipulation and coercion.[54] Both manipulation and coercion use illicit means to lead another to choose what he or she would otherwise not select. Manipulation involves wrongfully changing a person's understanding of a situation so that the person is motivated to do what the manipulator wishes and not what he or she would otherwise have chosen. Coercion goes one step further and involves deliberately using a severe threat of harm or force to control another.[55] During the screening process, consideration should be given to whether donors are being subjected to direct or indirect forms of manipulation or coercion.[56]

Some feminist critics maintain that women are necessarily subjected to coercive factors because they have been socialized to feel compelled to put the needs of others ahead of their own[57] and to view the value of their lives in reproductive terms. As noted in Section II.B.3.c, other feminists disagree[58] and find that reproductive technologies offer an opportunity for women to increase, rather than lose their freedom to direct their lives. They argue that women are the appropriate judges of what is conducive to their own well-being. We consider it important to bring this concern about possible manipulation of women who donate eggs out of the feminist literature into the clinical setting.

We maintain that health care professionals have a responsibility to safeguard potential donors from manipulative and coercive influences. Consequently, we recommend that those who screen potential donors should ascertain that these participants understand what the procedure involves and are not acting from overbearing manipulative or coercive influences.

At one center, as part of the screening process a bioethical evaluation of potential donors is carried out to determine whether donors 1) have been given sufficient information to understand to what they are consenting,

2) understand the risks involved, 3) have given a valid informed consent, and 4) have been subjected to coercion.[59] We believe that certain parts of this important endeavor should not be conducted until *after* the screening process has been completed. It is necessary to ascertain that donors are acting voluntarily and without coercion and to explore the voluntariness of the donors' decisions before they are admitted to a program. However, the other three parts of the evaluation, which relate to the adequacy of informed consent, should not be carried out until after donor screening has been completed. To ask for consent creates an understanding on the candidate's part that she has been accepted as a donor. It is unfair to create this expectation and then, in certain cases, to dash it.

Therefore, we recommend that evaluation of donors for voluntariness and freedom from coercion be carried out as part of the initial screening process. The informed consent of donors should not be solicited until after the screening process has been completed, a decision has been made to admit them to the program, and, as discussed below, they have received appropriate counseling.

(I). COMPENSATION AS A POTENTIALLY COERCIVE FACTOR

The question whether gamete donors should receive compensation is part of a larger concern about the commodification of human beings and their bodies made possible by our developing medical capabilities.[60] Those who are paid for their body products, some argue, will no longer be treated as persons deserving of respectful treatment, but as objects of commerce to be manipulated. Procreation will become assimilated to a manufacturing process and gametes will be viewed as products with a market value.[61] Respondents maintain that individuals have a right to decide what to do with their bodies and that they should be allowed to donate gametes for financial compensation as long as they are not exploited.[62] Even so, some of these respondents note, the value of non-commodification and the principle of the inalienability of the human person should be preserved during the process of gamete donation.[63]

The question of compensation arises with special force for egg donors, since egg donation is more risky and more troublesome for the donor than semen donation. Therefore, it seems only fair to compensate oocyte donors for their greater investment of time, risk, and degree of inconvenience. However, it is ethically objectionable to pay donors for their eggs, as this would open the door to unsavory commodification of the human body.[64] In one program, women who produced an ample supply of oocytes were paid $2,000, but those who produced very few oocytes were paid only $1,000.[65] Since both sets of women experienced similar degrees of inconvenience and risk, these disparate amounts of compensation appear to indicate they were paid for their eggs, rather than their time, risk, and inconvenience. This is ethically unacceptable. At IVF America-Boston, in contrast, if the cycle is canceled prior to retrieval, the donor receives a *pro rata* share of the stated compensation for the inconvenience and time lost from work that she has experienced.[66]

Compensation can become a factor bordering on the coercive for some egg donors.[67] For instance, students with large loans for college tuition may feel compelled to donate oocytes in order to repay those loans. One program offers donors barely enough to compensate for their time and inconvenience and excludes those in dire financial straits out of a concern about coercion.[68] This approach, while laudable in its attempt to avoid undue influences on donors, may deny some potential donors an opportunity to receive reasonable, but not excessive and coercive, compensation. When the amount of money offered for a procedure is not large in view of the time, risk, and inconvenience involved, compensation is unlikely to render the offer coercive. Donors should be reimbursed adequately for their assistance, and should not be over- or under-compensated.[69]

We recommend the approach taken in the Guidelines of the American Fertility Society (AFS) to compensate donors "for the direct and indirect expenses associated with their participation, their inconvenience and time, and to some degree, for the risk and discomfort undertaken."[70] Egg donation involves a more difficult, time consuming, and discomforting procedure than blood or sperm donation. Therefore, donors who wish to receive compensation for their time and inconvenience should be paid,[71] as long as payments are limited and not substantial. Programs should develop standard measures of reimbursement for all donors.

Some clinics allow women with a plentiful supply of oocytes who wish to undergo IVF, but who cannot afford it, to share their oocytes with women who are economically better off and unable to produce their own oocytes.[72] In return, the latter share the cost of the former's IVF cycle. This creates a difficult situation for women of modest means since they will not have access to IVF unless they donate eggs. Yet if they donate eggs to another woman, this may result in pregnancy for her, but not for them.[73] Moreover, they may have moral reservations about participating in third-party donations.

Some argue that this practice amounts to coercion of poor women. Women with a deep desire to have a child would not give up eggs that might produce that child but for the fact that this is the only option available to them. The inducement offered in this arrangement, critics claim, is an irresistible one that negates their voluntary choice. Those who would allow this practice respond that these women are not coerced, for they can freely choose to enter such shared arrangements or not. Indeed, they declare, it is coercive to deny them the choice of doing so. Although women who donate eggs under these circumstances run the risk of giving away eggs that could have produced children, they argue, this leaves them no worse off than they would have been otherwise.

Critics also maintain that this arrangement amounts to an indirect way of buying eggs.[74] Women receive a procedure that they would pay for had they the means; they use their eggs as a substitute for money. Respondents aver that such arrangements do not constitute a form of egg buying, since those who provide eggs receive no money. Moreover, if this were a case of egg buying, it would be expensive, for the amount that well-to-do women would have to pay to cover the costs of IVF for those whose eggs they use is considerably greater than the amount they would ordinarily pay an egg donor. Women who take part in this practice, they further note, are not treated differently from other egg donors; they, too, are paid for their time and inconvenience. Critics respond that to underwrite their IVF procedure in exchange for eggs is to treat their eggs as commodities that are sold for a price higher than that paid to ordinary egg donors. Both sides agree that the social and economic system that gives rise to such arrangements is flawed and raises basic questions about justice and access.

NABER members find ethically problematic those arrangements in which poor women donate eggs to those who are well-to-do in return for coverage of the cost of their own IVF procedure. Some members maintain that this practice should be rejected as an indirect form of egg—and ultimately, child—buying. Others see it as the lesser of two evils under our current health care system, in which those who are poor are at a major disadvantage, particularly with regard to infertility services.[75] These NABER members would reluctantly acquiesce in the practice under our current system of reimbursement. However, all NABER members agree that the practice should be discouraged.

Donors are not necessarily compensated for injuries they incur during the process of egg donation.[76] In the program cited earlier, some donors had to withdraw because of medical complications caused by the procedure.[77] Yet they received no compensation for their disabling condition. Such policies need to be reconsidered.

We recommend that oocyte programs purchase insurance to compensate donors who suffer injury or disability due to their participation in an oocyte donation program.

(II). FAMILIES AS A POTENTIALLY COERCIVE FACTOR

Eggs can be donated to sisters, cousins, daughters, and mothers. (See below, A.6. "Intrafamilial donation.") When family donors are involved, the pressure exerted by the family may reach the point of coerciveness. Potential donors may believe they have a duty to contribute to a relative's welfare by donating oocytes and yet may be reluctant to do so because of the risks and inconveniences. They may find their will overborne by the repeated importuning of family members.

We recommend that the possibility of coercion of potential donors who plan to provide oocytes for another member of their family be reviewed in each situation. Potential donors should receive careful counseling and should not be accepted into a program if it is ascertained that they are under undue influence from their families that they cannot overcome.[78]

d. Psychological screening of donors

Many programs also carry out psychological screening of potential donors. A 1991–92 survey of oocyte donation programs indicated that 78% of 62 programs required psychological screening of donors.[79] Of these, 79% used interviews, 43% personality assessment, and 28% other psychological tests. Those conducting the survey maintained that it was "unclear what the purpose of the screening is and what criteria are being established for the information gathered."[80] Although 78% of the programs required psychological screening, only 60% indicated that they had developed psychological criteria for rejecting ovum donors. Some programs accept only donors who are clearly free of psychological difficulties, whereas others accept donors who are less stable emotionally provided they have considered how their emotional make-up may have influenced their decision.[81]

One justification for the use of psychological tests for potential oocyte donors is to safeguard their mental health. Indeed, those who administer one program maintain that it can be therapeutic for donors who have suffered some previous reproductive loss, such as miscarriage or abortion, to provide oocytes for others.[82] Tests are generally used to identify those who are at risk for having serious emotional difficulties.[83] The well-being of the donor should be a primary consideration. However, the kind and degree of emotional difficulty that would disqualify potential donors needs to be spelled out more specifically. In one developed program, for instance, potential donors were screened by means of the Minnesota Multiphasic Personality Inventory and a screening interview.[84] During the interview, donor candidates were "asked about possible personal troubles such as emotional or physical abuse, abandonment, depression and anxiety, drug and alcohol use" and were also questioned about social support, religious or spiritual convictions, and sexual behavior. At team meetings, 27% of donor candidates who were screened in this way over a two-year period were rejected. It is not clear, however, on what grounds this was done and whether such factors as their social support and religious or spiritual convictions played an appropriate or inappropriate role in this decision. In general, the psychological criteria used for donor exclusion need to be stated more explicitly, explained, and justified.

A second reason for psychological testing of donors is to ensure that the oocyte donation program will function effectively. Psychological tests assist in determining whether candidates are sufficiently stable emotionally to make a firm commitment to the program.[85] This is a valid concern. If programs are to perform their roles, they need to have donors who will remain with them until egg donation has been completed.

We recommend that psychological screening measures for oocyte donors that are currently in use be analyzed for adequacy and effectiveness and that inter-center guidelines for psychological screening of potential oocyte donors

be included among those developed by the inter-center task force recommended above. Such guidelines should be geared to assisting potential oocyte donors to choose autonomously and protecting their well-being. Insofar as possible, clear psychological criteria for exclusion from egg donation should be set. Standards for evaluating probable donor persistence in the program also need to be established. However, it must be noted that donors retain the right to withdraw from the program at any time.

e. Social screening of donors

Little is known about the social screening of potential egg donors. At some centers, they are asked to discuss such matters as their motivation for donation, their future childbearing desires, and the attitudes of their family, friends, and significant others toward donation.[86] It is unclear from the literature whether such discussions are used strictly for counseling purposes or also to screen donors. The information available suggests that implicit, rather than explicit, social screening of potential oocyte donors is being carried out according to no acknowledged standards.

As with oocyte recipients, we recommend that social evaluation be distinguished from psychological evaluation as far as possible and that donor candidates be informed that interviews are being used for the purpose of screening. We further recommend that social screening of potential oocyte donors be limited to consideration of whether they would have adequate social support in their decision to contribute gametes to an oocyte donation program.

f. Donor partner interviews

A majority of oocyte donation programs (76%) in a 1991–92 survey indicated that the partners of oocyte donors influence the program's decision about whether to accept or reject donors.[87] Donor partners were required to be seen in 59% of reporting oocyte donation programs. They were interviewed alone in 19% of the programs and in the company of the donor in 57%. In 17% of the programs, the partner appeared to have influenced the decision whether to accept the donor. No reasons were given for taking account of the partners of donors during the screening process in these programs. Presumably those carrying out screening were concerned that partners might influence donors to withdraw during oocyte retrieval. This is a difficulty that should be discussed openly with donors and their partners during the screening process.

g. Screening repeat donors

Some women donate eggs on multiple occasions. While such donors are attractive to programs because they have gone through the procedure successfully on previous occasions, repeat exposure to oocyte donation may place them at increased risk. Moreover, the possibility of unknowing consanguineous marriages between siblings born of the eggs of one donor, while remote, remains a concern. Therefore, it is advisable to limit the number of times a donor is allowed to provide oocytes for her own sake and for that of children who might be born of her eggs.[88]

h. Rejection of donor candidates

Although it is not surprising, one study revealed that the overall satisfaction of rejected donors was significantly lower than that of accepted donors who completed the cycle.[89] This can be taken to indicate that care should be taken in communicating the decision to reject a donor candidate. When donors are excluded from oocyte donation programs, they should be given an explanation about why this decision has been made. Should they be excluded for medical or psychological reasons, they should be informed of this and referred to appropriate health care providers for treatment.

3. THE NEED FOR POST-SCREENING DONOR COUNSELING AND EDUCATION PRIOR TO GAINING INFORMED CONSENT

Further counseling and education of potential oocyte donors before they make a final commitment to donate oocytes provides them with the opportunity to consider facets of donation that they may have overlooked previously. They can review with qualified counselors such matters as how they will cope with having a genetically linked child whom they will not know or meet (if they are confidential donors), how they will relate to their family and others who know of their donation, what they will tell their existing children about their frequent doctor's visits, and how they will deal with necessary scheduling changes at work.[90]

Therefore, we recommend that potential oocyte donors who successfully complete the pre-donation screening evaluation receive additional counseling and education before they make a decision to donate oocytes.

Known donors ought to be informed that should information unexpectedly come to light during their screening that they do not want revealed to recipients, it will be withheld unless this would have a harmful effect on those recipients or the children that might be born of donors' gametes. Although the desire of donors for privacy should be respected, the welfare of recipients and children born of oocyte donation takes ethical precedence. If donors wish to have all information about themselves withheld from recipients, they should withdraw from consideration for the program.

Therefore, we recommend that donors should be advised at this stage that to minimize medical risk to recipients and the children-to-be, it is necessary to disclose certain sorts of nonidentifying information to recipients.

We further recommend that informed consent should be solicited from donors at this time after they have successfully completed the screening process, but before they are enrolled as oocyte donors. They should be given comprehensive and accurate information about the rigors, risks, side effects, and long-term physical and psychological effects of the procedure, the need for synchronicity, statements about their legal rights and responsibilities, an indication of who is responsible if the donor has complications, and information about the benefits to them and to the recipients of the procedure.[91]

We recommend that donors also be informed of the purpose for which their eggs will be used, such as for implantation or research. If they wish to set any conditions on the use of their oocytes within the limits set by law, they should be given the opportunity to state these. Administrators of the program should have the option to accept or reject these conditions. Should they accept them, the conditions should be binding on those carrying out the procedure.[92]

We further recommend that donors be given at least 24 hours to consider whether or not to sign the consent form for egg donation. The donor consent form should indicate that donors may withdraw consent at any time during their participation in the oocyte donation program before the donated oocytes have been used. When a donor who was to be compensated withdraws, she should be given appropriate compensation for her time and inconvenience up to the point of her withdrawal.

Donor counseling should continue through the entire donation procedure. Follow-up counseling should be employed for those who report any negative outcome of donation.[93]

4. MATCHING OOCYTE DONORS AND RECIPIENTS: AVOIDING DISCRIMINATION AND EUGENICS

Some oocyte recipients seek donors with particular characteristics they hope will be transmitted to a child born of the procedure. Oocyte donation programs generally try to respond to their reasonable requests.[94] Consequently, once donors are accepted into a program, information about them may be used to "match" them with oocyte recipients. Braverman et al. found that programs provided recipients with information about the donor's physical characteristics (56%), psychosocial make-up (38%), and other characteristics such as medical and genetic factors (47%).[95] Donors were matched on the basis of physical characteristics in 76% of oocyte donation programs and on the basis of such features as race, blood type, and age in 44%.

Matching in itself is not ethically suspect. Individuals make certain kinds of choices about the characteristics of those they include in their families without ethical opprobrium. For instance, one factor affecting the decision of couples to marry is that certain attributes of the other meet their personal preferences. Similarly, it is ethically acceptable to match the features of donors with features sought in a child when oocyte donation is carried out.

The use of matching in oocyte donation would become a matter of ethical concern if the set of individual decisions in their totality expressed prejudices that violated our notions of human dignity and equality. Such decisions, when taken collectively, could amount to a form of eugenics aimed at improving the human race by selective breeding. This would be contrary to the commitment of our society to recognize the intrinsic value of each person with his or her particular characteristics and to respect individual differences.

At present, there is no evidence that the use of matching by recipients of oocytes, taken collectively, constitutes a form of eugenics. Indeed, since the genetic traits usually sought are polygenic and multifactorial, it is unlikely that matching would be effective in producing individual traits in children.[96] To prohibit this practice would require coercive and intrusive inquiry into the motives of oocyte recipients that would constitute an unjustified violation of their privacy.

Therefore, we recommend that the use of matching be continued and that oocyte recipients be allowed to choose oocyte donors on the basis of information provided them about their features and background. We further recommend that lists of donor features currently used for matching purposes be reviewed by the inter-center task force suggested above and that the task force develop a standard list of characteristics of donors from which it is ethically acceptable for potential oocyte recipients to select. Until such a list is developed and adopted across the board by oocyte donation programs, lists of characteristics used by individual fertility centers and professionals for matching purposes should be set out in writing so that candidates for oocyte donation and recipients can know of these in advance.

5. USE OF KNOWN AND CONFIDENTIAL DONORS

Both known and stranger donors have provided eggs for women who cannot use their own. Donors whose identity is not revealed to gamete recipients are sometimes referred to as "anonymous" donors. This is not strictly correct, as they are known to health care professionals and administrators at the centers where they give their oocytes. Their identity, however, is kept hidden from all others. We believe it more apt to refer to such donors as "confidential" donors. Confidentiality should not be confused with secrecy. Confidentiality involves keeping the donor's identity hidden from others. Secrecy has to do with keeping the child's origins hidden from others. Although the fact that a child has been born of oocyte donation may be known to others, the identity of a person who contributed the egg from which the child resulted may be kept confidential. Or egg recipients may keep secret the fact that they have used oocyte donation and yet use an identified donor. Still, secrecy and confidentiality can overlap, as when a couple keeps the fact that they have used egg donation a secret and does not know the identity of the donor. A discussion of donor confidentiality, therefore, will sometimes involve a discussion of secrecy as well.

Oocyte donation programs are moving away from the use of known to confidential donors. When the procedure was first introduced in the mid-1980s, known donors were used almost exclusively because stranger donors were unwilling to undergo the risks of surgical laparoscopy.[97] With the advent of a less intrusive means of collecting eggs, ultrasound-guided transvaginal follicular aspiration, strangers became more willing to donate. By 1991, only 20% of 51 oocyte donation programs in the United States used known donors exclusively.[98] About 50% provided both known and confidential methods of donor participation, and approximately 30% relied exclusively on donors whose identity was kept confidential.

There has been considerable discussion of whether confidential or known donors should be used in both sperm and egg donation. Debate has turned on the needs, interests, and rights of donors, recipients, and resulting children.

a. Arguments in favor of the use of confidential donors

The primary reason for keeping the identity of donors confidential is consequential—this is likely to produce greater numbers of them.[99] Advocates of confidentiality believe that potential donors would be unwilling to participate were they identified out of concern that children born of their gametes might later intrude into their lives. Maintaining donor confidentiality is attractive to donors, according to its advocates, because it allows them to avoid parental responsibility for children born of their eggs.

Use of confidential donors also avoids some of the interpersonal difficulties that known donors may face. Within families, for example, when sister donates to sister, the donor may be uncertain about whether she is the aunt or the mother of the child born to her sister.[100] Some argue that donor confidentiality is also advantageous from the point of view of the rearing parents, for it protects the family from interference or harassment by the donor. Relations within the family, particularly between mother and child, might be damaged by the hovering presence of the known related donor.[101] Donor confidentiality allows the recipient couple to construct its own parental relation with the child.

Further, parents using gamete donation fear social stigmatization and ostracization should this become known. They want to make their family as "normal" as possible[102] and believe that using confidential donors allows recipients to appear fertile in the eyes of the world and to avoid the socially imposed shame of having their infertile condition recognized.

Some argue that the interests of the children require that the donor remain confidential. To reveal her identity would confuse the boundaries around parenthood for these children and cause them unresolvable identity conflicts.[103] They might experience bewilderment about their "real" mother if the donor were known.[104] Donor confidentiality, when paired with secrecy, is also seen as a way to protect children born of oocyte donation from social disapprobation.[105] It has been feared that should the mode of conception of these children become a matter of common knowledge, they would be socially isolated by their peers. Keeping the identity of the donor and the fact of donation secret protects children from this unwanted effect.

In summary, four main reasons have been given for donor anonymity: to maintain an adequate donor pool, to avoid outside interference with both rearing and donor families, to maintain satisfactory relations within the immediate and extended families of recipients, and to avoid social stigmatization of recipients and the resulting children.

b. Arguments in favor of the use of known donors

Arguments for the use of known donors center on the rights of children born of oocyte donation, as well as the needs and interests of donors, parents, and the children.

Although donors are entitled to privacy, they have certain responsibilities to children born of their eggs, proponents of openness maintain, because of their genetic connection with the child.[106] Fulfilling these requires that their identity be known by the recipients and that they reveal their past medical history and current medical condition. Identifying donors also avoids unrecognized incestuous unions among donor children.

Recent studies of semen donors suggest that donors themselves feel some sense of obligation toward children born of their gametes for these sorts of reasons. In a 1991 study, for example, nearly all semen donors indicated they were willing to have information about their medical and personal background revealed to the recipient family, and 60% were willing to be contacted by potential offspring when these children reached age 18.[107]

Donors are apparently not frightened away if their identity is revealed. When a law was passed in Sweden allowing identifying information about sperm donors to be made available to children born of AID when they reached age 18, the number of donors electing to enter the program decreased immediately after, but rose to its previous level a few months later.[108] When a policy of non-anonymity was adopted in France, there were sufficient sperm donors to meet the demand.[109] No reason has been advanced to explain why egg donors would respond in a different way were they known.

Donor confidentiality is usually part of a larger picture of secrecy about oocyte donation. Yet some argue that there is growing documentation of the negative effects of secrecy within the family.[110] In one study of semen donation, it was found that secrecy about participation in the procedure was abandoned when the relation between the rearing parents deteriorated.[111] The anxiety that results from evasiveness and fear of disclosure can create a significant barrier between parent and child, those advocating openness suggest.[112]

Moreover, secrecy in sperm donation, some maintain, only serves to delay the infertile man's acknowledgment of the pain and suffering that accompany his condition.[113] The same may be true of the infertile woman who turns to a confidential oocyte donor. If oocyte donation is kept secret and confidential donors are used, the recipient's concerns may not be addressed and her relation to her husband and child may be detrimentally affected.

Some parents prefer to know oocyte donors and their backgrounds.[114] The advantage of using a sister, cousin, or close friend as donor is that recipients can know a great deal about her medical, genetic, social, personal, and intellectual background. The personal and, at times, genetic link to the child that a known donor offers is preferred by many recipient parents.

Those who favor openness also argue that it wrongs the children to maintain donor confidentiality. Secrecy about an individual's origins places a lie at the center of family relationships. Children have a moral right to know about their mode of conception and their progenitors. One study of children conceived by sperm donation whose parents were open about this revealed that when the children were told of their origin they accepted this with equanimity.[115] Indeed, some were pleased about it, feeling they must be important to their parents since they went to such great lengths to have them. Even when children have difficulty in accepting the information, proponents of openness maintain, this is insignificant in comparison with the wrongness of deception. Children born of donation who have learned of their origins accidentally have been shocked and embittered.[116]

Some argue that donor confidentiality wrongs children because it denies them knowledge of their biological and family origins. One's biological inheritance and genealogy are significant social constructions essential to one's individual and social identity. Children need to know the basic circumstances under which they were conceived and the people who contributed to their creation.[117] To be able to view donors as people with specific interests, skills, and family histories enables these children to identify with their genetic heritage and develop a sense of self.[118]

In summary, the primary reasons given for confidential oocyte donation have to do with the moral obligations of donors to children who result from use of their gametes, the detrimental effects of anonymity and secrecy on the family, the right of children to know the truth, the need of children to know certain essential facts about the donor, and the importance to self-identity of knowledge of one's origins.

c. Using both known and confidential donors

The oocyte donor system has been guided by standards of professional practice, rather than by law.[119] These standards were designed, in part, to protect all involved from the onus imposed on egg donation by a society that is ambivalent about it. Fear of donor-assisted reproduction, some claim, has led to its stigmatization and fear of such stigmatization, in turn, has caused those receiving donated gametes to conceal this from others and to opt for anonymous donors. This dynamic of fear has resulted in a legal, social, and psychological vacuum in relation to donor-assisted reproduction that has further fueled the dynamic of fear.[120] Recently there have been signs of a movement toward greater openness about the use of oocyte donation and donors.[121] Consequently, we believe that this is an appropriate time to address the aura of fear and evasiveness that overhangs oocyte donation and to develop guidelines that allow a greater degree of information about donors to be made available to all parties.

The act of gamete donation creates certain obligations and responsibilities for both recipients and donors. Recipients owe donors a debt of gratitude for their contribution of gametes. They often partially repay this debt by compensating donors for their pain, time, and inconvenience. Some recipients may be willing to exhibit their gratitude more fully by providing donors who wish to know more about the families they assist with basic information about themselves. Recipients themselves may be interested in learning more about the donor and might view a mutual exchange of information as welcome.

Donors, too, incur a responsibility to the children born of their gametes. The donation of an oocyte involves the provision of a life-*giving* gamete, the very means whereby another human being is brought into existence. Because donors voluntarily and intentionally contribute their oocytes, they have certain responsibilities to the resulting child. They have an obligation to provide relevant and appropriate information about their medical and personal history that can be used in the child's health care. They also have a responsibility to provide sufficient information about themselves so that the child can avoid unknowing marriage with a sibling.

We find convincing the arguments in favor of providing recipients and children born of oocyte donation with information about the donor. This upholds the interest of the children in developing a more complete identity. We realize, however, that some donors may not want to reveal such information about themselves. Some maintain that requiring parents to tell children that they were conceived by means of a reproductive technology could amount to an unconstitutional infringement on their right to make decisions about childrearing.[122] This accords with other parts of our legal and ethical tradition that recognize the importance of allowing families to make decisions about personal matters according to their values and preferences with minimal intrusion by others.[123] We are concerned not only about the right of the child to know about his or her origins, but also about the potentially devastating effect of mandatory "truth dumping" on children born of gamete donation whose parents have kept their origins hidden. We also recognize that children have a stake in retaining their own privacy.

In order to promote the welfare of the children born of oocyte donation in their formative years and to accommodate their interest in learning of their genetic and social background when they reach the age of maturity and also to protect the privacy of donors, recipients, and children, we recommend the following requirements and options. Certain of these options would have to be chosen by two or three of the parties involved, who would then be "matched" with each other, in order to become operational.

(I). RECIPIENTS' AND PARTNERS' REQUIREMENTS AND OPTIONS:

(a). We recommend that recipients and their partners be offered the option of using either known or confidential oocyte donors. Rearing parents should make their own decision about this based on their judgment about which option will be more appropriate for their family. It is advisable to allow rearing parents to make this choice, as they are the ones who will have responsibility for the welfare of the child within the family setting. Some oocyte donation centers currently are organized to use only known or confidential donors and therefore would be unable to provide this option to recipients. We urge such centers to move toward a policy of offering both known and confidential donors to those seeking donated oocytes.

(b). We recommend that recipients be required to receive information about the donor's medical history and genetic health at the time of donation. When the donor's identity is to be kept confidential, this information should be nonidentifying.

(c). We recommend that recipients be given the option of receiving additional information about donors concerning such matters as their physical characteristics, including height, weight, eye and hair color; racial and ethnic background; occupation; education; and interests at the time of donation.

(II). DONORS' REQUIREMENTS AND OPTIONS:

(a). We recommend that donors be required to provide information about their medical history and genetic health to recipients of their oocytes at the time of donation and to children born of their oocytes at the request of those children when they reach age 18 or at any time up to that point with their parents' consent. Donors should have the option of providing either relevant identifying or nonidentifying information.

(b). We recommend that donors have the option of providing in writing additional information concerning such matters as their physical characteristics, including height, weight, eye and hair color; racial and ethnic background; occupation; education; and interests to recipients of their oocytes at the request of those recipients at the time of donation.

(c). We recommend that donors be required to provide additional information concerning such matters as their physical characteristics, including height, weight, eye and hair color; racial and ethnic background; occupation; education; and interests to children born of their oocytes at the request of those children when they reach age 18 or at any time up to that point with their parents' consent. Donors should have the option of providing either relevant identifying or nonidentifying information.

(III). CHILDREN'S OPTIONS:

(a). We recommend that when confidential donors are used, children born of their oocytes be given access to information about the medical history and genetic health of donors at the request of those children when they reach age 18 or at any time up to that point with their parents' consent. Donors should have the option of providing either relevant identifying or nonidentifying information.

(b). We recommend that additional information about such physical characteristics of the donor as height, weight, eye and hair color; racial and ethnic background; occupation; education; and interests be made available to children born of their oocytes at the request of those children when they reach age 18 or at any time up to that point with their parents' consent. Donors should have the option of providing either relevant identifying or nonidentifying information.

6. INTRAFAMILIAL DONATION

Some egg recipients wish to have family members provide them with eggs. One study indicates that among infertile couples seeking an oocyte donor, both husbands and wives prefer asking a sister, rather than a stranger.[124] A major benefit of intrafamilial oocyte donation is that the donor and recipient share a genetic connection with the child. This form of donation can also create close ties within the family that are satisfying to all involved.[125]

However, there is concern that not all intrafamilial donations are beneficial to the child, since the proximity of the donor increases the opportunities for intrafamilial conflict.[126] Disagreements might arise about the child's upbringing or relationship with the donor that could continue indefinitely due to the availability of the family. Concern that close familial ties might have harmful psychological consequences for the children led the United Kingdom to prohibit oocyte donations to family members until recently.[127] Such donations have been banned in Victoria, South Australia, and New South Wales, presumably on the same grounds.[128] To date, however, there is no evidence that intrafamilial oocyte donation creates major burdens for participants or harms for children born of it. Similar concerns have been raised about the welfare of children who enter "blended families," in which children from different marriages are reared in the same family unit. Yet here, too, there is no evidence that this is detrimental to the welfare of the children.[129] Therefore, we maintain that intrafamilial oocyte donation should be allowed.

When daughters donate oocytes to mothers, however, certain distinct ethical and medical questions arise. This arrangement has been looked upon favorably because it allows the mother to have a genetic tie to the child.[130] Yet the child born of this donation will be more closely related to the daughter than the mother, since half of the child's genetic make-up will be derived from the daughter.[131] This can leave the relationship between the participants in an ambiguous state, as the daughter will be both mother and sister to the child and the mother both mother and grandmother. Further, the donation of an oocyte by a daughter to her own mother and the fertilization of that oocyte by the daughter's father would be medically inadvisable, as the daughter and her father would share 50% of the same genome. Even though a careful family history would have been taken, this arrangement would run the risk of transmitting deleterious genetic traits.[132] Such an arrangement seems "unnatural" and incestuous to some and contrary to traditional conceptions of how families should function.

We recommend that those considering intrafamilial donation review their family situation to assess whether they will be brought closer together by egg donation or seriously divided. There may be forewarning that disagreements are likely to arise that would create difficulties and possibly lead to psychological harm to the children. Counselors should explore with participants issues that can arise for sisters, guilt and manipulation, the effect of the donation on the rest of the family, what to tell the child.[133] We recognize that the situation of intrafamilial donation represents one in which providers may decide that they must, in good conscience, refuse to provide this procedure. In such instances, they should attempt to find others who will.

SECTION IV

PUBLIC POLICY
AND THE USE OF
OOCYTE DONATION

A. QUESTIONS OF
REGULATION AND CONTROL

There is no explicit public policy in the United States directed toward some of the pressing ethical and social questions raised by oocyte donation at the present time. Legislation regulating the procedure is virtually non-existent and the courts are only beginning to hear cases in which this practice figures.[1] No national commission has been established to consider its ethical, social, legal, and policy implications and to craft guidelines for its use. The application of this technique is largely a matter of private discretion left to infertile people, egg donors, and health care professionals. As a result, practices vary from center to center, and information about the procedure is not readily available to many outside infertility clinics. Yet oocyte donation, as a way of creating children and families, touches basic issues about the sort of society in which we live and will create for future generations. It is among the new reproductive technologies that raise fundamental policy questions about the appropriate means for setting social priorities "and ultimately who decides and controls the use of genetic and reproductive technologies in a democratic society."[2]

There are at least four routes through which a greater degree of societal direction could be provided to address some of the ethical and policy issues raised by oocyte donation. Its use could be 1) subjected to direction through a framework of laws and regulations, 2) assessed by the courts on a case-by-case basis as conflicts arise, 3) governed by policies developed through a national forum in the public or private sector, 4) directed by guidelines crafted by health care professionals through their professional groups or through inter-oocyte donation center committees.[3] These routes are not mutually exclusive.

I. REGULATION BY LAW

Some other countries have imposed various sorts of legal restrictions on oocyte donation. Sweden and Norway have passed laws forbidding its use altogether. France allows the technology to be employed only for women who are of an age to procreate and have not reached menopause. The aim of such legal restrictions is to protect social values, as well as the health and well-being of oocyte recipients, donors, and the children who result from its use.

It is not clear whether broad legislation that imposed major restrictions on the use of oocyte donation in the United States would withstand judicial scrutiny, since the procedure involves reproduction and privacy, two interests that have been interpreted to be protected by the constitution.[4] Even limited attempts to restrict access to the procedure on grounds of the age of potential oocyte recipients could raise significant constitutional questions, not only about privacy, but about equal protection and discrimination on the basis of age and sex. Still, the fundamental reason for seeking greater regulation of oocyte donation would be to safeguard those who use it and those who result from it, a purpose that falls within the responsibilities of government. Therefore, regulation of certain aspects of the procedure in the United States to protect the health and welfare of adult and child citizens, to govern the quality of medical services offered, and to ensure the familial and personal privacy of the parties involved would arguably pass constitutional muster.

A step in this direction has already been taken on the national level with passage of the Fertility Clinic Success Rate and Certification Act of 1992.[5] This law requires assisted reproductive technology programs to provide their pregnancy success rates to the Secretary of Health and Human Services for publication and distribution to the states and the public on an annual basis. It also requires monitoring of these programs under the auspices of state medical agencies to ensure that their laboratories are operated adequately. Medical groups such as the American Fertility Society and the Society for Assisted Reproductive Technology supported the administrative regulations embodied in this law as significant and necessary advances for ensuring the quality of care, as did the national infertility consumer group, Resolve.[6] Additional federal legislation governing such new reproductive technologies as oocyte donation has not been forthcoming largely because family matters and reproduction have traditionally fallen within the purview of the states. Moreover, there is concern that because oocyte donation is an evolving technique, enacting laws to govern it at this point in time might prove premature and of limited and temporary use.[7]

2. REGULATION BY THE COURTS

Very few cases dealing with oocyte donation have been decided in the courts, and these have dealt only with the issue of whether the oocyte donor or recipient should be given the legal status of mother.[8] A disadvantage of using the common law process as a means of regulating oocyte donation is that it does not provide a way of developing a clear and consistent policy that can be known in advance. Common law rules and principles develop only after the fact when cases involving them are presented to courts. Those who use the new reproductive technologies, however, need principles for action in advance. When there are no precedents, people tend to be reluctant to go to court and instead develop strategic behavior designed to get around a problem without resolving it.

The courts themselves view state legislatures as more appropriate bodies to set policy in this area, since they are designed to foster democratic decision-making. Yet the role of the courts in crafting principles to guide the use of egg donation should not be dismissed out of hand. There is some movement of thinking from court decisions to legislatures so that court holdings in individual situations of conflict can, when taken collectively, enunciate areas of consensus that can be incorporated into laws and regulations. In this way, the courts have an indirect role in developing policy enacted by elected representatives in legislatures.

3. REGULATION BY PUBLIC AND/OR PRIVATE BODIES

In some countries, a nationally sponsored commission has reviewed the ethical and legal implications of such biomedical technologies as oocyte donation. In Canada, the Royal Commission on New Reproductive Technologies was established to review policies and practices in this area. It recommended establishment of a National Reproductive Technologies Commission to devise and enforce standards and monitoring devices for research and practice in the new reproductive technologies.[9] In Great Britain, a public regulatory body was put in place on the basis of a recommendation of the Warnock Committee, a public commission that reported to the British government in 1984.[10] The purpose of this regulatory authority is to develop specific accreditation requirements for medical centers and practitioners involved in providing assisted reproduction. Such national commissions serve to generate public awareness about the technologies and their application and to air public concerns about their use.

In the United States, public policy in this area has been at an impasse because the ethical issues that surround human reproduction are highly controversial. Some would prefer that a private sector group such as NABER develop reports and guidelines for the use of oocyte donation and other reproductive technologies, as such a body is not subject to political winds and interest groups to the same degree as are federally constituted bodies.[11] NABER was initially established by practitioners and their professional associations for this and related reasons as a result of a report of the Institute of Medicine of the National Academy of Sciences, and of the recommendation of others.[12] NABER is now financially independent of these associations and is under no obligation to give them special preference in its deliberations. The federal government could commission an independent group such as NABER to develop ethical guidelines for research and practice in oocyte donation and other methods of assisted reproduction. Or the government could establish a commission *de novo* to perform this and related functions. The advantage of a government-sponsored body is that it would have the authority and the wherewithal to carry out its regulatory functions.

4. SELF-REGULATION BY THE MEDICAL PROFESSION

In a time of rapidly advancing technological change and government inaction, and in the absence of a public forum for developing consensus, self-regulation by the medical profession has provided the only available route for regulation of the new reproductive technologies. Physicians have generally served as gatekeepers of techniques such as oocyte donation, providing it to infertile persons on the basis of professional standards of ethical practice and individual discretion. They and their associations have been able to affect the way in which oocyte donation is carried out in clinical practice and research to some degree because they have the power to censure members who depart from accepted standards. Informal and voluntary critiques by fellow infertility specialists have helped to guard against exploitation of those who are infertile.[13] Physicians have a variety of incentives for self-regulation, including the desire to uphold their professional integrity, the drive to provide high quality beneficial care to infertile patients, their tradition of self-regulation which is affected by the desire to avert state or federal intervention into the practice of medicine, and the concern to avoid lawsuits. Moreover, their firsthand experience with the practical problems that arise in the provision of oocyte donation gives them a firm basis for developing standards to direct its use.

A self-regulatory approach gives practitioners and their professional associations responsibility for crafting guidelines for oocyte donation that cover such matters as recipient and donor screening, age limits, and donor compensation. Institutional ethics committees specifically devoted to use of the new reproductive technologies established at some infertility centers have assisted medical professionals in developing such guidelines.[14] Physicians' professional associations also provide guidance to those in the field by developing policies regarding the practice of oocyte donation.[15]

While such self-imposed guidelines offer an important means of ensuring that oocyte donation is carried out in ways that take account of ethical and policy issues, they do not provide a sufficient regulatory force. Physicians typically are not in a position to perceive and address some of the overarching policy issues that the practice of oocyte donation raises and may therefore produce standards and guidelines that are incomplete. Guidelines developed at individual oocyte donation centers may vary and be inconsistent across the board. Moreover, the authority of medical professionals to enforce guidelines at centers other than their own is only indirect and limited. Additional controls beyond those capable of being provided by the medical profession therefore need to be instituted to address certain areas of the practice of oocyte donation that raise distinct ethical and policy questions.

B. RECOMMENDATIONS OF THE NATIONAL ADVISORY BOARD ON ETHICS IN REPRODUCTION

Greater regulation of the use of oocyte donation is needed to address pressing ethical and policy issues that this technology creates. Different issues require different avenues of regulation. In crafting recommendations for regulation, we are not faced with an either/or choice between new laws and professional self-regulation. Both the private and public sectors can provide ways in which to pursue such central values described at the beginning of this Report as the welfare of participants in this technology and the children who result from it. We maintain that immediate action is needed in the following areas.

I. LEGISLATION

The value that is placed on procreative privacy in the United States entails that any form of state regulation of oocyte donation adopted should not place the government in the position of controlling human reproduction. Yet the weight of the state is necessary in certain areas in which the use of oocyte donation raises significant ethical and policy issues affecting the parent-child relationship and the health and safety of participants and the resulting children.

a. The need for legislation to assign parenthood

Parenthood is traditionally understood as combining genetic, gestational (in the case of the mother), and rearing components. In oocyte donation, the genetic and gestational mother are separated. This can give rise to conflict about who should be considered the rearing mother of the child born of the procedure, the oocyte donor or recipient. Few states have addressed this question. As of this writing, only Oklahoma, Texas, Florida, North Dakota, and Virginia have passed legislation that assigns parentage to the oocyte recipient and her husband, provided both have consented to this in writing beforehand.[16] The Uniform Status of Children of Assisted Conception Act, a model act drafted by the National Conference of Commissioners on Uniform State Laws that could be adopted by state legislatures, states that "a donor is not a parent of a child conceived through assisted conception."[17] The donor of an oocyte would not be given the legal status of mother of the resulting child according to this act.

What reasons have been given for favoring the gestational or the genetic mother as the rearing mother of the child born of oocyte donation? It is necessary to consider which factors have the greatest moral weight in determining who ought to be responsible for the upbringing of the child.[18] Those who favor the gestational mother hold that the woman who bears the child has a "greater biological and psychological investment" in that child.[19] This argument focuses on what the gestational mother deserves because of her own investment in the child. It takes into account "the biological reality that the mother [gestating woman] at this point has contributed more to the child's development, and that she will of necessity be present at birth and immediately thereafter to care for the child."[20]

The alternative view maintains that genetics should be considered the overriding factor. One argument for this position is that since each individual has a unique set of genes, each person can be said to have a claim of ownership on what develops from his or her own genes. The child-centered position for assigning greater weight to the contribution of the genetic mother is that it is in children's best interest to be reared by parents to whom they are genetically related. S. Callahan argues, "A child who has donor(s) intruded into its parentage will be cut off from its genetic heritage and part of its kinship relations in new ways. . . . the psychological relationship of the child to its parents is endangered. . . . "[21]

While we maintain that both the genetic and gestational mother have responsibilities toward the child born of a donated gamete,[22] as was noted in the discussion of the use of confidential versus known donors in Section III, we do not find that the above considerations lead to a conclusion that favors the genetic mother over the gestational or vice versa in the context of oocyte donation. Many members of NABER believe that the intentions of both women when the procedure was initiated should govern and that therefore the primary responsibility for the care and upbringing of the child should rest with the gestational mother. This is the approach that has been taken by the few courts that have addressed this question.

In *Johnson v. Calvert*,[23] in which a surrogate gestational mother carried a child to term on behalf of the two genetic parents, the Supreme Court of California took the view that both the gestational and genetic mother could arguably be considered the child's "natural mother." Since a choice had to be made between the two, it held in favor of the genetic mother on grounds that it was the intention of all parties at the time of conception that the child would be reared by the genetic mother and father. In cases of oocyte donation, the court added, where a woman gives birth to a child formed from the egg of another woman with the intent to raise the child as her own, the gestational mother is the "natural mother" under California law. A New York case, in which a couple had used donated eggs to achieve the successful delivery of twins, followed the approach taken in *Johnson v. Calvert.*[24] After the birth of the children, the husband appealed for divorce and for their custody on grounds that he was the "only genetic and natural parent available" to them. The court, citing *Johnson v. Calvert,* held that the gestational mother was the "natural mother" of the children and was entitled to temporary custody of the children because this was what the parties had intended at the time of conception.

As the use of oocyte donation burgeons, there is a need to adopt laws that clarify the parentage of the resulting children. While this is an area largely governed by state law, many states thus far have not adequately addressed even artificial insemination (and some have not addressed it at all). Therefore, we recommend that states adopt laws that utilize a presumption that the gamete recipient, rather than the gamete donor, is recognized as the legal parent of the child born as a result of oocyte donation. State legislatures should not just stipulate, but should clarify the legal status and rights of all of those—parents, donors, children—who are involved in oocyte donation.[25]

b. The need for legislation on record keeping

Currently there are no laws requiring practitioners to keep permanent records about oocyte donors. The Fertility Clinic Success Rate and Certification Act of 1992 (P. L. 102–493) is directed toward such clear, preventable injuries as shoddy laboratory conditions and includes no provision for keeping records about donors, recipients, or children born of gamete donation. Yet there are sound ethical reasons for keeping such records and for enacting laws requiring this. As discussed in Section III of this Report, the interest of children in their personal and genetic identity is significant, as are the privacy interests of donors and recipients. These interests have a claim to recognition. They can be met by keeping nonidentifying medical and genetic histories of donors on record. This would allow children to know of their medical susceptibilities and genetic heritage and yet would retain the confidentiality of those donors who do not want their identity revealed.

This approach to gamete donation has been adopted in several other countries. For instance, a central registry relevant to gamete donation was established by law in England in 1989. Children born of gamete donation have access to the registry and to a certain amount of nonidentifiable medical and social information about the donor. They can, for example, ascertain from this information whether they are related to their prospective spouse. Assurances have been given that the name of the donor will never be divulged, even if the law were to be changed in the future.[26]

If such a network of registries were established across states in this country, it would provide for continuity and consistency in management of information, updating of information, easier access to information, greater security from death and disaster than when it is kept by individual physicians or institutions, a resource for research into trends associated with donor gamete programs, and a way of attaining state cooperation with the growing interstate and international exchange of donor gametes. While a major drawback of a centralized registration system is that it can allow unauthorized access to confidential information, it also allows the possibility of monitoring attempted invasions of privacy. On balance, we find that the advantages of such a system outweigh its disadvantages.

Therefore, we recommend that as a matter of law a centrally coordinated network of registries be established in the United States with permanent records containing medical, genetic, and certain social information about donors. Such registries would keep these records in either identifiable or coded form, depending on the option elected by oocyte donors, for the purpose of providing oocyte recipients and children born from donor oocytes with information about their medical history and genetic background at the age of maturity. Donors who do not wish to have their identity revealed should be granted confidentiality with the proviso that oocyte donation centers would be authorized to decode their records without publicly revealing their identity in the event that this were needed to address serious illness in children born of their oocytes. Before they agree to donate oocytes, donors should be informed that such nonidentifying coded records will be kept and that they may be decoded in certain circumstances.

We further recommend that oocyte donation centers be required to establish a standard record form on which to keep the above information to avoid variation in the quality and kind of information kept. The information should be appropriately protected and secured.

We also recommend that a voluntary registry be established under the auspices of the centrally coordinated network of registries in which oocyte recipients, donors, and children born of oocyte donation can exercise the options listed in Section III.

c) The need for regulation and monitoring of infertility centers

In the United Kingdom, a Voluntary Licensing Authority that was largely the product of infertility specialists in that country was converted into a state licensing authority by law. All centers that offer methods of assisted reproduction must meet the standards for licensing of the new Human Fertilisation and Embryology Authority. The Canadian Royal Commission, in recommending that a national regulatory body be established in that country to license and monitor centers providing assisted reproductive services, maintained:

[A] National Commission presents the only feasible response to the clearly demonstrated need and justified public demand for coherent, effective, and appropriate national regulation of new reproductive technologies. The field is developing too rapidly, the consequences of inaction are too great, and the potential for harm to individuals and to society is too serious to allow Canada's response to be delayed, fragmented or tentative.[27]

The situation may not be as urgent in the United States, as professional associations of physicians who offer infertility services have developed guidelines for what they view as ethical use of the new reproductive technologies. Even so, it is in the public interest to establish some structure for regulating the use of the new reproductive technologies that stands outside the medical profession, while working closely with it.

We recommend that serious and timely consideration be given in the United States to the establishment of a standing federal regulatory body to license infertility centers. This body would have responsibility and sufficient support for surveillance of infertility centers around the country for the purpose of regulating and accrediting the provision of services of assisted reproduction. This regulatory body should work closely with the inter-center task force recommended below to establish standards and criteria for such licensing.

2. SELF-REGULATION BY THE MEDICAL PROFESSION

Accelerated self-monitoring efforts are needed from the medical profession for the use of oocyte donation at infertility centers. Although some individual centers have developed specific, detailed guidelines for the provision of the procedure, there are no consistent guidelines that hold across centers. Fairness to potential oocyte recipients and donors requires that they be accorded similar treatment that meets high medical and ethical standards no matter where they receive treatment in the country. Consequently, there is a need for the development of inter-center guidelines concerning certain aspects of the provision of oocyte donation by relevant experts and laypeople who are drawn from within and without the clinical setting.

Therefore, we recommend that an inter-center task force composed of qualified physicians, nurses, and counselors who are experienced in the provision of oocyte donation, as well as consumers, patient representatives, ethicists, lawyers, and other relevant persons be established through a cooperative effort by those involved in oocyte donation programs. It is appropriate to delegate this function to such a task force to ensure that guidelines are based on clinical realities and that the needs and concerns of those who are affected by such guidelines are addressed. This task force would be charged with developing specific, detailed guidelines for the screening of oocyte donors and recipients, for the content of consent forms, for compensation arrangements, and for practices on confidentiality. We would hope that the guidelines and recommendations given in this NABER Report would be of assistance to this body as it develops detailed recommendations for practice. Periodic updating of guidelines developed by this task force should be carried out by that body.

NOTES TO PART C

INTRODUCTION

1. A. D. Hard, "Artificial Impregnation," *Medical World* 27 (1909): 136; H. Rohleder, *Test Tube Babies* (New York: Vantage Press, 1930); A. T. Gregoire, R. C. Mayer, "The Impregnators," *Fertility and Sterility* 16 (1965): 130–33.

2. Paul Ramsey, "Shall We Reproduce?" *Journal of the American Medical Association* 220 (1972): 1346–50 and 1480–85.

3. Medical Research International, The American Fertility Society Special Interest Group, "In Vitro Fertilization/Embryo Transfer in the United States: 1987 Results from the IVF-ET Registry," *Fertility and Sterility* 51 (1989): 13–20.

4. Society for Assisted Reproductive Technology, The American Fertility Society, "Assisted Reproductive Technology in the United States and Canada: 1991 Results from the Society for Assisted Reproductive Technology/American Fertility Society Registry," *Fertility and Sterility* 59 (1993): 956–62.

5. Judith Bernstein, Mara Brill, Susan Levin, Machelle Seibel, Sharon Steinberg, "Implementation of Ovum Donation Technology: Start-up Decisions, Challenges, and Problems," in *Technology and Infertility: Clinical, Psychosocial, Legal and Ethical Aspects,* ed. Machelle M. Seibel, Judith Bernstein, Ann A. Kiessling, and Susan R. Levin (New York: Springer-Verlag, 1993), pp. 329–36.

6. Zev Rosenwaks, "Donor Eggs: Their Application in Modern Reproductive Technologies," *Fertility and Sterility* 47 (1987): 895–909.

SECTION I. ETHICAL QUESTIONS RAISED BY OOCYTE DONATION AND VALUES INFORMING THIS REPORT

1. Leon Kass, *Toward a More Natural Science* (New York: Free Press, 1985), p. 101.

2. "Instruction on Respect for Human Life in Its Origin and on the Dignity of Procreation, March 10, 1987," in *Medical Ethics: Sources of Catholic Teaching,* ed. Kevin O'Rourke and Philip Boyle (St. Louis, MO: The Catholic Health Association of the United States, 1989), p. 161.

3. Elio Sgreccia, "Moral Theology and Artificial Procreation in Light of Donum Vitae" in *Gift of Life: Catholic Scholars Respond to the Vatican Instruction*, ed. Edmund Pellegrino, John Collins Harvey, John P. Langen (Washington, DC: Georgetown University Press, 1990), p. 130.

4. "Instruction on Respect for Human Life in Its Origin and on the Dignity of Procreation. 1987," in O'Rourke and Boyle, p. 57.

5. Leon Kass, "New Beginnings in Life," in *The New Genetics and the Future of Man*, ed. Michael Hamilton (Grand Rapids, MI: Eerdmans, 1972), pp. 53-56.

6. Paul Ramsey, *Fabricated Man* (New Haven: Yale University Press, 1970), pp. 38-39.

7. Kass, *Toward a More Natural Science*, p. 109.

8. Ramsey, *Fabricated Man*, p. 131.

9. Oliver O'Donovan, *Begotten or Made?* (Oxford, England: Clarendon Press, 1984), pp. 1-13.

10. Paul Lauritzen, *Pursuing Parenthood: Ethical Issues in Assisted Parenthood* (Bloomington: Indiana University Press, 1993), p. 9.

11. Janet Dickey McDowell, "Ethical Implications of In Vitro Fertilization," in *On Moral Medicine: Theological Perspectives in Medical Ethics*, ed. Stephen E. Lammers and A. Verhey (Grand Rapids, MI: Eerdmans, 1987), pp. 335-36.

12. Richard McCormick, "Naturalness and Conjugal Gametes," *Annals of the New York Academy of Sciences* 541 (1988): 664-67.

13. Hessel Bouma III, Douglas Diekema, Edward Langrak, Theodore Rottman, Allen Verhey, *Christian Faith, Health, and Medical Practice* (Grand Rapids, MI: Eerdmans, 1989), pp. 193-94.

14. Richard A. McCormick, "Ethical Considerations of the New Reproductive Technologies," *Fertility and Sterility* 46, Supplement 1 (1986): 82.

15. Lauritzen, *Pursuing Parenthood*, p. 71.

16. Rabbi Moses Tendler, personal communication.

17. See Cynthia B. Cohen, "Parents Anonymous," in *New Ways of Making Babies: The Case of Egg Donation*, ed. Cynthia B. Cohen (Bloomington: Indiana University Press, 1996), this volume.

18. Lisa Sowle Cahill, "What is the 'Nature' of the Unity of Sex, Love and Procreation? A Response to Elio Sgreccia," *Gift of Life: Catholic Scholars Respond to the Vatican Instruction*, ed. Edmund Pellegrino, John Collins Harvey, John P. Langen (Washington, DC: Georgetown University Press, 1990), p. 144.

19. Lisa Sowle Cahill, "The Ethics of Surrogate Motherhood: Biology, Freedom, and Moral Obligation," *Journal of Law, Medicine, and Health Care* 16 (1988): 65-71.

20. Bouma, p. 196.

21. Daniel Callahan, "Bioethics and Fatherhood," *Utah Law Review* 3 (1992): 735-46; see also, Daniel Callahan, "Opening the Debate?: A Response to the Wiklers," *Milbank Quarterly* 69 (1991): 43.

22. Ruth Chadwick, "Having Children: Introduction," in *Ethics, Reproduction, and Genetic Control*, ed. Ruth Chadwick (London: Croom Helm, 1987), pp. 3-43; see also Sue Martin, "What about the Child?" *Second Opinion* 17 (1992): 95-98.

23. A. Raoul-Duval, H. Letur-Konirsch, R. Frydman, "Anonymous Oocyte Donation: A Psychological Study of Recipients, Donors and Children," *Human Reproduction* 7 (1992): 51-54.

24. John A. Robertson, "Ethical and Legal Issues in Human Egg Donation,"

Fertility and Sterility 52 (1989): 355; see also John A. Robertson, "Legal Uncertainties in Human Egg Donation," in *New Ways of Making Babies: The Case of Egg Donation,* ed. Cynthia B. Cohen (Bloomington: Indiana University Press, 1996), this volume.

25. Linda S. Williams, "Biology or Society? Parenthood Motivation in a Sample of Canadian Women Seeking In Vitro Fertilization," in *Issues in Reproductive Technology I: An Anthology,* ed. Helen Bequaert Holmes (New York and London: Garland Publishing, 1992), pp. 261-74.

26. Elizabeth Bartholet, "In Vitro Fertilization: The Construction of Infertility and of Parenting," in *Issues in Reproductive Technology I: An Anthology,* ed. Helen Bequaert Holmes (New York and London: Garland Publishing, 1992), pp. 253-60.

27. Margarete Sandelowski, "Compelled to Try: The Never Enough Quality of Conceptive Technology," *Medical Anthropology Quarterly,* New Series, 5, 1991, pp. 29-45.

28. Gena Corea, *The Mother Machine* (New York: Harper and Row, 1985); see also Ruth Macklin, "What Is Wrong with Commodification?" in *New Ways of Making Babies: The Case of Egg Donation,* ed. Cynthia B. Cohen (Bloomington: Indiana University Press, 1996), this volume.

29. Robyn Rowland, "Women as Living Laboratories: The New Reproductive Technologies," in *The Trapped Woman,* ed. Josefina Figueira-McDonough and Rosemary Sarri (Newbury Park: Sage, 1987), pp. 81-111.

30. Alison Jagger, *Feminist Politics and Human Nature* (New Jersey: Rowman and Allanheld, 1983, p. 132) as quoted in Jean Bethke Elshtain, "The New Eugenics and Feminist Quandaries," *Lutheran Forum* 23(1992): 20-29; see also Marjorie Maguire Shultz, "Reproductive Technology and Intent-Based Parenthood: An Opportunity for Gender Neutrality," *Wisconsin Law Review* 1990 (1990): 297-398.

31. E. Freeman, M. Boxer, K. Rickels, R. Tureck, and L. Mastroianni, "Psychological Evaluation and Support in a Program of in Vitro Fertilization and Embryo Transfer," *Fertility and Sterility* 43 (1985): 48-52.

32. Sandra Evans, "The Other Side of Adoption," *Washington Post,* Health Section, January 18, 1994, p. 11.

33. "Developments in the Law," *Harvard Law Review,* 103 (1990): 1519, 1554.

34. Joan Hollinger, "From Coitus to Commerce: Legal and Social Consequences of Noncoital Reproduction," *Journal of Law Reform* 18 (1985): 865-932.

35. Christine Overall, *Ethics and Human Reproduction: A Feminist Analysis* (Boston: Allen and Unwin, 1987), p. 143.

SECTION II. ETHICAL AND POLICY ISSUES RELATED TO OOCYTE RECIPIENTS IN THE CLINICAL SETTING

1. Zev Rosenwaks, "Donor Eggs: Their Application in Modern Reproductive Technologies," *Fertility and Sterility* 47 (1987): 895-909.

2. Ibid.

3. Mark V. Sauer, Richard J. Paulson, and Rogerio A. Lobo, "A Preliminary Report on Oocyte Donation: Extending Reproductive Potential to Women over 40," *New England Journal of Medicine* 323 (1990): 1157-60.

4. Mark V. Sauer and Richard J. Paulson, "Understanding the Current Status of

Oocyte Donation in the United States: What's Really Going on Out There?" *Fertility and Sterility* 58 (1992): 16-18; John Leeton, "Patient Selection for Assisted Reproduction," *Balliere's Clinical Obstetrics and Gynaecology* 6 (1992): 217-27; Mark V. Sauer, Richard J. Paulson, and Rogerio A. Lobo, "Reversing the Natural Decline in Human Fertility: An Extended Clinical Trial of Oocyte Donation to Women of Advanced Reproductive Age," *Journal of the American Medical Association* 269 (1992): 1275-79.

5. D. Schwartz, M. J. Mayaux, and Federation CECOS, "Female Fecundity as a Function of Age: Results of Artificial Insemination in 2,193 Nulliparous Women with Azoospermic Husbands," *New England Journal of Medicine* 306 (1982): 404-406.

6. Rosenwaks, "Donor Eggs," p. 902; Sauer, "Reversing the Natural Decline," p. 1278; Mark V. Sauer, Richard J. Paulson, Rogerio A. Lobo, "Pregnancy after Age 50: Application of Oocyte Donation to Women after Natural Menopause," *Lancet* 341 (1993): 321-23; Paul F. Serhal and Ian L. Craft, "Oocyte Donation in 61 Patients," *Lancet* 1 (1989): 1185-97.

7. Leeton, "Patient Selection for Assisted Reproduction," p. 217; Sauer, "Reversing the Natural Decline," p. 1276.

8. Andrea M. Braverman and Ovum Donor Task Force of the Psychological Special Interests Group of the American Fertility Society, "Survey Results on the Current Practice of Ovum Donation," *Fertility and Sterility* 59 (1993): 1216-20.

9. Braverman, "Survey Results," p. 1218; Sauer, "Understanding the Current Status," p. 17.

10. Lynne S. Wilcox and William D. Mosher, "Use of Infertility Services in the United States," *Obstetrics and Gynecology* 82 (1993): 122-27.

11. Sauer, "Understanding the Current Status," p. 17.

12. Norma J. Wikler, "Society's Response to the New Reproductive Technologies: The Feminist Perspective," *Southern California Law Review* 59 (1986): 1043-57.

13. Martin M. Quigley, Robert L. Collins, and Leslie R. Schover, "Establishment of an Oocyte Donor Program: Donor Screening and Selection," *Annals of the New York Academy of Sciences* 626 (1991): 445-51.

14. Judith Bernstein, Mara Brill, Susan Levin, Machelle Seibel, Sharon Steinberg, "Implementation of Ovum Donation Technology: Start-up Decisions, Challenges, and Problems," in *Technology and Infertility: Clinical, Psychosocial, Legal and Ethical Aspects*, ed. Machelle M. Seibel, Judith Bernstein, Ann A. Kiessling, and Susan R. Levin (New York: Springer-Verlag, 1993), pp. 329-36.

15. Jacqueline A. Bartlett, "Psychiatric Issues in Non-Anonymous Oocyte Donation," *Psychosomatics* 32 (1991): 733-37.

16. Iain T. Cameron, Peter A. W. Rogers, Catriona Caro, Jayne Harman, David L. Healy, and John F. Leeton, "Oocyte Donation: A Review," *British Journal of Obstetrics and Gynaecology* 96 (1989): 893-99.

17. Richard W. Tureck, Celso-Ramon Garcia, Luis Blasco, and Luigi Mastroianni, Jr., "Perioperative Complications Arising after Transvaginal Oocyte Retrieval," *Obstetrics and Gynecology* 81 (1993): 590-93.

18. Mark V. Sauer and Richard J. Paulson, "Human Oocyte and Pre-Embryo Donation: An Evolving Method for the Treatment of Female Infertility," *American Journal of Obstetrics and Gynecology* 163 (1990): 1421-24.

19. Medical Research International, The American Fertility Society Special Inter-

est Group, "In Vitro Fertilization/Embryo Transfer in the United States: 1988 Results from the IVF-ET Registry," *Fertility and Sterility* 53 (1990): 13–20.

20. Society for Assisted Reproductive Technology, "Assisted Reproductive Technology in the United States and Canada: 1991 Results from the Society for Assisted Reproductive Technology/American Fertility Society Registry," *Fertility and Sterility* 59 (1993): 956–62.

21. Sauer, "Human Oocyte and Pre-Embryo Donation," p. 1421.

22. Mark V. Sauer, Richard J. Paulson, Thelma M. Macaso, Mary Francis-Hernandez, Rogerio A. Lobo, "Establishment of a Nonanonymous Donor Oocyte Program: Preliminary Experience at the University of Southern California," *Fertility and Sterility* 52 (1989): 433–36.

23. Howard Blanchette, "Obstetric Performance of Patients after Oocyte Donation," *American Journal of Obstetrics and Gynecology* 168 (1993): 1803–1809.

24. Mary Anne Rossing, Janet R. Daling, Noel S. Weiss, Donald E. Moore, Steven G. Self, "Ovarian Tumors in a Cohort of Infertile Women," *New England Journal of Medicine* 331 (1994): 771–76; R. Spirtas, S. C. Kaufman, N.J. Alexander, "Fertility Drugs and Ovarian Cancer: Red Alert or Red Herring?" *Fertility and Sterility* 59 (1993): 291–93; A. S. Whittemore, R. Harris, J. Halpern, "The Collaborative Ovarian Cancer Group Characteristics Relating to Ovarian Cancer Risk: Collaborative Analysis of 12 US Case-control Studies. 1. Methods," *American Journal of Epidemiology* 136 (1992): 1175–83; S. Fishel, P. Jackson, "Follicular Stimulation for High Tech Pregnancies: Are We Playing It Safe?" *British Medical Journal* 299 (1989): 309–11.

25. Alice S. Whittemore, "The Risk of Ovarian Cancer after Treatment for Infertility," *New England Journal of Medicine* 331 (1994): 805–806.

26. Ibid.

27. Louis Keith, Jose A. Lopez-Zeno, Barbara Luke, "Triplet and Higher Order Pregnancies," *Contemporary Ob/Gyn* June, 1993, pp. 36–50.

28. Paulo Serafini, Jeffrey Nelson, Shelley B. Smith, Ana Richardson, Joel Batzofin, "Oocyte Donation Program at Huntington Reproductive Center: Quality Control Issues," in *New Ways of Making Babies: The Case of Egg Donation,* ed. Cynthia B. Cohen (Bloomington: Indiana University Press, 1996), this volume.

29. S. Sabourin, J. Wright, C. Duchesne, S. Belisle, "Are Consumers of Modern Fertility Treatments Satisfied?" *Fertility and Sterility* 56 (1991): 1084–90; L. Jill Halman, Antonia Abbey, Frank M. Andrews, "Why Are Couples Satisfied with Infertility Treatment?" *Fertility and Sterility* 59 (1993): 1046–54.

30. Halman, "Why Are Couples Satisfied with Infertility Treatment?" pp. 1050–51.

31. David H. Barad, Brian L. Cohen, "Oocyte Donation at Montefiore Medical Center, Albert Einstein College of Medicine," in *New Ways of Making Babies: The Case of Egg Donation,* ed. Cynthia B. Cohen (Bloomington: Indiana University Press, 1996), this volume.

32. Richard E. Blackwell, Bruce R. Carr, R. Jeffrey Chang, Alan H. DeCherney, Arthur F. Haney, William R. Keye, Robert W. Rebar, John A. Rock, Zev Rosenwaks, Machelle M. Seibel, Michael R. Soules, "Are We Exploiting the Infertile Couple?" *Fertility and Sterility* 48 (1987): 735–39.

33. Patricia M. McShane, "Oocyte Donation Service at IVF America-Boston," in *New Ways of Making Babies: The Case of Egg Donation,* ed. Cynthia B. Cohen

(Bloomington: Indiana University Press, 1996), this volume; Nancy A. Klein, Gretchen Sewall, Michael R. Soules, "Donor Oocyte Program at the University of Washington Medical Center," in *New Ways of Making Babies: The Case of Egg Donation,* ed. Cynthia B. Cohen (Bloomington: Indiana University Press, 1996), this volume.

34. Susan Levin, "Psychological Evaluation of the Infertile Couple," in *Technology and Infertility: Clinical, Psychosocial, Legal and Ethical Aspects,* ed. Machelle M. Seibel, Judith Bernstein, Ann A. Kiessling, and Susan R. Levin (New York: Springer-Verlag, 1993), pp. 289–96.

35. Braverman, "Survey Results," p. 1218.

36. Levin, "Psychological Evaluation," pp. 293–94.

37. Ibid., p. 291.

38. Sauer, "Understanding the Current Status of Oocyte Donation," p. 17.

39. Braverman, "Survey Results," p. 1217.

40. Bernstein, "Implementation of Ovum Donation Technology," p. 332; Braverman, "Survey Results," p. 1219.

41. Blackwell, "Are We Exploiting the Infertile Couple?" p. 736.

42. Rosenwaks, "Donor Eggs," p. 895.

43. Ibid.

44. American Fertility Society, "Guidelines for Gamete Donation: 1993," *Fertility and Sterility* 59, Supplement 1 (1993): 5S–9S.

45. Carson Strong, "Genetic Screening in Oocyte Donation: Ethical and Legal Aspects," in *New Ways of Making Babies: The Case of Egg Donation,* ed. Cynthia B. Cohen (Bloomington: Indiana University Press, 1996), this volume.

46. Daniel Navot, Zev Rosenwaks, "Ovum Donation," in *Infertility: A Comprehensive Text,* ed. Machelle M. Seibel (Norwalk, Connecticut: Appleton and Lange, 1991), pp. 513–24.

47. Carson Strong, "Genetic Screening in Oocyte Donation: Ethical and Legal Aspects," this volume.

48. Janet G. Raymond, "Reproductive Gifts and Gift Giving: The Altruistic Woman," *Hastings Center Report* 20 (1990): 7–11 at 8.

49. See Section I of this Report, "Ethical Questions Raised by the Use of Oocyte Donation," sub-section on Women; see also Rosalind Petchesky, "Reproductive Freedom: Beyond a Woman's Right to Choose," *Signs* 5 (1980): 661–85.

50. Dorothy E. Roberts, "The Future of Reproductive Choice for Poor Women and Women of Color," *Women's Rights Law Reporter* 12 (1990): 59–67 at 62.

51. Wikler, "Society's Response to the New Reproductive Technologies," pp. 1049–50; See Rosemarie Tong, "Toward a Feminist Perspective on Gamete Donation and Reception Policies," *New Ways of Making Babies: The Case of Egg Donation,* ed. Cynthia B. Cohen (Bloomington: Indiana University Press, 1996), this volume.

52. Susan Sherwin, *No Longer Patient: Feminist Ethics and Health Care* (Philadelphia: Temple University Press, 1992), p. 126.

53. Nadine Taub, "Introduction. A Symposium on Reproductive Rights: The Emerging Issues," *Women's Rights Law Reporter* 7 (1982): 169.

54. Klein, Sewall, Soules, "Donor Oocyte Program at the University of Washington Medical Center," this volume.

55. Braverman, "Survey Results," p. 1218; Sauer, "Establishment of a Nonanonymous Donor Oocyte Program," p. 434.

56. Serafini, Nelson, Smith, Richardson, Batzofin, "Oocyte Donation Program at Huntington Reproductive Center," this volume.

57. Braverman, "Survey Results," p. 1219.

58. Alice D. Domar, Machelle M. Seibel, "Emotional Aspects of Infertility," in *Infertility: A Comprehensive Text,* ed. Machelle M. Seibel (Norwalk, CT: Appleton and Lange, 1991), pp. 23–35.

59. Leeton, "Patient Selection," p. 219.

60. Navot, "Ovum Donation," p. 522.

61. Leeton, "Patient Selection," p. 219; Levin, "Psychological Evaluation," p. 293.

62. Jerome H. Check, Nowroozi Kosrow, Eytan R. Barnea, Kathryn J. Shaw, Mark V. Sauer, "Successful Delivery after Age 50: A Report of Two Cases as a Result of Oocyte Donation," *Obstetrics and Gynecology* 81 (1993): 835–36.

63. Anne Waldschmidt, "Against Selection of Human Life—People with Disabilities Oppose Genetic Counseling," *Issues in Reproductive and Genetic Engineering* 5 (1992): 155–67.

64. Joan H. Hollinger, "From Coitus to Commerce: Legal and Social Consequences of Noncoital Reproduction," *Journal of Law Reform* 18 (1985): 865–90.

65. Christine Overall, *Ethics and Human Reproduction: A Feminist Analysis, Reproductive Rights and Access to the Means of Reproduction* (Boston: Allen and Unwin, 1987), p. 186.

66. Bernstein, "Implementation of Ovum Donation Technology," p. 332.

67. Idem; Levin, "Psychological Evaluation of Infertile Couples," p. 293; Patricia P. Mahlstedt, Dorothy A. Greenfeld, "Assisted Reproductive Technology with Donor Gametes: The Need for Patient Preparation," *Fertility and Sterility* 52 (1989): 908–14.

68. Mahlstedt, "Assisted Reproductive Technology," pp. 912–13.

69. Bernstein, "Implementation of Ovum Donation Technology," p. 334.

70. Mahlstedt, "Assisted Reproductive Technology," p. 909; Hossam I. Abdalla, "Ethical Aspects of Oocyte Donation," *British Journal of Obstetrics and Gynaecology* 101 (1994): 567–70.

71. Andrea L. Bonnicksen, "Private and Public Policy Alternatives in Oocyte Donation," in *New Ways of Making Babies: The Case of Egg Donation,* ed. Cynthia B. Cohen (Bloomington: Indiana University Press, 1996), this volume; Bernstein, "Implementation of Ovum Donation Technology," pp. 332–34.

72. Halman, "Why Are Couples Satisfied with Infertility Treatment?" p. 1052.

73. Braverman, "Survey Results," p. 1218.

74. Sauer, "Establishment of a Nonanonymous Donor Oocyte Program," pp. 433, 436.

75. Domar and Seibel, "Emotional Aspects of Infertility," pp. 23–25.

76. Dorothy A. Greenfeld, Michael P. Diamond, Alan H. DeCherney, "Grief Reactions Following In-vitro Fertilization Treatment," *Journal of Psychosomatic Obstetrics and Gynaecology,* 8 (1988): 169–74.

77. Halman, "Why Are Couples Satisfied with Infertility Treatment?" p. 1052.

78. Domar and Seibel, "Emotional Aspects of Infertility," p. 33.

79. Margarete Sandelowski, "Compelled to Try: The Never Enough Quality of Conceptive Technology," *Medical Anthropology Quarterly* 5 (1991): 31.

80. M. V. Sauer, B. R. Ary, and R. J. Paulson, "The Demographic Characterization of Women Participating in Oocyte Donation: A Review of 300 Consecutively Performed Cycles," *International Journal of Gynecology and Obstetrics* 45 (1994): 147–51.

81. Sauer, "Understanding the Current Status of Oocyte Donation," p. 17.

82. Nancy A. Klein, Gretchen Sewall, Michael R. Soules, "Donor Oocyte Program at the University of Washington Medical Center," this volume.

83. Patricia M. McShane, "Oocyte Donation Service at IVF America-Boston," this volume; IVF America-Boston, "Medical Departmental Operating Guidelines," Fourth Edition, May, 1993, Sec. 23, p. 1.

84. Serafini, Nelson, Smith, Richardson, Batzofin, "Oocyte Donation Program at Huntington Reproductive Center," this volume; Abdalla, "Ethical Aspects of Oocyte Donation," p. 568.

85. R. L. Naeye, "Maternal Age, Obstetric Complications and the Outcome of Pregnancy," *Obstetrics and Gynecology* 61 (1983): 210–16; A. Friede, W. Baldwin, P. H. Rhodes, J. W. Buehler, L. T. Strauss, "Older Maternal Age and Infant Mortality in the United States," *Obstetrics and Gynecology* 72 (1988): 152–57.

86. Martin M. Quigley, "The New Frontier of Reproductive Age," *Journal of the American Medical Association* 268 (1992): 1320–21.

87. Editorial, "Too Old to Have a Baby?" *Lancet* 341 (1993): 344–45.

88. Ibid., p. 345.

89. Ibid.

90. Ezra Davidson, Jr., M. D., personal communication.

91. Blanchette, "Obstetric Performance of Patients after Oocyte Donation," p. 1806.

92. Lori B. Andrews, "When Baby's Mother Is Also Grandma—and Sister: Commentary," *Hastings Center Report* 15 (1985): 29–30.

93. Royal Commission on New Reproductive Technologies, *Proceed with Care* (Ottawa: Minister of Government Services, 1993), pp. 588–89.

94. Sauer, "Reversing the Natural Decline," p. 1278.

95. American Fertility Society, "Guidelines," 5S–9S.

96. *Law and Ethics of AID and Embryo Transfer: Ciba Foundation Symposium* (Amsterdam: Elsevier, 1973), p. 27.

97. Sauer, "Understanding the Current Status of Oocyte Donation," p. 17.

98. Sauer, "Reversing the Natural Decline," p. 1278.

99. Maureen McGuire and Nancy J. Alexander, "Artificial Insemination of Single Women," *Fertility and Sterility* 43 (1985): 182–84.

100. Daniel Wikler and Norma J. Wikler, "Turkey-Baster Babies: The Demedicalization of Artificial Insemination," *Milbank Quarterly* 69 (1991): 5–40 at 7.

101. U.S. Congress, Office of Technology Assessment, *Artificial Insemination: Practice in the United States: Summary of a 1987 Survey—Background Paper,* OTA-BP-BA-48 (Washington, DC: U.S. Government Printing Office, 1988), p. 9.

102. Sidney Callahan, "The Ethical Challenge of the New Reproductive Technology," in *Medical Ethics: A Guide for Health Professionals,* ed. John F. Monagle, David C. Thomasma (Rockville, MD: Aspen, 1988), pp. 26–37; Barbara Dafoe Whitehead, "Dan Quayle Was Right," *Atlantic* 271 (1993):47–84.

103. McGuire, "Artificial Insemination of Single Women," p. 182.

104. Callahan, "The Ethical Challenge of the New Reproductive Technology," p. 29.

105. Ibid., p. 34.

106. Susan Golombok and John Rust, "The Warnock Report and Single Women: What about the Children?" *Journal of Medical Ethics* 12 (1986): 185–88.

107. Mary Warnock, *A Question of Life: The Warnock Report on Human Fertilisation and Embryology* (London: Basil Blackwell, 1985).

108. Ross D. Parke, *Fathers* (Cambridge, MA: Harvard University Press, 1981); Shirley M. H. Hanson and Frederick W. Bonett, *Dimensions of Fatherhood* (Beverly Hills, CA: Sage Publications, 1985).

109. McGuire, "Artificial Insemination of Single Women," p. 182; Carson Strong and Jay S. Schinfeld, "The Single Woman and Artificial Insemination by Donor," *Journal of Reproductive Medicine* 29 (1984): 293-99.

110. Strong, "The Single Woman," p. 294; R. B. Zajonc, "Family Configurations and Intelligence," *Science* 192 (1976): 227-31.

111. Golombok, "The Warnock Report and Single Women," p. 188.

112. Ibid.

113. McGuire, "Artificial Insemination of Single Women," p. 182.

114. McGuire, "Artificial Insemination of Single Women," p. 182; Strong, "The Single Woman," p. 294.

115. B. G. Cashion, "Female-Headed Families: Effect on Children and Clinical Implications," *Journal of Marital and Family Therapy* 8 (1992): 77-86.

116. McGuire, "Artificial Insemination of Single Women," p. 182; R. Weiss, "Growing Up a Little Faster," *Journal of Social Issues* 35 (1979): 97-103.

117. Golombok, "The Warnock Report," p. 187.

118. Wikler, "Turkey-Baster Babies," p. 7; Golombok, "The Warnock Report," p. 188; Strong, "The Single Woman," p. 296.

119. C. Pies, "Lesbians and the Choice to Parent," in F. W. Bozertt and M. B. Sussman, eds., *Homosexuality and Family Relationships* (New York: Harrington Park, 1990), pp. 137-54.

120. McGuire, "Artificial Insemination of Single Women," pp. 183-84; Strong, "The Single Woman," p. 295; A. Brewaeys, H. Olbrechts, P. Devroey, A. C. Van Steirteghem, "Counselling and Selection of Homosexual Couples in Fertility Treatment," *Human Reproduction* 4 (1989): 850-53; P. J. Falk, "Lesbian Mothers: Psychosocial Assumptions in Family Law," *American Psychologist* 44 (1989): 941-47.

121. Falk, "Lesbian Mothers," p. 946; D. J. Kleber, R. J. Howell, and A. L. Tibbits-Kleber, "The Impact of Parental Homosexuality in Child Custody Cases: A Review of the Literature," *Bulletin of the American Academy of Psychiatry and Law* 14 (1986): 81-87.

122. Editors of the Harvard Law Review, *Sexual Orientation and the Law* (Cambridge, MA: Harvard University Press, 1990).

123. R. Green, "The Best Interests of the Child with a Lesbian Mother," *Bulletin of the American Association for Psychiatry and Law* 10 (1982): 7-15; Charlotte J. Patterson, "Children of Lesbian and Gay Parents," *Child Development* 63 (1992), 1025-42; R. Green, J. B. Mandel, M. E. Hovedt, J. Gray, L. Smith, "Lesbian Mothers and Their Children: A Comparison with Solo Parent Heterosexual Mothers and Their Children," *Archives of Sexual Behavior* 15 (1986): 167-84.

124. McGuire, "Artificial Insemination of Single Women," p. 183.

125. M. Kirkpatrick, C. Smith, R. Roy, "Lesbian Mothers and Their Children: A Comparative Survey," *American Journal of Orthopsychiatry* 51 (1981): 545-54; S. Golombok, A. Spencer, M. Rutter, "Children in Lesbian and Single-Parent House-

holds: Psychosexual and Psychiatric Appraisal," *Journal of Psychology and Psychiatry* 24 (1983): 551-72.

126. McGuire, "Artificial Insemination of Single Women," p. 184; Golombok, "The Warnock Report," p. 188; Brewaeys, "Counselling and Selection of Homosexual Couples," p. 852; Kirkpatrick, "Lesbian Mothers," p. 545; Golombok, Spencer, "Children in Lesbian and Single-Parent Households," p. 561; R. Green, "Sexual Identity of 37 Children Raised by Homosexual or Transsexual Parents," *American Journal of Psychiatry* 135 (1978): 692-98; J. S. Gottman, "Children of Gay and Lesbian Parents," in F. W. Boztt and M. B. Sussman, eds., *Homosexuality and Family Relations* (New York: Harrington Park, 1990), pp. 177-96.

127. McGuire, "Artificial Insemination of Single Women," p. 183; Brewaeys, "Counselling and Selection of Homosexual Couples," p. 852; Charlotte J. Patterson, "Children of the Lesbian Baby Boom: Behavioral Adjustment, Self Concepts, and Sex-Role Identity," in B. Greene and G. Herek, eds., *Contemporary Perspectives on Gay and Lesbian Psychology: Theory, Research and Applications* (Beverly Hills, CA: Sage. In press).

128. Patterson, pp. 1029.

129. Lori Andrews and Ami S. Jaeger, "Legal Aspects of Infertility," in *Infertility: A Comprehensive Text*, ed. Machelle M. Seibel (Norwalk, CT: Appleton and Lange, 1991), pp. 539-50; Patterson, "Children of Lesbian and Gay Parents," pp. 1036-38.

130. Texas S. B. No. 512, 73rd Leg., R. S. (1993).

131. D. S. Kaiser, "Artificial Insemination: Donor Rights in Situations Involving Unmarried Recipients," *Journal of Family Law* 26 (1987-88): 795-96.

132. Bartha M. Knoppers and Sonia LeBris, "Recent Advances in Medically Assisted Conception: Legal, Ethical and Social Issues," *American Journal of Law and Medicine* 17 (1990): 329-61.

133. Walter Wadlington, LL. B., personal communication.

134. See Patricia M. McShane, "Oocyte Donation Service at IVF America-Boston," this volume.

135. *Smedes v. Wayne State University,* E. D. Michigan, filed July 16, 1980.

136. Wikler, "Turkey-Baster Babies," p. 8.

137. Barad, Cohen, "Oocyte Donation at Montefiore Medical Center, Albert Einstein College of Medicine," this volume.

SECTION III. ETHICAL AND POLICY ISSUES RELATED TO OOCYTE DONORS IN THE CLINICAL SETTING

1. Mark V. Sauer and Richard J. Paulson, "Human Oocyte and Preembryo Donation: An Evolving Method for the Treatment of Infertility," *American Journal of Obstetrics and Gynecology* 163 (1990): 1421-24.

2. Martin M. Quigley, Robert L. Collins, and Leslie R. Schover, "Establishment of an Oocyte Donor Program: Donor Screening and Selection," *Annals of the New York Academy of Sciences* 626 (1991): 445-51.

3. P. R. Braude, M. V. Bright, C. P. Douglas, P. J. Milton, R. E. Robinson, J. G. Williamson, and J. Hutchison, "A Regimen for Obtaining Mature Human Oocytes

from Donors for Research into Human Fertilization in Vitro," *Fertility and Sterility* 42 (1984): 34–38.

4. M. Power, R. Baber, H. Abdalla, A. Kirkland, T. Leonard, and J. W. W. Studd, "A Comparison of the Attitudes of Volunteer Donors and Infertile Patient Donors on an Ovum Donation Programme," *Human Reproduction* 5 (1990): 352–55.

5. Andrea M. Braverman and Ovum Donor Task Force of the Psychological Special Interests Group of the American Fertility Society, "Survey Results on the Current Practice of Ovum Donation," *Fertility and Sterility* 59 (1993): 1216–20; David H. Barad, Brian L. Cohen, "Oocyte Donation Program at Montefiore Medical Center, Albert Einstein College of Medicine," in *New Ways of Making Babies: The Case of Egg Donation,* ed. Cynthia B. Cohen (Bloomington: Indiana University Press, 1996), this volume; Patricia M. McShane, "Oocyte Donation Service at IVF America-Boston," in *New Ways of Making Babies: The Case of Egg Donation,* ed. Cynthia B. Cohen (Bloomington: Indiana University Press, 1996), this volume.

6. M. V. Sauer, B. R. Ary, and R. J. Paulson, "The Demographic Characterization of Women Participating in Oocyte Donation: A Review of 300 Consecutively Performed Cycles," *International Journal of Gynecology and Obstetrics* 45 (1994): 147–51; Roberta Lessor, Nancyann Cervantes, Nadine O'Connor, Jose Balmaceda, Ricardo H. Asch, "An Analysis of Social and Psychological Characteristics of Women Volunteering to Become Oocyte Donors," *Fertility and Sterility* 59 (1993): 65–71; Mark V. Sauer and Richard J. Paulson, "Oocyte Donors: A Demographic Analysis of Women at the University of Southern California," *Human Reproduction* 7 (1992): 726–28.

7. Susan Edelman, "Egg-donor Programs Raise Questions," *The Record,* Hackensack, New Jersey, February 7, 1993, pp. A1, A12–13.

8. Elizabeth Heitman and Mary Schlachtenhaufen, "The Differential Effects of Race, Ethnicity, and Socioeconomic Status on Infertility and Its Treatment: Ethical and Policy Issues for Oocyte Donation," in *New Ways of Making Babies: The Case of Egg Donation,* ed. Cynthia B. Cohen (Bloomington: Indiana University Press, 1996), this volume.

9. Nancy A. Klein, Gretchen Sewall, Michael R. Soules, "Donor Oocyte Program at the University of Washington Medical Center," in *New Ways of Making Babies: The Case of Egg Donation,* ed. Cynthia B. Cohen (Bloomington: Indiana University Press, 1996), this volume.

10. Barad, Cohen, "Oocyte Donation Program at Montefiore Medical Center, Albert Einstein College of Medicine," this volume; Quigley, "Establishment of an Oocyte Donor Program," pp. 446–47; Mark V. Sauer, Richard J. Paulson, Rogerio A. Lobo, "Pregnancy after Age 50: Application of Oocyte Donation to Women after Natural Menopause," *Lancet* 341 (1993): 321–23.

11. Mark V. Sauer, Richard J. Paulson, Thelma M. Macaso, Mary Francis-Hernandez, Rogerio A. Lobo, "Establishment of a Nonanonymous Donor Oocyte Program: Preliminary Experience at the University of Southern California," *Fertility and Sterility* 52 (1989): 433–36.

12. John A. Robertson, "Technology and Motherhood: Legal and Ethical Issues in Human Egg Donation," *Case Western Reserve Law Review* 39 (1988–89): 1–38.

13. Braverman, "Survey Results," p. 1217.

14. Mark V. Sauer and Richard J. Paulson, "Understanding the Current Status of

Oocyte Donation in the United States: What's Really Going on Out There?" *Fertility and Sterility* 58 (1992): 16–18.

15. Braverman, "Survey Results," p. 1218.

16. Machelle M. Seibel and Ann Kiessling, "Compensating Egg Donors: Equal Pay for Equal Time?" *New England Journal of Medicine* 328 (1993): 737.

17. Michael Feinman, David Barad, Ivan Szigetvari, Steven G. Kaali, "Availability of Donated Oocytes from an Ambulatory Sterilization Program," *Journal of Reproductive Medicine* 34 (1989): 441–43.

18. Braverman, "Survey Results," p. 1218.

19. Barad, Cohen, "Oocyte Donation Program at Montefiore Medical Center, Albert Einstein College of Medicine," this volume; Klein, Sewall, Soules, "Donor Oocyte Program at the University of Washington Medical Center," this volume; Quigley, "Establishment of an Oocyte Donor Program," p. 449; Power, "A Comparison of Attitudes," p. 354.

20. Lessor, "An Analysis of Social and Psychological Characteristics," p. 67.

21. Quigley, "Establishment of an Oocyte Donor Program," p. 449.

22. Power, "A Comparison of Attitudes," p. 353.

23. Jacqueline A. Bartlett, "Psychiatric Issues in Non-Anonymous Oocyte Donation," *Psychosomatics* 32 (1991): 733–37.

24. Lessor, "An Analysis of Social and Psychological Characteristics," p. 67.

25. Edelman, "Egg-donor Programs Raise Questions," p. A12.

26. Feinman, "Availability of Donated Oocytes," p. 442.

27. Ibid.

28. Ibid.

29. D. Navot, A. Relou, A. Birkenfield, R. Rabinowitz, A. Brzezinski, E. J. Margalioth, "Risk Factors and Prognostic Variables in the Ovarian Hyperstimulation Syndrome," *American Journal of Obstetrics and Gynecology* 159 (1988): 210–15.

30. Edelman, "Egg-donor Programs Raise Questions," p. A13.

31. Ibid., p. A12.

32. J. Riegler, A. Weikert, "Product Egg: Egg Selling in an Austrian IVF Clinic," *Reproductive and Genetic Engineering* 1 (1988): 221–23.

33. Edelman, "Egg-donor Programs Raise Questions," p. A13.

34. Ibid.

35. Mark V. Sauer, Richard J. Paulson, "Mishaps and Misfortunes: Complications that Occur in Oocyte Donation," *Fertility and Sterility* 61 (1994): 963–65.

36. Rita Arditti, "Egg Retrieval," *Encyclopedia of Childbearing: Critical Perspectives,* edited by Barbara Katz Rothman (Phoenix, AZ: Oryx Press, 1993), pp. 119–20.

37. Mary Anne Rossing, Janet R. Daling, Noel S. Weiss, Donald E. Moore, Steven G. Self, "Ovarian Tumors in a Cohort of Infertile Women," *New England Journal of Medicine* 331 (1994): 771–76.

38. Royal Commission on New Reproductive Technologies, *Proceed with Care* (Ottawa: Minister of Government Services, 1993), pp. 591–92.

39. Donald Rieger, "Gamete Donation: An Opinion on the Recommendations of the Royal Commission on New Reproductive Technologies," *Canadian Medical Association Journal* 151 (1994): 1433–35.

40. L. R. Schover, R. I. Collins, M. M. Quigley, J. Blankenstein, G. Kanoti, "Psychological Follow-up of Women Evaluated as Oocyte Donors," *Human Reproduction* 6 (1991): 1487–91.

41. Power, "A Comparison of Attitudes," p. 353; Schover, "Psychological Follow-up," p. 1489.

42. A. Raoul-Duval, H. Letur-Konirsch, R. Frydman, "Anonymous Oocyte Donation: A Psychological Study of Recipients, Donors and Children," *Human Reproduction* 7 (1992): 51-54.

43. R. J. Paulson, R. P. Marrs, "Ovulation Stimulation and Monitoring for in Vitro Fertilization," *Current Problems in Obstetrics Gynecology and Infertility* 9 (1986): 497-99.

44. Ibid.

45. Richard J. Paulson, "*In Vitro* Fertilization and Other Assisted Reproductive Techniques," *Journal of Reproductive Medicine* 38 (1993): 261-68.

46. Richard W. Tureck, Celso-Ramon Garcia, Luis Blasco, and Luigi Mastroianni, Jr., "Perioperative Complications Arising after Transvaginal Oocyte Retrieval," *Obstetrics and Gynecology* 81 (1993): 590-93.

47. Klein, Sewall, Soules, "Donor Oocyte Program at the University of Washington Medical Center," this volume.

48. American Fertility Society, "Guidelines for Oocyte Donation," "Minimal Genetic Screening for Gamete Donors," in "Guidelines for Gamete Donation: 1993," *Fertility and Sterility* 59 (1993): 5S-7S, 9S; Daniel Navot, Zev Rosenwaks, "Ovum Donation," in *Infertility: A Comprehensive Text,* ed. Machelle M. Seibel (Norwalk, CT: Appleton and Lange, 1991), pp. 513-24.

49. Lori B. Andrews, Ami S. Jaeger, "Legal Aspects of Infertility," in *Infertility: A Comprehensive Text,* ed. Machelle M. Seibel (Norwalk, CT: Appleton and Lange, 1991), pp. 539-49.

50. Braverman, "Survey Results," p. 1218.

51. American Fertility Society, "Guidelines for Oocyte Donation," p. 6S.

52. Sauer, "Pregnancy after Age 50," p. 322; Schover, "Psychological Follow-up," pp. 1487-88.

53. Tom L. Beauchamp and James F. Childress, *Principles of Biomedical Ethics* (New York: Oxford University Press, 1989), p. 106.

54. Joel Feinberg, *Harm to Self* (New York: Oxford University Press, 1986), p. 189.

55. Beauchamp and Childress, p. 107.

56. McShane, "Oocyte Donation Service at IVF America-Boston," this volume.

57. Janet Raymond, "Of Eggs, Embryos and Altruism," *Reproductive and Genetic Engineering* 1 (1981): 282-83.

58. See Rosemarie Tong, "Toward a Feminist Perspective on Gamete Donation and Reception Policies," in *New Ways of Making Babies: The Case of Egg Donation,* ed. Cynthia B. Cohen (Bloomington: Indiana University Press, 1996), this volume.

59. Quigley, "Establishment of an Oocyte Donor Program," p. 447.

60. Ruth Macklin, "What Is Wrong with Commodification?" in *New Ways of Making Babies: The Case of Egg Donation,* ed. Cynthia B. Cohen (Bloomington: Indiana University Press, 1996), this volume; John A. Robertson, "Legal Uncertainties in Human Egg Donation," in *New Ways of Making Babies: The Case of Egg Donation,* ed. Cynthia B. Cohen (Bloomington: Indiana University Press, 1996), this volume.

61. Paul Lauritzen, *Pursuing Parenthood* (Bloomington: Indiana University Press, 1993), p. 15; see Rosemarie Tong, "Toward a Feminist Perspective on Gamete Donation and Reception Policies."

62. Robertson, "Technology and Motherhood," pp. 29-33.

63. Bartha M. Knoppers and Sonia LeBris, "Recent Advances in Medically Assisted Conception: Legal, Ethical and Social Issues," *American Journal of Law and Medicine* 17 (1990): 329-61.

64. Macklin, "What Is Wrong with Commodification?" this volume.

65. Edelman, p. A12.

66. McShane, "Oocyte Donation Service at IVF America-Boston," this volume.

67. P. J. Parker, "Motivation of Surrogate Mothers: Initial Findings," *American Journal of Psychiatry* 140 (1983): 117-18.

68. Schover, "Psychological Follow-up," p. 1490.

69. Andrea L. Bonnicksen, "Private and Public Policy Alternatives in Oocyte Donation," in *New Ways of Making Babies: The Case of Egg Donation,* ed. Cynthia B. Cohen (Bloomington: Indiana University Press, 1996), this volume.

70. American Fertility Society, "Guidelines for Oocyte Donation," p. 6S.

71. Margaret Radin, "Market Inalienability," *Harvard Law Review* 100 (1987): 1845-1937 at 1915-1918.

72. For example, Jerome H. Check, H. Ali Askari, Charlene Fisher, Luann Vanaman, "The Use of a Shared Donor Oocyte Program to Evaluate the Effect of Uterine Senescence," *Fertility and Sterility* 61 (1994): 252-56.

73. McShane, "Oocyte Donation Service at IVF America-Boston," this volume.

74. Gail Vines, "Double Standards for Egg and Sperm Donors," *New Scientist* 143 (1994): 8.

75. Dan Brock, "Funding New Reproductive Technologies: Should They Be Included in Health Insurance Benefit Packages?" in *New Ways of Making Babies: The Case of Egg Donation,* ed. Cynthia B. Cohen (Bloomington: Indiana University Press, 1996), this volume.

76. Robertson, "Legal Uncertainties in Human Egg Donation," this volume.

77. Edelman, p. A12.

78. Jonathan Glover, *Ethics of New Reproductive Technologies: The Glover Report to the European Commission* (DeKalb: Northern Illinois University Press, 1989), pp. 42-43.

79. Braverman, "Survey Results," p. 1218.

80. Ibid., p. 1219.

81. Schover, "Psychological Follow-up," p. 1489; Lessor, "An Analysis of Social and Psychological Characteristics," p. 69.

82. Schover, "Psychological Follow-up," p. 1489.

83. Judith Bernstein, Mara Brill, Susan Levin, Machelle Seibel, Sharon Steinberg, "Implementation of Ovum Donation Technology: Start-up Decisions, Challenges, and Problems," in *Technology and Infertility: Clinical, Psychosocial, Legal and Ethical Aspects,* ed. Machelle M. Seibel, Judith Bernstein, Ann A. Kiessling, and Susan R. Levin (New York: Springer-Verlag, 1993), pp. 329-36.

84. Lessor, "An Analysis of Social and Psychological Characteristics," p. 66.

85. Bernstein, "Implementation of Ovum Donation Technology," p. 332.

86. Ibid.

87. Braverman, "Survey Results," p. 1218.

88. Robertson, "Technology and Motherhood," pp. 27-28.

89. Schover, "Psychological Follow-up," p. 1489.

90. Paulo Serafini, Jeffrey Nelson, Shelley B. Smith, Ana Richardson, Joel Batzofin,

"Oocyte Donation Program at Huntington Reproductive Center: Quality Control Issues," in *New Ways of Making Babies: The Case of Egg Donation*, ed. Cynthia B. Cohen (Bloomington: Indiana University Press, 1996), this volume.

91. Bonnicksen, "Private and Public Policy Alternatives in Oocyte Donation," this volume.

92. Knoppers and LeBris, "Recent Advances," p. 356.

93. Schover, "Psychological Follow-up," p. 1491.

94. Klein, Sewall, Soules, "Donor Oocyte Program at the University of Washington Medical Center," this volume

95. Braverman, "Survey Results," p. 1218.

96. Sherman Elias and George J. Annas, "Social Policy Considerations in Noncoital Reproduction," *Journal of the American Medical Association* 255 (1986): 62-68.

97. Martin M. Quigley, "Screening Providers of Gametes and Embryos," in *Emerging Issues in Biomedical Policy: An Annual Review*, Volume I, ed. Robert H. Blank, Andrea L. Bonnicksen (New York: Columbia University Press, 1992), pp. 238-51.

98. Seibel, "Compensating Egg Donors," p. 737.

99. American Fertility Society, "Guidelines for Oocyte Donation," p. 5S; Mary Warnock, *A Question of Life: The Warnock Report on Human Fertilisation and Embryology* (New York, NY: Basil Blackwell, 1985), p. 37.

100. Glover, *Ethics of New Reproductive Technologies*, p. 41.

101. Family Law Council, *Creating Children: A Uniform Approach to the Law and Practice of Reproductive Technology in Australia* (Canberra: Australian Government Publishing Service, 1985).

102. Robert D. Nachtigall, "Secrecy: An Unresolved Issue in the Practice of Donor Insemination," *American Journal of Obstetrics and Gynecology* 168 (1993): 1846-51; Rona Achilles, "Donor Insemination: The Future of a Public Secret," *The Future of Human Reproduction*, ed. Christine Overall (Toronto: Women's Press, 1989), pp. 105-19.

103. Patricia P. Mahlstedt, Dorothy A. Greenfeld, "Assisted Reproductive Technology with Donor Gametes: The Need for Patient Preparation," *Fertility and Sterility* 52(1989): 908-14.

104. Raoul-Duval, "Anonymous Oocyte Donation," p. 51.

105. Paul Lauritzen, *Pursuing Parenthood: Ethical Issues in Assisted Reproduction* (Bloomington: Indiana University Press, 1993), p. 85.

106. James Lindemann Nelson, "Parental Obligations and the Ethics of Surrogacy: A Causal Perspective," *Public Affairs Quarterly* 5 (1991): 49-61.

107. Patricia P. Mahlstedt, Kris A. Probasco, "Sperm Doors: Their Attitudes toward Providing Medical and Psychological Information for Recipient Couples and Donor Offspring," *Fertility and Sterility* 56 (1991): 747-53.

108. Erica Haimes, "Recreating the Family? Policy Considerations Relating to the 'New' Reproductive Technologies," in *The New Reproductive Technologies*, ed. M. McNeil, I. Varcoe, S. Yearley (New York, NY: St. Martin's Press, 1990), pp. 154-72.

109. Simone B. Novaes, "Semen Banking and Artificial Insemination by Donor in France: Social and Medical Discourse," *International Journal of Technology Assessment in Health Care* 2 (1986): 92.

110. Lauritzen, *Pursuing Parenthood,* pp. 84–88.

111. Annette Baran and Reuben Pannor, *Lethal Secrets* (New York, N Y: Warner Books, 1989).

112. Mahlstedt, "Assisted Reproductive Technology with Donor Gametes," pp. 910–11.

113. Nachtigall, "Secrecy," p. 87.

114. Mark V. Sauer, Ingrid A. Rodi, Michelle Scrooc, Maria Bustillo, John E. Buster, "Survey of Attitudes Regarding the Use of Siblings for Gamete Donation," *Fertility and Sterility* 49 (1988): 721–22.

115. R. Snowden, G. D. Mitchell, E. M. Snowden, *Artificial Reproduction: A Social Investigation* (London: 1983), p. 98.

116. Robyn Rowland, "The Social and Psychological Consequences of Secrecy in Artificial Insemination by Donor (AID) Programmes," *Social Science and Medicine* 21 (1988): 395.

117. The National Bioethics Consultative Committee, *Reproductive Technology: Record Keeping and Access to Information, Birth Certificates and Birth Records of Offspring Born as a Result of Gamete Donation. Final Report to Australian Health Ministers,* August, 1989.

118. Mahlstedt, "Assisted Reproductive Technology with Donor Gametes," p. 911.

119. Haimes, "Recreating the Family?" p. 98.

120. Mahlstedt, "Assisted Reproductive Technology with Donor Gametes," p. 911.

121. Barad, Cohen, "Oocyte Donation Program at Montefiore Medical Center, Albert Einstein College of Medicine," this volume.

122. Lori B. Andrews, "Legal and Ethical Aspects of New Reproductive Technologies," *Clinical Obstetrics and Gynecology* 29(1986): 190–204.

123. Cynthia B. Cohen, "Parents Anonymous," in *New Ways of Making Babies: The Case of Egg Donation,* ed. Cynthia B. Cohen (Bloomington: Indiana University Press, 1996), this volume.

124. Sauer, "Survey of Attitudes," p. 722.

125. Robertson, "Technology and Motherhood," p. 22.

126. Serafini, Nelson, Smith, Richardson, Batzofin, "Oocyte Donation Program at Huntington Reproductive Center," this volume.

127. Voluntary Licensing Authority for Human *In Vitro* Fertilization and Embryology, *Second Report,* 1987, p. 8.

128. Victoria Committee to Consider the Social, Ethical, and Legal Issues Arising from In Vitro Fertilisation and Embryology, *Report on Donor Gametes in IVF,* 1983; South Australia Working Party on In Vitro Fertilization and Artificial Insemination by Donor, *Report,* 1984, p. 28; Victoria. Infertility (Medical Procedures) Act, No. 10163, 1986, 1739–43.

129. Robertson, "Ethical and Legal Issues," pp. 357–58.

130. Lori B. Andrews, "When Baby's Mother Is Also Grandma—and Sister," *Hastings Center Report* 15 (1985): 29–30.

131. Hans Tiefel, "When Baby's Mother Is Also Grandma—and Sister," *Hastings Center Report* 15 (1985): 30–31.

132. Paul McDonough, M. D., personal communication.

133. Bernstein, "Implementation of Ovum Donation Technology," p. 333.

SECTION IV. PUBLIC POLICY AND THE USE OF OOCYTE DONATION

1. John A. Robertson, "Legal Uncertainties in Human Egg Donation," in *New Ways of Making Babies: The Case of Egg Donation*, ed. Cynthia B. Cohen (Bloomington: Indiana University Press, 1996), this volume.

2. Robert H. Blank, *Regulating Reproduction* (New York: Columbia University Press, 1990), p. 170.

3. Andrea L. Bonnicksen, "Private and Public Policy Alternatives in Oocyte Donation," in *New Ways of Making Babies: The Case of Egg Donation*, ed. Cynthia B. Cohen (Bloomington: Indiana University Press, 1996), this volume.

4. John A. Robertson, "Technology and Motherhood: Legal and Ethical Issues in Human Egg Donation," *Case Western Reserve Law Review* 39(10) (1988–89): 1–38; Andrea Bonnicksen, "Private and Public Policy Alternatives in Oocyte Donation," this volume.

5. Fertility Clinic Success Rate and Certification Act of 1992. P. L. 102–493 (October 24, 1992).

6. Hearings on H. R. 3940 before the Subcommittee on Health and the Environment of the Committee on Energy and Commerce, 102nd Congress, Second Session (February 27, 1992).

7. Andrea Bonnicksen, "Private and Public Policy Alternatives in Oocyte Donation," this volume.

8. John A. Robertson, "Legal Uncertainties in Human Egg Donation," this volume.

9. Royal Commission on New Reproductive Technologies, *Proceed with Care*, 2 vols. (Ottawa: Minister of Government Services, 1993).

10. Mary Warnock, *A Question of Life: The Warnock Report on Human Fertilisation and Embryology* (London: Basil Blackwell, 1985).

11. Cynthia B. Cohen and Elizabeth Leibold McCloskey, "Private Bioethics Forums: Counterpoint to Government Bodies," *Kennedy Institute of Ethics Journal* 4 (1994): 283–89.

12. *Medically Assisted Conception: An Agenda for Research*. Report of a Study by a Committee of the Institute of Medicine, National Research Council (Washington, DC: National Academy Press, 1989).

13. Richard E. Blackwell, Bruce R. Carr, R. Jeffrey Chang, Alan H. DeCherney et al., "Are We Exploiting the Infertile Couple?" *Fertility and Sterility* 48 (1987): 735–39; Michael R. Soules, "The In Vitro Fertilization Pregnancy Rate: Let's Be Honest with One Another," *Fertility and Sterility* 43 (1985): 511–513.

14. Andrea M. Braverman and Ovum Donor Task Force of the Psychological Special Interests Group of the American Fertility Society, "Survey Results on the Current Practice of Ovum Donation," *Fertility and Sterility* 59 (1993): 1216–20.

15. Ethics Committee of the American Fertility Society, Ethical Considerations of the New Reproductive Technologies. *Fertility and Sterility* 53, Suppl. 2 (1990):1S-109S.

16. Okla. Stat. Ann. Tit. 10, Sec. 544 (1991); Tex. S. B.512, 73rd Leg., R. S. (1993); S.2082, 1993 Reg.Sess., 1993 Florida Laws; Va. Code Ann. #20-158 (Miche Supp. 1994); N. D. Cent. Code #14-18-01 to #14-18-04 (1994); see John A. Robertson, "Legal Uncertainties in Human Egg Donation," this volume.

17. Uniform Status of Children of Assisted Conception Act, 9B U. L. A. Suppl. 87 (1988), section 4a.

18. Ruth Macklin, "Artificial Means of Reproduction and Our Understanding of the Family," *Hastings Center Report* 21 (1991): 5–11.

19. Sherman Elias and George J. Annas, "Noncoital Reproduction," *Journal of the American Medical Association* 255 (1986): 67.

20. George J. Annas, "Death without Dignity for Commercial Surrogacy: The Case of Baby M," *Hastings Center Report* 18 (1988): 21–24.

21. Sidney Callahan, "The Ethical Challenge of the New Reproductive Technology," in John F. Monagle and David C. Thomasma, eds., *Medical Ethics: A Guide for Health Care Professionals* (Frederick, MD: Aspen Publishers, 1987), pp. 26–37.

22. Cynthia B. Cohen, "Parents Anonymous," in *New Ways of Making Babies: The Case of Egg Donation,* ed. Cynthia B. Cohen (Bloomington: Indiana University Press, 1996), this volume.

23. *Johnson v. Calvert,* 5 Cal 4th 84, 104, 851 P2d 776, 789. cert denied US, 114 SCt 206.

24. *McDonald v. McDonald,* 91–08907 Supreme Court of New York, Appellate Division, Second Department, 1994 N.Y. App. Div. LEXIS 1463.

25. Lori B. Andrews, "Legal and Ethical Aspects of New Reproductive Technologies," *Clinical Obstetrics and Gynecology* 29 (1986): 190–204.

26. A. Templeton, "Gamete Donation and Anonymity," *British Journal of Obstetrics and Gynecology* 98 (1991): 343–45.

27. Royal Commission, p. xxxv.

CONTRIBUTORS

David H. Barad is Associate Professor at the Albert Einstein College of Medicine in the Bronx, New York. He is Director of the Division of Reproductive Endocrinology in the Department of Obstetrics and Gynecology at the Montefiore Medical Center. Dr. Barad has served on many hospital and medical school committees and is a lecturer for both the clinical and preclinical curriculums at the Albert Einstein College of Medicine. He has published extensively in the field of reproductive endocrinology and has achieved a national and international reputation in that discipline.

Joel Batzofin is a Diplomate of the American Board of Obstetrics and Gynecology. Born and raised in South Africa, Dr. Batzofin attended medical school in Johannesburg and completed a residency in OB-GYN at Harvard Medical School in Boston, Massachusetts. He completed a fellowship in Reproductive Endocrinology and Infertility and Reproductive Andrology, both at Baylor College of Medicine, in Houston, Texas. In 1988 he co-founded Huntington Reproductive Center in Pasadena. Dr. Batzofin's research interests are endometriosis, laser surgery, and male infertility in assisted reproductive treatments.

Andrea L. Bonnicksen is Professor of Political Science at Northern Illinois University, where she teaches courses in biomedical and biotechnology policy. She is author of *In Vitro Fertilization: From Laboratories to Legislatures* and *Civil Rights and Liberties: Principles of Interpretation*. She is coeditor, with Robert Blank, of *Emerging Issues in Biomedical Policy*, a three-volume series, and is book review editor for *Politics and the Life Sciences*. Her research interests include the policy implications of reproductive and genetic technologies. In 1990–91 she was a Rockefeller Foundation Fellow at the University of Texas Medical Branch, studying genetics and public policy.

Dan W. Brock is Professor of Philosophy and Biomedical Ethics, as well as Director of the Center for Biomedical Ethics in the School of Medicine, Brown University. He was Staff Philosopher in 1981–82 on the President's Commission for the Study of Ethical Problems in Medicine where he worked on the Commission's reports on informed consent, life-sustaining treatment, and access to health care. He also served on the 1993 White

House Task Force on National Health Reform. Dr. Brock has published many papers in biomedical ethics as well as in moral and political philosophy, and is coauthor with Allen Buchanan of *Deciding for Others: The Ethics of Surrogate Decision Making*, and author of *Life and Death: Philosophical Essays in Biomedical Ethics*.

Lisa Sowle Cahill is Professor of Christian Ethics at Boston College. She is Associate Editor of the *Journal of Medicine and Philosophy* and of the *Journal of Religious Ethics*. Her most recent book is *Sex, Gender, and Christian Ethics* (forthcoming).

Brian L. Cohen is an Associate Professor in the Division of Reproductive Endocrinology of the Department of Obstetrics and Gynecology at the Albert Einstein College of Medicine/Montefiore Medical Center. Dr. Cohen is also the Coordinator of the Resident Training Program in Obstetrics and Gynecology at the Albert Einstein College of Medicine/Montefiore Medical Center.

Cynthia B. Cohen is Senior Research Fellow at the Kennedy Institute of Ethics at Georgetown University and Adjunct Associate of the Hastings Center. She is the former Executive Director of the National Advisory Board on Ethics in Reproduction, has served as Associate for Ethical Studies at The Hastings Center, and has chaired the Philosophy Department at the University of Denver. She has published extensively in the field of medical ethics.

Elizabeth Heitman is Assistant Professor of Humanities and Technology in Health Care at the University of Texas School of Public Health in Houston. She is also Associate Editor of the *International Journal of Technology Assessment in Health Care*.

Nancy A. Klein is Medical Director of the In Vitro Fertilization Program at the University of Washington Medical Center and is Assistant Professor in the Division of Reproductive Endocrinology and Infertility at the University of Washington's Department of Obstetrics and Gynecology. In 1991–93 she was Fellow in the Division of Reproductive Endocrinology and Infertility at the University of Texas Health Science Center in San Antonio.

Patricia M. McShane is a board-certified reproductive endocrinologist and expert in treating infertile couples. She is Vice President Medical Affairs of IVF America, Inc., and Medical Director of the IVF America Program-Boston. Dr. McShane is a Diplomate of both the American Board of Obstetrics and Gynecology and its Division of Reproductive Endocrinology. She is a Fellow of the American College of Obstetrics and Gynecology, and a member of the Society of Reproductive Endocrinologists and the American Society for Reproductive Medicine. She has served as President of the Boston Fertility Society, and Director of the In Vitro Fertilization Program at Brigham and Women's Hospital. Her professional experience also includes positions as Assistant Professor of Obstetrics and Gynecology at Harvard Medical School and as researcher in reproductive immunology in collaboration with the Department of Medicine at Harvard. Dr. McShane has published and lectured extensively on the subjects of infertility and new reproductive technologies.

Ruth Macklin is Professor of Bioethics at Albert Einstein College of Medicine in New York City. She has been teaching and conducting research in bioethics for more than 20 years, is author of ten books, and has more than 120 publications in professional journals, as well as articles in magazines and newspapers for general audiences. An elected member of the Institute of Medicine of the National Academy of Sciences, Dr. Macklin is a consultant to national and international organizations, including the World Health Organization. In 1994 she was appointed by President Bill Clinton to the Advisory Committee on Human Radiation Experiments, a panel investigating radiation experiments conducted during the Cold War and sponsored by the U.S. government. Her current research concentrates on ethics and reproductive health.

Thomas H. Murray is Professor of Biomedical Ethics and Director of the Center for Biomedical Ethics in the School of Medicine, Case Western Reserve University. He is a founding editor of the journal *Medical Humanities Review* and is on the editorial boards of *Human Gene Therapy*, *Social Science and Medicine*, and *The Physician and Sportsmedicine*. He is an elected fellow of The Hastings Center and of the Environmental Health Institute. He serves as a member of the U.S. Olympic Committee's Sports Medicine Committee, and is a past member and founder of the Working Group on Ethical, Legal and Social Issues to the National Institutes of Health Center for Human Genome Research, and Chair of its Task Force on Genetics and Insurance. Dr. Murray is author of over 150 publications. He is past President of the Society for Health and Human Values, on the Executive Committee of the Association for Practical and Professional Ethics, and on the Board of Directors of the American Society for Law, Medicine, and Ethics. His most recent book is *The Worth of the Child*.

Jeffrey R. Nelson is a reproductive endocrinologist specializing in the treatment of infertility. Dr. Nelson attended medical school at the Texas College of Osteopathic Medicine in Ft. Worth, Texas, and is a member of the American College of Osteopathic Obstetricians and Gynecologists. Following his residency in Obstetrics and Gynecology, Dr. Nelson completed a fellowship in Reproductive Endocrinology and Infertility at Pennsylvania Hospital in conjunction with the Philadelphia Fertility Institute. Dr. Nelson became an associate of Huntington Reproductive Center in 1992. His current research interests include sonographic uterine imaging techniques and advanced operative endoscopy.

Ana Richardson is a member of the American Society for Reproductive Medicine and the Association of Reproductive Health Professionals. She served for many years as a labor and delivery nurse prior to her work in reproductive medicine. She is currently working with third-party assisted reproduction cycles at the Huntington Reproductive Center in Pasadena, California.

John A. Robertson is the Thomas Watt Gregory Professor of Law at the University of Texas School of Law at Austin. A Fellow of The Hastings Center, he has served on a federal Task Force on Organ Transplantation, on the National Institutes of Health Panel on Fetal Tissue Transplantation Research, and on the Ethics Committee of the American Fertility Society. He is author of *The Rights of the Critically Ill* and has written widely on law and bioethics issues, including reproductive rights, organ transplantation, and human experimentation. His most recent book is *Children of Choice: Freedom and the New Reproductive Technologies*.

Mary Schlachtenhaufen, J.D., is completing her Ph.D. in Religious Studies at Rice University, Houston.

Paulo D. Serafini is a Diplomate of the American Board of Obstetrics and Gynecology and is board certified in reproductive endocrinology and infertility. He is founder of the *in vitro* fertilization program at the University of California, Irvine, and Associate Director of Reproductive Medicine at Cedars-Sinai Medical Center in Los Angeles. He is currently a codirector of Huntington Reproductive Center in Pasadena. Dr. Serafini's areas of research are physiopharmacology of induced folliculogenesis and interventional ultrasonography.

Gretchen Sewall earned her Bachelor of Science in Nursing from Seattle University and her Master in Social Work from the University of Washington. Since 1991, she has been the Coordinator and counselor of the Donor Egg Program at the University of Washington Medical Center Fertility and Endocrine Center.

Shelley B. Smith is a practicing psychotherapist in Los Angeles. In addition to her private practice, she has been a counselor at the acclaimed Southern California Counseling Center where she specializes in working with families. She has been instrumental in initiating and running "Good Beginnings," a Cedars-Sinai Medical Center program focusing on parents who have undergone neonatal loss. She runs a couples' infertility group and works with men and women who have been impacted by this issue and has recently been working with several reproductive endocrinologists to establish an innovative new "Egg Donor" program for infertile women.

Michael R. Soules is Professor and Director of the Division of Reproductive Endocrinology and Infertility at the University of Washington School of Medicine in Seattle. He is President of the Society of Reproductive Endocrinologists, Chair of the Resident Education Committee of the American Society for Reproductive Medicine, and a member of the editorial board of *Fertility & Sterility*.

Carson Strong is a professor in the Department of Human Values and Ethics at the University of Tennessee College of Medicine. He is author of *Ethics in Reproductive and Perinatal Medicine* (forthcoming) and coauthor of *A Casebook of Medical Ethics*.

Rosemarie Tong is the Thatcher Professor in Philosophy and Medical Humanities at Davidson College, North Carolina. She is author of *Feminine and Feminist Ethics*, *Women, Sex and the Law*, and *Feminist Thought: A Comprehensive Introduction*. She is also coeditor of *Feminist Philosophies: Problems, Theories, and Applications*, coauthor of *Controlling Our Reproductive Destiny: A Technological and Philosophical Perspective*, and has published numerous articles in the area of medical humanities and ethics.

INDEX